Evidence-Based
Psychotherapy

Evidence-Based
Psychotherapy

Where Practice and
Research Meet

Edited by
Carol D. Goodheart
Alan E. Kazdin
Robert J. Sternberg

American Psychological Association • Washington, DC

Published by
American Psychological Association
750 First Street, NE
Washington, DC 20002
www.apa.org

To order
APA Order Department
P.O. Box 92984
Washington, DC 20090-2984
Tel: (800) 374-2721; Direct: (202) 336-5510
Fax: (202) 336-5502; TDD/TTY: (202) 336-6123
Online: www.apa.org/books/
E-mail: order@apa.org

In the U.K., Europe, Africa, and the Middle East, copies may be ordered from
American Psychological Association
3 Henrietta Street
Covent Garden, London
WC2E 8LU England

Typeset in Goudy by Stephen McDougal, Mechanicsville, MD

Printer: Sheridan Books, Ann Arbor, MI
Cover Designer: Naylor Design, Washington, DC
Technical/Production Editor: Genevieve Gill

The opinions and statements published are the responsibility of the authors, and such opinions and statements do not necessarily represent the policies of the American Psychological Association.

Library of Congress Cataloging-in-Publication Data

Evidence-based psychotherapy : where practice and research meet / edited by Carol D. Goodheart, Alan E. Kazdin, and Robert J. Sternberg.
    p. cm.
  Includes bibliographical references and index.
  ISBN 1-59147-403-5
  1. Evidence-based psychiatry. I. Goodheart, Carol D. II. Kazdin, Alan E. III. Sternberg, Robert J.
  [DNLM: 1. Psychotherapy—methods. 2. Evidence-Based Medicine—methods.
3. Professional Practice. WM 420 E9227 2006]
  RC455.2.E94E9557 2006
  616.89—dc22   2005027816

British Library Cataloguing-in-Publication Data
A CIP record is available from the British Library.

Printed in the United States of America
First Edition

To all the dedicated practitioners and researchers who strive to make psychotherapy an effective, meaningful, and healing experience.

CONTENTS

CONTRIBUTORS

Michael E. Addis, PhD, Department of Psychology, Clark University, Worcester, MA

Andrea Archer, BA, Department of Psychology, Brigham Young University, Provo, UT

David H. Barlow, PhD, Center for Anxiety and Related Disorders, Boston University, Boston, MA

Jean A. Carter, PhD, Independent Practice, Washington, DC

Lillian Comas-Díaz, PhD, Transcultural Mental Health Institute, Washington, DC

Elena J. Eisman, EdD, Massachusetts Psychological Association, Wellesley

Amanda Fabbro, BA, Department of Psychology, University of Connecticut, Storrs

Carol D. Goodheart, EdD, Independent Practice, Princeton, NJ

Jonathan D. Huppert, Center for the Treatment and Study of Anxiety, University of Pennsylvania School of Medicine, Philadelphia

Alan E. Kazdin, PhD, Child Study Center, Yale University School of Medicine, New Haven, CT

Michael J. Lambert, PhD, Department of Psychology, Brigham Young University, Provo, UT

Geoffrey M. Reed, PhD, Practice Directorate, American Psychological Association, Washington, DC

Robert J. Sternberg, PhD, School of Arts and Sciences, Tufts University, Medford, MA

Sandra J. Tanenbaum, PhD, Division of Health Services Management and Policy, School of Public Health, The Ohio State University, Columbus

Steven J. Trierweiler, PhD, Program for Research on Black Americans, Research Center for Group Dynamics, Institute for Social Research, University of Michigan, Ann Arbor

John R. Weisz, PhD, Judge Baker Children's Center, Harvard University, Boston, MA

ACKNOWLEDGMENTS

We thank our patients, colleagues, supervisors, supervisees, teachers, and students who have enriched our understanding of psychotherapy over the years. We appreciate and applaud the contributors to this volume who have extended the dialogue on evidence-based practice to cast important distinctions and to bridge differences in thoughtful ways. We are especially grateful to Cheri Stahl for her good-natured and unflagging administrative support throughout the project.

Evidence-Based
Psychotherapy

INTRODUCTION

CAROL D. GOODHEART AND ALAN E. KAZDIN

What's in a name? This is a book about evidence-based practice (EBP). In a short span of time, psychology has seen the term *empirically validated treatment* evolve into *empirically supported treatment*, and further into *evidence-based treatment* (EBT). The concept of *empirically supported relationships* has been incorporated into the discussions about psychotherapy, and further consideration has led to the rise of the umbrella term *evidence-based practice*. The terms used vary within and among different countries. Terms are not perfectly interchangeable, because each time someone does the analysis to identify evidence-based treatments, the criteria are slightly different. No doubt the terms will continue to change as psychologists learn more, whether the discipline continues to look toward medicine as its model or forges its own path.

DEFINITIONS AND SCOPE

Although the connotations of these terms overlap, the distinction between EBT and EBP is more than a matter of semantics and is useful conceptually. EBP is a larger concept than any one treatment. EBP integrates all scientific evidence and clinical information that is used to guide and improve psychotherapy processes, interventions, therapeutic relationships, and outcomes. *Psychotherapy* is another term that encompasses more than any one treatment; evidence-based psychotherapy implies a coherent and clinically expert process of assessment, case formulation, identification of goals, treatment planning, alliance building, research-informed intervention, monitoring of progress, adjustments as needed, and termination—all in the context of collaboration with the client (or parent, guardian, or caretaker of the client). Therefore, we have chosen to focus the book on the larger constructs of EBP and psychotherapy. EBTs are a part of this picture and are included, of course, but the scope is intended to be broader to address far-reaching and important questions about EBP. There is a growing body of literature on the EBP movement, as well as different conclusions drawn about its merits and the uses and misuses of the concepts within health care service systems. This literature and varying points of view on the current state of knowledge about psychology practice are discussed in the chapters to follow.

Within health care, the term *patient* refers to the person, couple, family, or group receiving psychotherapy services. In psychology, the term *client* has a long tradition of use to refer to recipients. Further, some authors have reason to refer to recipients of care as *consumers* or *persons*. For the purposes of this book, the terms are synonymous, and contributors have made their own choices.

The subtitle of the book reflects a critical aspect of the evidence for psychotherapy: "where practice and research meet." Discussions about EBP generate high interest and strong opinions because the stakes are high. EBP has become a meeting ground for a wide range of clinicians, researchers, educators, and public policy professionals. They come together, sometimes to listen and learn and sometimes to clash, because they are all participants in how EBP is defined and shaped. Debates within the discipline center on the nature of evidence and the utility of drawing on multiple theories and methods; the relative importance of different types of research; the predominance of common factors in psychotherapy; the role of clinical expertise; the weight and interaction among client characteristics, clinician characteristics, relationship factors, and treatment factors, all of which contribute to psychotherapy outcomes; and the impact and interaction of such important client dimensions as comorbid conditions and multisymptom presentations, developmental level, personality, age, gender, ethnicity and culture, socioeconomic status, physical health status, and idiosyncratic risk factors. Within psychology and other health disciplines, the movement has been described as a "culture war" in which those involved in clinical practice and research are battling over what treatment approaches to use and on what basis (Messer, 2004). By now, many psychologists and professionals from other disciplines who are involved in delivery or investigation of clinical services are familiar with the disagreements and the entrenched positions. However, we believe it is nonetheless productive and fruitful to begin a reality-based progressive dialogue among mental health professionals affected by the EBP movement. It is time for all of us to consider the views of professionals who work in areas of research or service delivery different from our own. Therefore, *Evidence-Based Psychotherapy: Where Practice and Research Meet* offers distinctive perspectives, seeks common ground, and reveals the areas where there are legitimate differences, unanswered questions, and promising avenues by which we may improve psychotherapy.

ORGANIZATION AND CHAPTER THEMES

The chapters are grouped into three sections, with the editors' bridge comments in between the sections. Part I presents the practice perspective, Part II the research perspective, and Part III the perspectives on training, policy, and the need for caution based on selected themes from the chapters. There are discussions of the evolution of the EBP movement in all three sections of the book from the somewhat differing vantage points of practice, science, and policy. The editors recognize that perspectives overlap and issues intermingle. Chapters are placed in sections according to authors' primary work and role identification; however, there are several that might easily have been placed in a different section.

Part I

Chapter 1 (Geoffrey M. Reed and Elena J. Eisman) orients the reader with a broad conceptual discussion of the history of the EBP movement, a consideration of evidence in relationship to organized systems of health care delivery, and the specific impact of large systems' decisions on psychological practice. Chapter 2 (Carol D. Goodheart) defines EBP, discusses differences between the endeavors of practice and science, summarizes the multiple streams of evidence valuable to practitioners, and presents the role of clinical expertise. Chapter 3 (Jean A. Carter) proposes the integration of theoretical pluralism and technical eclecticism as essential to effective psychological practice in real-world clinical situations, which are often rapidly evolving and complex. Chapter 4 (Lillian Comas-Díaz) shows how psychotherapy is mediated by culture and suggests that effective multicultural psychotherapy uses clinical expertise to balance scientifically sound treatments with cultural relevance. The author's focus, unique in the book, is on exploration of the role of culture in the therapeutic relationship.

Part II

Chapter 5 (Michael J. Lambert and Andrea Archer) begins the research section by reviewing the research evidence on the effectiveness of psychotherapy (a recurrent theme in earlier chapters) and the implications of the research for practice, future studies, and the funding of psychotherapy. The chapter addresses specific questions: Do clients make clinically meaningful changes? Do they maintain their gains? Do some deteriorate? Chapter 6 (Jonathan D. Huppert, Amanda Fabbro, and David H. Barlow) presents a history of the EBP movement as a context in which to review the evidence for the efficacy and clinical utility of psychological treatments. The authors offer suggestions for improving EBP by delineating areas of potential benefit and collaboration. Chapter 7 (Alan E. Kazdin) discusses the need for systematic evaluation in clinical practice, offers useful steps for practitioners and an illustrative case example, highlights clinical and research issues that must be addressed to provide an adequate foundation for evaluation, and presents aspects of clinical training that may have the unintended consequence of undermining evaluation. Chapter 8 (John R. Weisz and Michael E. Addis) acknowledges profound differences between the worlds of researchers and clinicians, but the authors build on the premise that researchers and clinicians share important common goals, too. They propose complementary bridging activities, such as extending treatments tested in research settings into clinical practice settings both for testing under representative community conditions and for routine use when effective.

Part III

Chapter 9 (Steven J. Trierweiler) focuses on graduate education in psychology, as rooted in scientific traditions, and calls for the integration of scientific facts and local clinical situations. He proposes to push the methodological ideas of both science and practice until they can no longer be seen as separate. The question then becomes, How can good science and good practice converge in ways that will be genuinely helpful to clients? Chapter 10 (Sandra J. Tanenbaum) is a broad conceptual discussion of EBP in the context of public policy. The author describes three important working hypotheses of the EBP movement and suggests enlarging the terms of debate, as well as demonstrating the ramifications of the current terms of debate. Chapter 11 (Robert J. Sternberg) identifies key issues and differences from the chapters and offers a set of cautions.

CONVERGENCE AND DIVERGENCE OF VIEWS

This volume includes a broader range of clinical researchers, clinical practitioners, clinical educators, and public policy advocates than one normally finds keeping company. Areas of agreement and disagreement are implicit within and across some of the chapters and sections and are explicit for others. They are outlined here for readers to consider in advance.

Convergence

Implicit in all of the chapters is the fact that psychological practice is founded on science. Psychologists are trained in scientific methods and attitudes, which is a particular strength of psychology among mental-health–related disciplines. Contributors have common ground as social scientists. Although they have different methods and work settings, all form hypotheses, develop interventions, and evaluate progress—scientific processes that represent common training. All recognize the importance of being sensitive to individual client characteristics and preferences and tailoring care to the person. All are committed to the improvement of clients' lives through good psychological research and practice.

Psychotherapies that span many theoretical orientations have been identified as efficacious. The convergent evidence for this conclusion is based on hundreds of studies involving thousands of clients conducted over more than half a century. This conclusion is discussed in multiple chapters.

The Institute of Medicine (IOM; 2001) definition of EBP is accepted throughout health care, and the American Psychological Association (APA) definition of evidence-based practice in psychology, which closely follows the IOM definition, was agreed on by all members of the diverse group of psychologist scientists, practitioners, public health analysts, consumer advocates, and health economists who formed the APA Presidential Task Force on EBP (APA, 2005). The Council of Representatives approved and adopted the Task Force definition and policy document recommendations without change. Four contributors to this volume were members of the APA Task Force: David H. Barlow, Jean A. Carter, Carol D. Goodheart (Chair), and Geoffrey M. Reed (Professional Staff). This is of interest because the Task Force members represented distinctive views and expertise, yet they achieved consensus on a complex set of concerns about EBP that are reflected similarly in this volume in the discussion of areas of potential convergence and rapprochement.

No one would dispute that the practice environment is changing rapidly and markedly. On the one hand, there has been an explosion of clinically relevant research aimed at improving treatments, as well as gains in basic neuroscience. On the other hand, EBP is a movement toward accountability for the health care dollars spent and as such is closely associated with private and public insurance program requirements pertaining to authorization and reimbursement of treatment. The lack of consensus and coordination in the marketplace results in inconsistent requirements and the potential for mismanagement and negative impact on clients and mental health professionals.

Divergence

It is not clear whether the EBP movement is good for clients or for psychology. Opinions vary depending on whether the definition of EBP is broad or is restrictive. Although many psychologists agree with the IOM and the APA definitions in principle, they disagree about what the actual implementation of EBP looks like in practice. Philosophical worldview differences concerning EBP among contributors, and in the discipline as a whole, are reflected in a central tension between those who believe that to obtain positive therapeutic outcomes, *either*

- best practice entails *starting with a diagnosed disorder* and applying an EBT package; other evidence is sought only when an EBT is not available or is not working; this may be characterized as the use of a hierarchical system of treatment, in line with the hierarchy of research evidence *or*
- best practice entails *starting with the client*, establishing a therapeutic relationship, and developing a treatment plan from research evidence on interventions, common factors, human development, psychopathology, individual and group differences, and other relevant research topics; this may be characterized as the use of a heterarchical system, in line with the need for multiple strands of research and clinical information to tailor treatment for a particular client.

Many, perhaps most, psychologists do not fit neatly into these opposing positions and fall somewhere on a continuum between the two views. There is agreement on the interest and priority of improving client care. There is disagreement on the extent to which conclusions from research ought to be applied to and constrain clinical practice and the extent to which practitioners can genuinely identify client needs and apply the best or more appropriate combination of treatments based on that evaluation. Among the strengths of this book are that it clarifies key issues and points of overlap among different perspectives and cautions against polarizing views about the priorities of clinical work and research.

OPPORTUNITIES FOR RAPPROCHEMENT

The initial step in reaching a rapprochement of practitioner and scientist positions is clarifying the points of convergence and divergence as well as the diversity of different perspectives. There is no single practitioner or scientist view, and that is a critical point of departure for moving forward. Clearly there is agreement on such matters as the high priority of client care, the importance of professional training, and reliance on research whenever possible as a guide to intervention. Key aspects of the different positions among practitioners and scientists are not close enough to form a good basis for compromise or reconciliation beyond this level of abstraction.

Psychotherapy is designed to change lives, subjective experience, and adaptive functioning. Research is designed to show differences among various treatments where they exist and to understand the bases for these differences and the factors that influence outcome. These different priorities and foci do not connect very well, and one ought not to be surprised about this. On the clinician side, there is interest in identifying what the client's needs are in relation to treatment and indeed life, what procedures are appropriate, and how the treatment can be tailored to the individual needs of that client. The scientist is likely to view these as subjective and without the bases that would permit replicability across therapists. On the scientist side, randomized controlled trials, multiple measures to evaluate outcome, and results that compare groups and show statistically significant differences are taken as unequivocally relevant to clinical work. The practitioner is more likely to see the findings as useful information, but not necessarily relevant to help the client sitting across from the therapist with complex problems that have not really been studied. Findings are not a replacement for reasoned judgment about what should be applied to a specific case. Also, average (mean) differences that were statistically significant over time in a study or between groups may reflect changes that may not have really helped clients in a palpable way. As a consequence, research studies are not axiomatic guides for what to do in treatment. There is little direct evidence that can help the clinician. Meta-analyses and the effect sizes they use as their metric may show that this or that treatment is better than the rest, but is it better in ways that actually make a difference or help clients? Clinicians, scientists, clients, agents of third-party payers, policymakers, and even book editors would love to know. No meta-analysis (to our knowledge) has accomplished that feat.

Can science and practice views be reconciled? We believe so, but not by illusory solutions such as adding a dash (e.g., scientist–practitioner) and saying psychology has a training model that serves both. Perhaps we can begin with the premise that psychologists by training are scientists and share an appreciation for replicable evidence and careful assessment. The almost exclusive focus on group research and controlled trials, as currently conceived and executed, provides an unnecessary constraint on reaching common ground. We need to have findings that at once address and are relevant to the lives of individuals (clients in clinical practice) and that meet the desiderata of research. There is a point of rapprochement that in some ways may be the best of both worlds, namely, qualitative research. Qualitative research focuses on the rich experience of individuals and meets the standards of scientific research. In qualitative research, as in psychotherapy, the experience of the individual is the focus and is richly elaborated. The rich assessments would provide the basis for systematically examining the problems of the clients before, during, and after treatment and might even be used to guide decision making in a replicable fashion. Is the client benefiting from treatment? Is his or her life changed in any ways or in any important way? These questions can be answered scientifically and in a way that helps individual clients. Clinical practice can be put on firmer scientific footing in ways to help clients. Science can remain on scientific footing but become more directly relevant and useful to clinicians and to clients. Efforts to reach a rapprochement require clarification of the different views and many perspectives that different parties bring to the table. The many contributions that follow convey multiple opportunities for rapprochement in relation to doing psychotherapy, conducting research, and providing training to professionals.

REFERENCES

American Psychological Association. (2005). *Report of the 2005 Presidential Task Force on Evidence-Based Practice.* Retrieved October 24, 2005, from http://www.apa.org/practice/ebpstatement.pdf

Institute of Medicine. (2001). *Crossing the quality chasm: A new health system for the 21st century.* Washington, DC: National Academies Press.

Messer, S. B. (2004). Evidence-based practice: Beyond empirically supported treatments. *Professional Psychology, 35,* 580–588.

I

THE PRACTICE
PERSPECTIVE

1

USES AND MISUSES OF EVIDENCE: MANAGED CARE, TREATMENT GUIDELINES, AND OUTCOMES MEASUREMENT IN PROFESSIONAL PRACTICE

GEOFFREY M. REED AND ELENA J. EISMAN

The evidence-based practice (EBP) movement as it has developed in the United States can best be understood in the context of contemporary patterns of organized health care delivery. This chapter explores the background and history of EBP at a systems level as they affect psychological health care services. We examine how EBP reinforces a certain set of attributions about health professionals and how these attributions are institutionalized in treatment guidelines, practice standards, and authorization and reimbursement models. Many of our examples are drawn from Massachusetts, which we use as a case study in EBP implementation. Massachusetts consistently ranks second in managed care penetration in the United States, just behind California (Henry J. Kaiser Family Foundation, 2005) and has been a bellwether state for many of the changes in organized health care delivery. Currently, a variety of public and private sector initiatives based on the premises of EBP promise to have a major impact on psychologists and other practitioners in Massachusetts and augur changes soon to occur in other parts of the country.

MANAGED CARE AND EVIDENCE-BASED PRACTICE AS A PUBLIC IDEA

Managed care expanded rapidly during the 1970s and 1980s following the enactment by the U.S. Congress of the Health Maintenance Organization (HMO) Act of 1973 (Pub. L. 93-222; see DeLeon, VandenBos, & Bulatao, 1991). At that time, there was considerable concern about rapidly growing health care costs following the passage during the 1960s of Medicare, Medicaid, and other legislation intended to expand health care coverage. Managed care advocates argued that fee-for-service indemnity health plans provided incentives to health care professionals and facilities to provide expensive and excessive diagnostic and treatment services. In contrast, they said, HMOs would reward the maintenance of health and the prevention of illness. Managed care proponents believed that the components of effective treatment were generally well understood. Therefore, HMOs could easily identify and eliminate unnecessary services, achieving substantial cost savings without sacrificing the quality of care. Health professionals could not be trusted to do this because of their profit motive to provide unnecessary care.

The competence of health professionals to determine what services should be provided was further challenged by Wennberg (1984), who found significant unexplained variation in the rates of specific medical procedures for given health conditions among otherwise similar populations in different geographic locations. This and subsequent small area variation studies were "widely interpreted to mean that physicians were uncertain about the value of alternative treatments and that their actions were consequently influenced by clinically extraneous factors such as tradition and convenience" (Tanenbaum, 1999, p. 758). The growing managed care movement adopted this perspective with enthusiasm. Health care professionals were portrayed as major causes of waste, inefficiency, and needless expense, and this portrayal was used as a further justification for the transfer of control and decision-making authority from the physician to the health plan through a variety of initiatives intended to reduce demand, limit access, reduce practice variation, and standardize care (Reed, McLaughlin, & Newman, 2002). Health systems and health plans developed increasingly specific rules—medical necessity criteria, standards, guidelines, practice parameters, critical pathways, best practices—to govern the provision of care by health professionals.

The emphasis on standardizing and regulating professional behavior also received substantial federal support. Congress established the Agency for Health Care Policy and Research (AHCPR) in 1989; a central part of its charge was to develop practice guidelines for physicians and other health care providers (AHCPR, 1993a). During the 1990s, National Institutes of Health (NIH) agencies, under congressional pressure to demonstrate their practical contribution to U.S. health care, launched a series of "technology transfer" initiatives to disseminate research-based treatments to the field. Although the rhetoric of EBP had not yet matured, these efforts were generally based on the assumption that the major challenges in improving health care quality and reducing health care costs included teaching health care professionals to use research-based treatments properly and developing appropriate strategies to ensure that they were doing so. Managed care organizations offered a promising vehicle for implementing these changes.

Managed care, however, soon developed an image problem. As it turned out, trimming the fat and waste helped to stabilize health care costs briefly but did not address the underlying drivers of escalating costs. Managed care companies used increasingly restrictive measures to hold costs down, resulting in high levels of tension with health professionals, increased scrutiny from regulators, and increasingly negative views among consumers (Keckley, 2003). By 1997, movie audiences across America broke into cheers as Helen Hunt's character in *As Good as It Gets* (Johnson & Brooks, 1997), struggling to obtain adequate medical treatment for her young son, finally cursed managed care in frustration. At around the same time, EBP was gaining currency as what Tanenbaum (2003) described as a "public idea," meaning an idea that both describes a public problem and suggests the wisdom of a particular response. Tanenbaum cited Gusfield (1981), who described how drunk drivers became the focus of transportation safety efforts when a public idea cast them as the essential public threat on U.S. highways. The idea that drunk drivers cause accidents is not untrue, but accidents also have many other causes. A public idea focuses attention on one aspect of a complex problem and calls for logical solutions to it. Although these solutions may indeed be helpful, the true usefulness of a public idea is in creating the appearance of wise public policy and the opportunity for public satisfaction in taking action, even though it may contribute to a false sense of security that the problem is being addressed adequately.

Health care policymakers are indeed faced with a complex reality. It is undeniable that there are major structural problems in the U.S. health care system. Approximately 15% of the U.S. population is uninsured (U.S. Census Bureau, 2004). An even higher percentage have no mental health benefits, and only about half of those who do have mental health benefits have them at what could be considered to be reasonable levels (Maxfield, Achman, & Cook, 2004). The United States spends more per capita on health care than any other industrialized nation and does not provide demonstrably better care (World Health Organization, 2001). The future costs of Medicare promise to create unacceptable burdens for the next generation unless there are significant reductions in benefits. State budgets have been sorely strained over the past few years, attributed in part to the growing cost of health care, particularly Medicaid. Overall, the problems with the U.S. health care system seem intractable. Vested interests oppose any specific solutions, and health care costs continue to rise.

In the face of these problems, the American public has been offered the idea that the essential problem with the health care system is uninformed practice, which could be resolved if health care professionals practiced in ways more consistent with research findings. EBP is premised on the need for the lay management of professional behavior, which has been a central operating principle of managed care. Keckley (2003) proposed that EBP can be a mechanism for managed care to improve its image among stakeholders and members. EBP can be "the fundamental basis for managing cost as well as quality" (p. 3), in large part by providing a basis for coverage limitations and denials. This time, however, these practices can be framed in the language of science. In psychology, this perspective has been given legitimacy by academically based clinical researchers who support the view that the essential problem in health care services is the inadequate application of the research literature by clinicians and who suggest that their own research provides a superior basis for services if clinicians would only follow it (e.g., Beutler, Moleiro, & Talebi, 2002; Chorpita et al., 2002; Lampropoulos & Spengler, 2002; Nathan & Gorman, 1998).

Tanenbaum (2003) pointed out that EBP's potency as a public idea is based in part on its powerful rhetoric:

> It is, in fact, a rhetorical triumph, for who can argue with evidence? Critics of EBP literally have nothing to call themselves or their position; it is not evidence, but the limitations of certain evidence hierarchies they oppose. . . . Moreover, the rhetoric of evidence-based practice raises an important question in the listener's mind: If EBP is the introduction of evidence into practice, how have clinicians been practicing all along? What is there besides evidence? Even if the public never gets specifics, however, it should be clear to them that clinicians are in the wrong. (p. 294)

THE SELECTIVE USE OF EVIDENCE

The assertion that there is a lack of evidence supporting current psychological practice can be made only on the basis of a narrow and highly selective reading of the literature. A large body of evidence, including hundreds of studies going back to the 1930s and dozens of meta-analyses, indicates the following:

1. Psychotherapy is generally effective, with positive outcomes reported for a wide variety of theoretical orientations and treatment techniques.

2. Although there is some variability across disorders, the effects of psychotherapy are generally as good as or superior to the effects of psychotropic medications for all but the most severely disturbed patients.
3. The outcomes of psychotherapy are substantial across a variety of relevant areas, including psychiatric symptoms, interpersonal functioning, social role performance, and occupational functioning.
4. Psychotherapy is relatively efficient in producing its effects.
5. The outcomes of psychotherapy are likely to be maintained over time, particularly in contrast to the effects of psychotropic medications (see Lambert & Ogles, 2004, for a review).
6. Psychotherapy may offset the costs of medical services by reducing hospital stays and other medical expenses (see Chiles, Lambert, & Hatch, 1999, for a review).

Unfortunately, this body of evidence does not rank highly on the "hierarchy of evidence" that the evidence-based movement has taken as its foundation (Sackett, Straus, Richardson, Rosenberg, & Haynes, 2000). To be truly "evidence based," an intervention must have been tested in multiple efficacy studies. The greatest weight is accorded to evidence from studies using the "gold standard" methodology of randomized controlled trials (RCTs). In mental health, proponents of EBP have adopted evidentiary criteria that not only include RCTs as the highest form of evidence but also add the existence of a standardized treatment manual and its application to a study sample with a specific mental health condition as prerequisites for being considered evidence based (Chambless et al., 1996). This effectively excludes many treatments that are widely used in the community. Even a casual glance at the lists of evidence-based psychological treatments indicates that these are overwhelmingly behavioral or cognitive–behavioral treatment modalities. However, this conclusion arises from the confounding of the evidentiary criteria with the characteristics of the treatments they are used to assess (Tanenbaum, 2005; Westen, Novotny, & Thompson-Brenner, 2004).

In this way, some approaches to treatment are legitimized and others are delegitimized (Tanenbaum, 2003). Although this was clearly not the intention of those who developed them, the lists contribute to the underestimation and even devaluation of the body of professional knowledge in the field of psychology by health policymakers and commercial health care organizations. Westen and colleagues (2004) described widespread confusion in the literature, sometimes explicit and sometimes implicit, between treatments that have been empirically disconfirmed and those that have not been tested using methods that fit the evidentiary criteria of EBP. In a similar way, there is also confusion between treatments that have been tested by researchers using these methods and "best available" treatments. For example, we researchers do not in fact know that cognitive–behavior therapy and interpersonal therapy are the most effective psychological treatments for depression. What we know is that these manualized, brief treatments are easier to test using RCT methodologies than other widely used forms of treatment. In fact, there has been virtually no research comparing experimental treatments with treatments as provided by clinicians in the community, so there is almost no direct evidence that treatments that appear on the lists of evidence-based treatments yield outcomes that are superior to those in clinical practice (Westen et al., 2004).

DEPROFESSIONALIZING THE PROFESSIONAL

The greatest omission in EBP's consideration of the scientific basis for psychological interventions concerns factors related to the therapist and the nature of the treatment relationship, which have repeatedly been found to be among the strongest and most consistent predictors of psychotherapy outcomes (Lambert & Okiishi, 1997; Norcross & Hill, 2004). This omission is consistent with managed care's emphasis on placing external controls on the behavior of health professionals as the primary vehicle for improving health care. One of the major effects of managed care has been to undermine the view of the individual healing relationship as central to care by decontextualizing health care services, moving away from therapeutic relationships and toward health-related service encounters (Gutek, 1995). Based on the industrial principles of the assembly line, health care has been broken down into smaller and smaller discrete units of service offered by generic providers.

Managed care's interest in prescribing and standardizing the behavior of health professionals interacts synergistically with a major conceptual shift that is supported by EBP's evidentiary criteria. EBP criteria that require that treatments be manualized to be considered and that accord the greatest weight to RCTs (which generally include the use of a treatment manual) lead to the view of treatment manuals as constitutive of psychological treatments rather than as exemplars or laboratory analogues of them (Westen et al., 2004). EBP proponents encourage consumers to seek the specified manualized treatments because they have met "basic scientific standards of effectiveness" (American Psychological Association [APA], Division 12, Society of Clinical Psychology, 2004), in contrast to the unmanualized treatments that are widely practiced in the community. State mental health systems and private health plans are formulating lists of evidence-based treatments with the goal of making the implementation of these manualized treatments as they have been tested the basis for reimbursement policies (e.g., Carpinello, Rosenberg, Stone, Schwager, & Felton, 2002; Chorpita et al., 2002; see also Tanenbaum, 2005). Such policies appear to view mental health professionals as technicians or "paraprofessionals who cannot—and should not—exercise clinical judgment in selecting interventions or interpreting the data of clinical observation" (Westen et al., 2004, p. 639). When health care professionals object to these requirements, they are often portrayed as antiscientific or simply unwilling to change their behavior. Health professionals' resistance is regularly cited as the major barrier to implementation of EBP in clinical settings (e.g., Keckley, 2003).

This debate is being played out in Massachusetts, where some managed care companies have instituted credentialing standards for specific treatments deemed to be evidence based. In one carve-out plan, practitioners credentialed in dialectical behavior therapy (Linehan, 1993) and programs certified in providing motivational interviewing for substance abuse problems (Miller & Rollnick, 2002) receive a higher reimbursement rate than other health professionals and programs. We believe that in the near future practitioners in other states are more likely to see similar financial incentives for specific treatments considered evidence based rather than outright prohibitions against others, but such restrictions are increasingly likely over time. For example, legislation recently passed in Oregon requires that within 3 years, 75% of state-funded mental health and substance abuse services be considered evidence based (Oregon Office of Mental Health and Addiction Services, 2004).

EVIDENCE-BASED PRACTICE AS A BASIS FOR HEALTH CARE SERVICES

Substantial resources are being devoted to programs aimed at increasing practitioner adoption of research-based services. For example, a major joint initiative of the National Institute of Mental Health (NIMH) and the Substance Abuse and Mental Health Services Administration (SAMHSA) focuses on promoting and supporting the implementation of evidence-based mental health treatment practices in state mental health systems (e.g., see NIH, 2004). The goal of the NIMH portion of the initiative is to foster research on the most effective and feasible methods for implementing EBP in state clinical practice settings. The SAMHSA portion of the initiative goes further by providing direct support to states and localities that are ready for and committed to adopting EBP.

However, as a method for determining what treatments will be provided to whom, EBP as it currently exists gives rise to considerable concern. In the context of populations such as children and severely mentally ill persons, there is a tremendous need for interventions but relatively few treatments that meet the most narrowly defined criteria of evidence because of the difficulties associated with such documentation (e.g., people who cannot consent often cannot be randomized). There is also concern that patient samples enrolled in clinical trials are different from those seen in clinical practice on dimensions that moderate outcomes. For example, a comparison of schizophrenic and bipolar clinical trial samples with patients of a nationally representative sample of psychiatrists participating in the American Psychiatric Association's Practice Research Network (PRN) found that over one third of the schizophrenic PRN patients and over half of the bipolar PRN patients would have been ineligible to participate in clinical trials (Zarin, Young, & West, 2005). PRN patients were highly likely to have comorbid conditions that would have excluded them from clinical trials and tended to be on combinations of medications not allowed in clinical trial protocols. It is possible that deviation from "evidence-based" practices among the PRN patients was entirely appropriate given their differences from research samples.

There is virtually no evidence to support the underlying assumption that implementation of EBP will improve health care services and outcomes or reduce health care costs, except to the extent that it serves to restrict access to care. Nonetheless, state-level initiatives to date are clearly based on the assumption that restricting psychological treatments to those that appear on approved lists will result in cost savings, as these are presumed to be most efficient and therefore cost-effective. In fact, in the Oregon legislation cost-effectiveness is included in the definition of evidence-based services (Oregon Office of Mental Health and Addiction Services, 2004). Although cost is a legitimate factor to consider in treatment selection, confounding how well a treatment works with how much it costs is particularly dangerous (see Stricker et al., 1999).

When EBP is used as a basis for restricting access to treatment or prescribing particular forms of treatment, many questions should be addressed: What is the evidence that various forms of EBT are superior to other forms of mental health treatments more commonly practiced in the community among the relevant clinical population? What is the evidence of long-term impact of one treatment over another in a real-life clinical population? What is the evidence that holding a certificate in delivering a particular form of EBP has a greater impact on client outcomes than other characteristics of the health professional? How are consumer values and preferences (e.g., treatment acceptability) accounted for in the availability of treatment alternatives, and how has the rapidly growing consumer movement provided input to these policies? What are the relevant criterion measures one should use for evaluating treatment success? Should they be based on symptoms or on functional status? Should they relate to just the abatement of the presenting problem or include such things as improvements in quality of life? These questions generally go unanswered in the EBP discussion, and we believe that the psychology profession should not condone treatment restrictions or treatment prescriptions by health plans in the absence of such answers.

Indeed, a broader view of the evidence suggests that a *higher* rate of mental health services should be provided than is currently the case. The onset of mental health disorders is typically early in life (Kessler, Berglund, Demler, Jin, & Walters, 2005). These disorders are often chronic in nature and have a pervasive impact on functioning and development, thereby contributing heavily to worldwide disability and associated costs (World Health Organization, 2001). Many of those with even severe mental heath problems fail to receive any treatment at all (WHO World Mental Health Survey Consortium, 2004). In the United States, among persons who eventually make treatment contact, the average delay from the onset of a disorder to entry into treatment ranges from 5 to 23 years, depending on the disorder (Wang, Berglund, et al., 2005). Fewer than one third of patients with mental health disorders receive treatment that meets even minimal standards for treatment adequacy (Wang, Lane, et al., 2005). The proportion of patients receiving adequate care is lowest among those who receive treatment for mental health conditions in primary care settings (12.7%) and highest among those who receive care in specialty mental health settings (48.3%). The costs and consequences of failing to provide adequate mental health care are cumulative across the life span, both for the individual and for society. If the goal of EBP is actually to improve U.S. health care, we in the psychology profession would do well to replace the current discussion of which techniques are better and how practitioners can be made to apply them with one that focuses on how we can best deliver treatment to the population in need and thereby increase the population impact of services for mental health disorders.

EVIDENCE-BASED PRACTICE AND THE PHARMACOLOGICAL BIAS

The evidentiary criteria for EBP that have been most widely promoted in mental health (see Chambless et al., 1996) were patterned after Food and Drug Administration guidelines for the approval of new drugs (see Wampold, Lichtenberg, & Waehler, 2002). These methodologies remain most ideally suited to pharmacological research. Even manualized psychotherapies are far more difficult, expensive, and time consuming to test using RCT methodologies than are medications, and the research funding available for studies of psychological interventions is dwarfed by the millions and millions of dollars that drug companies and the federal government pour into RTCs of new pharmaceutical products, both in directly sponsored clinical trials and through grants to biomedical researchers. Negative results are routinely suppressed by pharmaceutical companies and rarely published by scientific journals, leading to a distorted picture of the relative evidentiary support for psychological and pharmacological interventions, given that EBP criteria often equate strength of evidence for a particular intervention with the number of RCTs published in the scientific literature that support it.

This distortion is consistent with the inclinations of health plans and payers, who tend to view medication as a quick fix and less expensive than psychotherapy, in spite of evidence to the contrary. For example, the notion that medications have effects in treating depression superior to those of psychotherapy became the central premise of a generation of treatment guidelines (AHCPR, 1993b; American Psychiatric Association, 2000), with psychotherapy recommended only after repeated treatment failures on medication. Although depressed persons are more likely now than in the past to be identified, they are proportionately more likely to be given medication (Olfson et al., 2002), in spite of the fact that multiple studies have demonstrated that psychological treatment is equally effective even in the treatment of severe depression (DeRubeis et al., 2005). Further, the effects of psychological treatment are long lasting, in contrast to those of medication (Hollon et al., 2005; Hollon, Stewart, & Strunk, in press), suggesting that psychological interventions are more cost-effective in the long run. Surveys across a variety of disorders indicate that when consumers are given a choice, they prefer psychological interventions to pharmacological ones (e.g., Hazlett-Stevens et al., 2002; Zoellner, Feeny, Cochran, & Pruitt, 2003), raising questions about the extent to which consumers are actually being given a choice of treatments.

This type of bias can be seen in Massachusetts in a program intended to increase children's access to the mental health services. The Children's Mental Health Task Force (CMHTF), sponsored by the Massachusetts chapter of the American Academy of Pediatrics, was created to make recommendations for addressing gaps in services. The CMHTF brought together members of multiple professional associations (including Eisman, the second author of this chapter), representatives of facilities that treat children, insurers, regulators, researchers, legislators, consumer groups, educators, and criminal justice and social service professionals. Now in its 4th year of existence, this group has supported major regulatory and legislative efforts to improve access to all forms of children's mental health services.

Over the past year, the CMHTF has supported an initiative to address the fact that the average wait for an appointment with a child psychiatrist in the Central Massachusetts area is 6 months. Pediatricians indicated that they were often uncomfortable with prescribing psychotropic medications for children and adolescents and that they would welcome consultation in this area. Psychiatrists were contracted to provide on-call telephone consultation to pediatricians in central Massachusetts regarding medication recommendations, with rapid face-to-face contact available for children needing to be seen by a psychiatrist. This program was so popular among the medical community that $2.5 million was allocated in the state budget to expand this program statewide. The CMHTF raised little question about whether the evidence base justified this emphasis on the use of psychotropic medications in children and adolescents. Some of the group, including the second author

(Eisman) and other psychologists, advocated for an integrated consultation approach, and the task force officially supported this position. However, the program clearly focuses on pharmacological treatment and has devoted minimal focus to providing consultation about other treatment options.

Preliminary implementation findings presented to the clinical advisory group of the Massachusetts Behavioral Health Partnership, the entity administering this program, show a decreasing frequency of calls from pediatricians to consultant psychiatrists, which may indicate that pediatricians are becoming more comfortable in prescribing psychoactive medications. Although the statewide expansion of the program was reviewed because of the recent controversy in the media regarding the use of antidepressants in adolescents, it is now proceeding using the same model and has received high praise from the medical community.

Given the general lack of data about the effectiveness of antidepressant medications in children and adolescents and the substantial concerns about such use that have been raised recently, it appears that there are different standards of evidence for pharmacological treatments than for psychological ones. However, there are some signs of a backlash against the overuse of psychotropic medications. The United Kingdom's National Institute for Clinical Excellence (2004) recently issued a guideline recommending that antidepressant medications not be used as a first line of treatment for mild depression because the cost–benefit ratio is likely to be poor. The report indicates that psychotherapy is a preferable alternative in these cases, although in our view it does not make this recommendation as clearly as the evidence warrants. In addition, the U.S. Food and Drug Administration (2005) recently began requiring manufacturers of all antidepressant drugs to include in their labeling a boxed warning and expanded warning statements that alert health care providers to an increased risk of suicidal inclinations in children and adolescents being treated with these medications. Whether these recommendations and requirements will result in increased rates of nonpharmacological treatment remains to be seen.

THE MOVE TO OUTCOMES

A recent survey conducted by the APA Practice Directorate (2004) asked practicing psychologists to report on a specific treatment session with an individual patient selected at random from their practice. Over two thirds of those psychologists who were seeing a patient with a known substance abuse problem reported that they were using one of several treatments considered to be evidence based for substance abuse during that specific session. (Other practitioners may also have been using these treatments, just not in the session on which they were asked to report.) However, it is difficult to assess exactly what a practitioner means when he or she reports using "motivational interviewing" or "relapse prevention." To address this issue, some authors have recommended the use of fidelity measures to ensure that practitioners are providing the treatment as specified in the manual.

However, we believe that efforts on the part of health plans to police the specific forms of treatment that practitioners provide (including the use of fidelity measures) are likely to be costly, inefficient, and ineffective. There are many legitimate reasons for variations even within an overall approach to treatment, and variations in response to patient characteristics and behaviors can be associated with positive outcomes (Anderson & Strupp, 1996; Beutler et al., 2002; Norcross & Hill, 2004). Moreover, it is doubtful that managed care companies would wish to assume the liability that would be associated with directing health care at this level of specificity. Instead, we believe that health plans will increasingly require that psychologists and other mental health professionals be able to document the outcomes of the treatment they provide, regardless of what therapeutic techniques they use.

Although discussions of outcomes measurement and its possibilities predate the broad discussion of EBP in the field of psychology, they are closely related ideas. We believe that, like EBP, outcomes measurement has now become a "public idea," and we see it as the next wave that will have a major effect on the profession. Outcomes measurement has been positioned as a vehicle for being able to "pay for performance" to ensure value for money spent, a concept that both payers and the public find highly attractive. This is particularly the case in relation to mental health services, which have always been poorly understood. It is extremely important that organized psychology recognize the movement to outcomes-based practice that is already taking place and work toward two ends: (a) to ensure that policies governing how outcome measures are implemented, analyzed, and interpreted are based on sound principles of both measurement and health care and (b) to ensure that individual practitioners are positioned to provide evidence for their practices in ways that appropriately reflect the experiences of their patients and the goals of their treatments. It is here that we believe that psychology should be placing a substantial portion of its energy as a field.

In principle, the assessment of outcomes could offer substantial benefit to health systems, practitioners, and consumers. Theoretically, outcomes assessment can support the identification of best practices and help to ensure that health care quality does not suffer in the interests of cost containment. To do this, a system would need to include the evaluation of access, treatment quality, and costs and to make it possible to use this information in clinically meaningful ways in real time within the system. Such a system would help the individual health professional identify the types of patients with whom he or she tends to have most success and evaluate the best techniques to use with specific types of patients. It would support quality improvement initiatives across the whole system by facilitating the examination of which care processes are associated with the best patient outcomes.

And it could reduce costs by eliminating the need for case-specific benefits management, because practitioners with good records of outcomes would in essence have proved their effectiveness with the actual patient population they are being paid to treat. Unfortunately, the outcomes measures and information infrastructure that are currently available fall short of being able to fully support such programmatic applications, and the manner in which they are currently being implemented within the context of managed care threatens to undermine their potential usefulness for quality improvement. To explore these issues, we now turn to our case study.

MANAGED CARE AND OUTCOMES IN MASSACHUSETTS

As noted, the rate of managed care penetration in Massachusetts is among the highest in the country. Moreover, in the Boston area, all but one of the major insurance companies, including the state Medicaid program, have carved out their services to for-profit managed behavioral health care organizations (MBHOs). These companies are characterized by intensive utilization management processes, and some require treatment authorization as frequently as every four sessions. Several of the largest MBHOs have initiated systems of provider profiling, comparing each provider's length of treatment by diagnosis with system averages. Most recently, Massachusetts has witnessed the proliferation of requirements related to outcomes measurement.

The first system to initiate the requirement that mental health professionals collect outcomes measures was the Massachusetts Behavioral Health Partnership (hereafter referred to as "the Partnership"), the state Medicaid mental health managed care carve out. For a decade, the state had included a provision in the Partnership's contracts that it begin to assess patient-level outcomes of the services it provides, but aside from several small-scale studies, the Partnership had not done so. Under pressure from the state Executive Office of Human Services, in the summer of 2003 the Partnership finally proposed to begin requiring that providers begin using outcomes measures with Medicaid behavioral health patients entering treatment after a certain date. The Partnership issued a list of 19 outcomes measures and announced that it would begin requiring providers to select one or more instruments from among them to assess the outcomes of all services other than medication management and psychological assessment. The Partnership did not propose that providers share these data with the Partnership. Rather, they wanted providers to be responsible for their own quality improvement process and to develop their own way of analyzing, synthesizing, and interpreting the data. The Partnership's directive gave providers 4 months to select instruments from the list. They would have another 7 months to implement use of the instruments, begin providing feedback to consumers, and begin integrating outcomes assessments into treatment plans. Within another

3 months, they were to integrate outcomes assessments into practice management and perform basic analyses of outcomes scores (Massachusetts Behavioral Health Partnership, 2004).

The Massachusetts Mental Health Coalition, representing the professional and consumer communities, expressed concern about the adequacy of the Partnership's plan for professional education, selection of instruments, and the lack of specificity regarding data analysis and interpretation. Other issues the Coalition raised included the lack of outcomes instruments in the public domain; the high cost of using proprietary instruments; and the high indirect costs of time spent on training and administration, scoring, and interpretation of the outcomes measures. The Partnership had already implemented an across-the-board fee cut of 2% earlier that year, and providers began to refer to the outcomes initiative as an unfunded mandate. In partial response to the Coalition's advocacy, the Partnership found money to restore the pay cut and to offer a small fee increase to offset partially the professional time needed to implement the measures. The Partnership agreed on a single proprietary outcomes measure, the Treatment Outcome Package (Kraus, Seligman, & Jordan, 2005), and the Partnership agreed to pay the per administration fee for the use and scoring of this measure for some providers. However, if providers take advantage of this offer, the Partnership will collect, analyze, and own the data. One set of questions still unresolved is how those data will be analyzed and interpreted and who will be consulted as part of this process.

In 2004, Magellan Health Services, the largest MBHO in the country and the holder of the mental health carve-out plan for the Blue Cross Blue Shield of Massachusetts HMO product, notified Massachusetts providers that it had contracted with Polaris Health Systems to use the Polaris–MH instrument (Grissom, Lyons, & Lutz, 2002; Sperry, Brill, Howard, & Grissom, 1996) as a basis for both case management by the MBHO and quality improvement initiatives on the part of the professional. At the time of this writing, Magellan is doing pilot testing of the Polaris–MH system in large practice settings. Magellan is also soliciting small groups and individual providers to participate in pilot testing of a new one-page fax-back version. All data are to be submitted to Magellan for analysis.

At about the same time, United Behavioral Health announced that they would be using an outcomes measure. Unlike the other companies, however, they plan to send an instrument directly to the consumer to fill out and return to the company. Finally, another MBHO, PacifiCare Behavioral Health, Inc., is now entering the Massachusetts marketplace after taking over the mental health carve out for a health plan that had been in receivership. PacifiCare plans to use the outcomes measurement system in Massachusetts that it is already using in other parts of the country. The client is to fill out the Life Status Questionnaire (LSQ), a 30-item instrument based on the Outcome Questionnaire (Lambert et al., 1996). The clinician is to administer the LSQ to the patient after the first, third, and fifth sessions and every five sessions thereafter.

It is clear that patient-level outcomes assessment represents a trend among managed care companies. There has been a good deal of alarm among professional associations in Massachusetts in response to four different plans for outcomes assessment springing up within 1 year. We believe that appropriately designed, properly implemented outcomes measurement systems have the potential to support health system and practitioner improvement and thereby help consumers. An emerging body of research demonstrates that providing clinicians with timely feedback on treatment effectiveness can have beneficial effects, particularly by reducing the rate of treatment failure (see Lambert, 2005). However, for feedback to cause positive change, it must be tailored to the needs and preferences of clinicians and must target an important goal of clinicians (Sapyta, Riemer, & Bickman, 2005). There are real questions about the extent to which the various outcomes initiatives being implemented in Massachusetts meet these conditions. Further, the requirement by each MBHO that mental health professionals use a different outcomes assessment strategy, with different administration schedules, promises to create both an enormous administrative problem for practitioners and conceptual confusion in the broader system. All of these outcomes technologies purport to assess similar constructs but use different measures and methodologies, making it unclear whether comparisons can be made among them. There are also significant differences in terms of how each strategy may impinge on the treatment relationship, how data are owned, and how outcomes will be reported to health professionals.

In addition, several major issues relate more generally to the use of outcomes measures as evidence and how that evidence will be collected, analyzed, interpreted, and acted on in health care settings. The model originally proposed by the Partnership was most supportive of professional autonomy in that health care professionals were to choose their own measures; own their own data; and be responsible for its analysis, interpretation, and reporting. However, there were also significant problems. The field of outcomes measurement is largely a proprietary enterprise. There are few widely used instruments in the public domain, and the costs associated with implementing the measures that are currently considered state of the art may be substantial. These include costs per individual administration, as well as costs associated with purchase of the initial measurement kit, computer scoring programs, and training in the use of the instrument. There are also costs of professional time for training, data review, and writing of quality improvement plans; practitioners lose income when they cannot provide billable services while they are engaged in these other activities. Organized delivery systems and larger group practices would benefit from economies of scale in implementing an outcomes system. However, the Massachusetts Psychological Association calculated that for an individual practitioner who treats some

Medicaid clients in a small private practice, direct and indirect costs based on the Partnership's original requirements would total approximately $3,000 during the 1st year, equivalent to a 17% cut in reimbursement.

There may also be questions about the validity of some of these measures as a basis for the types of decisions that health care systems wish to make. Health care systems should be held accountable for ensuring that the outcomes measures used meet accepted scientific standards for test development and are used for the purposes for which their validity has been demonstrated. When a previously validated instrument is modified or implemented in a different manner, the new version should be empirically demonstrated to be equivalent to the validated one, or new validation studies should be done. When measures designed to assess therapy outcomes are used to make decisions about patient acuity or need for treatment, the validity of the measures for these purposes should be demonstrated. These measures should also be validated with respect to criterion variables important to consumers and purchasers, such as functional status. If a health system purports to value evidence-based treatment, then all such validity information should be made available on request. Health systems' claims to be using evidence-based processes will be more persuasive to the extent that those who monitor outcomes measurement strategies and perform validation studies of the use of these measures do not have a financial stake in either the health system or the instruments.

In general, psychologists are better prepared than other mental health professionals for these new outcomes initiatives because of their background in statistics, measurement, and assessment. Nonetheless, psychologists may require substantial training in the selection, use, analysis, and interpretation of unfamiliar measures. Practitioners will also need a sophisticated understanding of various instruments to select those that are the most appropriate for their own practices or for particular clients (e.g., someone adjusting to a diagnosis of cancer vs. a patient with bulimia nervosa). In most of the initiatives described, data are to be provided to the MBHO, where they will be analyzed and interpreted. This would suggest an even greater need for training among MBHO employees—most of whom are unlikely to have doctoral training in psychology—who will be interpreting data and using it to make treatment decisions.

IMPLICATIONS FOR THE EMPLOYMENT ENVIRONMENT

In the short term, it appears that practitioners participating in the third-party payment system are likely to experience increasing pressure to describe their work in terms that are consistent with the various lists of evidence-based treatments. Over the next few years, we expect that differential rates of payment for treatments deemed evidence based (with varying criteria by state and by system) will be increasingly common. We also expect legislation at the state level that encourages or mandates these practices in state systems. These changes may increase legal risks for professionals providing treatments that have not been tested using particular methodologies and therefore do not meet whatever definition of EBP is being used. More slowly, there are likely to be increasingly explicit attempts to restrict practitioners' ability to provide forms of treatment that do not appear on the lists. As described in this chapter, we have substantive and substantial disagreements with aspects of the framework for evaluating evidence that is currently dominant within the EBP movement. We believe that it is important for organized psychology to continue to challenge these limitations and to advance a broader conceptualization of evidence. At the same time, it may be prudent for practitioners to be prepared to document their knowledge of those treatments being promulgated as evidence based that fall within their scope of practice. Although it is likely to be impractical for MBHOs to require specific certification in each of these treatments, they may require documentation of participation in relevant continuing education programs.

We also believe that national and state-level professional associations should consider how they can assist their members in responding to the increasing demand to document outcomes. This requirement is particularly difficult for independent practitioners, because they do not have the technological infrastructure, personnel support, and economies of scale that facilitate the collection, analysis, and benchmarking of data in organized health care systems. There is a great need for national and state-level advocacy related to models and policies regarding how outcomes systems are conceptualized; who will pay for their direct and indirect costs; and how data are collected, analyzed, interpreted, and applied. Again, however, we believe that there is a pragmatic need for practitioners to begin responding to the trend by considering what type of outcomes assessments may fit best with their practices, values, and needs rather than waiting until these larger questions are resolved by others. It is possible that every health plan will begin requiring their own sets of measures, as we have seen to date in Massachusetts, which would create enormous confusion in the practice community. It is also possible that in the long run, health plans will prefer to shift the considerable administrative burden for data collection and reporting to the practitioner, as was the Partnership's original plan. If that occurs, the use of outcomes measures may be one requirement for network membership. With the growth of defined contribution plans and other forms of what is being called "consumer-based" health care, outcomes measures will likely become even more important as a key basis for consumer choices among coverage options. Practitioners will need to be prepared to compete on this basis.

The burden of increasing requirements based on EBP—on top of those already imposed by managed care—is likely to cause practitioners who have the option of doing so to flee the third-party payment system in favor of a less restrictive and more lucrative self-pay and boutique practice environment. It is noticeable that the discussion on the professional listservs we monitor has shifted from questions about how to gain access to provider panels to questions about how to maintain a "managed care–free" practice. The proportion of psychologists who do not participate in any managed care panels and do no billing of insurance companies appears to be increasing within professional psychology, as it has also in psychiatry and other medical specialties. As health professionals, we are sympathetic to this movement but are also concerned that in the aggregate it will restrict private sector psychology practice to those who are willing and able to pay for services out of pocket. This population will be served by only so many practitioners, and although many may aspire to be among that elite, this cannot be the solution for the majority. In locating itself outside the reimbursement system, psychology also risks being disenfranchised by it. Many clients who pay directly for treatment in turn seek reimbursement from their health plans through a point of service option, and they are likely to stop coming if their health plans begin refusing to pay under this benefit for treatment provided by psychologists who cannot demonstrate an evidence base for their services.

Although clearly there will be problems that need to be addressed as these developments play out, this shift may create a significant opportunity for organized psychology to influence the conceptualization and design of a comprehensive outcomes measurement system. In anticipation of these developments, both the American Psychological Association Practice Organization and state psychological associations are beginning to test ways in which national and state-level professional associations can assist practitioners in developing the infrastructure needed to assess and track outcomes as part of their practices and make such information available to consumers.

CONCLUSION

In this chapter we have attempted to describe the implications and uses of EBP in the context of organized health care delivery. In general, EBP can be seen as a public idea that locates the blame for the problems in the current health care system in arbitrary and uninformed practice by health professionals and suggests that the solution lies in changing their practices in ways that are consistent with research findings. The evidentiary criteria that have been promulgated to evaluate mental health treatments are also being used to provide a justification for the lay management of professional behavior that has been a central operating principle of managed care. These criteria lead to an underestimation of the body of professional knowledge in the field of psychology, in part because the criteria are confounded with the characteristics of what is being evaluated.

These criteria and the resulting lists of treatments do not provide a sufficient basis for health services design and health care policy. Although EBP initiatives in mental health are widely touted and are currently receiving substantial support from federal and state governments, there is little evidence that their implementation will improve services and outcomes or reduce costs at a systems level, except to the extent that they serve to restrict access. There is also a basis for concern that the evidentiary criteria of EBP will contribute to an existing bias toward pharmacological rather than psychological interventions. Available data do not justify restricting patient choice among generally accepted treatments, reimbursing specific treatments at preferential rates, or compelling practitioners to use particular approaches. Such policies are inconsistent with the public interest in that mental health disorders are dramatically undertreated and contribute substantially to disease burden, in contrast to the concerns about overutilization that are at the heart of managed care.

We believe that over the next few years the current discussion about EBP will be reflected in an increasing requirement among health plans and payers that psychologists and other mental health professionals be able to document the outcomes of the treatment they provide. There are serious issues surrounding the conceptualization and implementation of outcomes measurement systems that should be the focus of advocacy and development efforts by organized psychology at both the state and federal levels. At the same time, we recommend that practitioners begin serious consideration of how outcomes assessments may fit best with their practices, values, and needs and of which of the available measures may fit best with the patient populations with whom they work.

Psychology, with its historical focus on science as a partner to practice, is well positioned to lead these developments. However, unless we successfully integrate science and practice in the service of demonstrable quality care in the current environment, we will lose any disciplinary advantage. We need to hold policymakers, consultants, and health plans accountable for providing evidence that their practices support quality of care rather than serving to restrict access, limit treatment options, and disenfranchise providers. As psychologists, we need to maintain a watchful eye on the misuse of science, just as we are admonished to keep that same watchful eye on the misuse of practice that is not supported by evidence.

REFERENCES

Agency for Health Care Policy and Research. (1993a). *Clinical practice guideline development* (AHCPR Publication No. 93-0023). Rockville, MD: U.S. Department of Health and Human Services.

Agency for Health Care Policy and Research. (1993b). *Depression in primary care: Vol. 2. Treatment of major depression* (Clinical Practice Guideline No. 5, AHCPR Publication No. 93-0551). Rockville, MD: U.S. Department of Health and Human Services.

American Psychiatric Association. (2000). Practice guideline for the treatment of patients with major depressive disorder (revision). *American Journal of Psychiatry, 157*(Suppl.), 1–45.

American Psychological Association, Division 12, Society of Clinical Psychology. (2004). *A guide to beneficial psychotherapy.* Retrieved November 23, 2004, from http://www.apa.org/divisions/div12/rev_est/index.html

American Psychological Association, Practice Directorate. (2004). *PracticeNet survey: Psychological treatment of substance abuse.* Retrieved January 11, 2005, from http://www.apapracticenet.net/results/SubstanceAbuse2003

Anderson, T., & Strupp, H. H. (1996). The ecology of psychotherapy research. *Journal of Consulting and Clinical Psychology, 64,* 776–782.

Beutler, L. E., Moleiro, C., & Talebi, H. (2002). How practitioners can systematically use empirical evidence in treatment selection. *Journal of Clinical Psychology, 58,* 1199–1212.

Carpinello, S. E., Rosenberg, L., Stone, J., Schwager, M., & Felton, C. J. (2002). New York State's campaign to implement evidence-based practices for people with serious mental disorders. *Psychiatric Services, 53,* 153–155.

Chambless, D. L., Sanderson, W. C., Shoham, V., Johnson, S. B., Pope, K. S., Crits-Christoph, P., et al. (1996). An update on empirically validated therapies. *The Clinical Psychologist, 49,* 5–18.

Chiles, J. A., Lambert, M. J., & Hatch, A. L. (1999). The impact of psychological intervention on medical offset: A meta-analytic review. *Clinical Psychology: Science and Practice, 6,* 204–220.

Chorpita, B. F., Yim, L. M., Donkervoet, J. C., Arensdorf, A., Amundsen, M. J., McGee, C., et al. (2002). Toward large-scale implementation of empirically supported treatments for children: A review and observations by the Hawaii empirical basis to services task force. *Clinical Psychology: Science and Practice, 9,* 165–190.

DeLeon, P. H., VandenBos, G. R., & Bulatao, E. Q. (1991). Managed mental health care: A history of the federal policy initiative. *Professional Psychology: Research and Practice, 22,* 15–25.

DeRubeis, R. J., Hollon, S. D., Amsterdam, J. D., Shelton, R. C., Young, P. R., Salomon, R. M., et al. (2005). Cognitive therapy vs. medications in the treatment of moderate to severe depression. *Archives of General Psychiatry, 62,* 409–416.

Grissom, G., Lyons, J., & Lutz, W. (2002). Standing on the shoulders of a giant: Development of an outcome management system based on the dose model and phase model of psychotherapy. *Journal of Psychotherapy Research, 12,* 397–412.

Gusfield, J. R. (1981). *The culture of public problems: Drinking, driving, and the symbolic order.* Chicago: University of Chicago Press.

Gutek, B. A. (1995). *The dynamics of service: Reflections on the changing nature of customer/provider interactions*. San Francisco: Jossey-Bass.

Hazlett-Stevens, H., Craske, M. G., Roy-Birne, P. P., Sherbourne, C. D., Stein, M. B., & Bystritsky, A. (2002). Predictors of willingness to consider medication and psychosocial treatment for panic disorder in primary care patients. *General Hospital Psychiatry, 24*, 316–321.

Henry J. Kaiser Family Foundation. (2005). *HMO penetration rate, 2003*. Retrieved January 26, 2005, from http://www.statehealthfacts.org/cgi-bin/healthfacts.cgi?action=compare&category=Managed+Care+%26+Health+Insurance&subcategory=HMOs&topic=HMO+Penetration+Rate

Hollon, S. D., DeRubeis, R. J., Shelton, R. C., Amsterdam, J. D., Salomon, R. M., O'Reardon, J. P., et al. (2005). Prevention of relapse following cognitive therapy versus medications in moderate to severe depression. *Archives of General Psychiatry, 62*, 417–422.

Hollon, S. D., Stewart, M. O., & Strunk, D. (in press). Cognitive behavior therapy has enduring effects in the treatment of depression and anxiety. *Annual Review of Psychology*.

Johnson, B. (Producer), & Brooks, J. L. (Director/Producer). (1997). *As good as it gets* [motion picture]. United States: Sony Pictures.

Keckley, P. H. (2003). *Evidence-based medicine and managed care: Applications, challenges, opportunities—Results of a national program to assess emerging applications of evidence-based medicine to medical management strategies in managed care*. Nashville, TN: Vanderbilt University Center for Evidence-Based Medicine.

Kessler, R. C., Berglund, P., Demler, O., Jin, R., & Walters, E. E. (2005). Lifetime prevalence and age-of-onset distributions of *DSM–IV* disorders in the National Comorbidity Survey Replication. *Archives of General Psychiatry, 62*, 593–602.

Kraus, D. R., Seligman, D., & Jordan, J. R. (2005). Validation of a behavioral health treatment outcome and assessment tool designed for naturalistic settings: The Treatment Outcome Package. *Journal of Clinical Psychology, 61*, 285–314.

Lambert, M. J. (2005). Emerging methods for providing clinicians with timely feedback on treatment effectiveness: An introduction. *Journal of Clinical Psychology, 61*, 141–144.

Lambert, M. J., Hansen, N. B., Umphress, V. J., Lunnen, K., Okiishi, J., Burlingame, G. M., et al. (1996). *Administration and scoring manual for the Outcome Questionnaire (OQ 45.2)*. Wilmington, DE: American Professional Credentialing Services.

Lambert, M. J., & Ogles, B. M. (2004). The efficacy and effectiveness of psychotherapy. In M. J. Lambert (Ed.), *Bergin and Garfield's handbook of psychotherapy and behavior change* (pp. 139–193). New York: Wiley.

Lambert, M. J., & Okiishi, J. C. (1997). The effects of the individual psychotherapist and implications for future research. *Clinical Psychology: Science and Practice, 4*, 66–75.

Lampropoulos, G. K., & Spengler, P. M. (2002). Introduction: Reprioritizing the role of science in a realistic version of the scientist–practitioner model. *Journal of Clinical Psychology, 58*, 1195–1197.

Linehan, M. M. (1993). *Cognitive–behavioral treatment of borderline personality disorder*. New York: Guilford Press.

Massachusetts Behavioral Health Partnership. (2004, May). *Quality Alert #10: Clinical Outcomes Management Protocol*. Retrieved January 11, 2005, from http://www.masspartnership.com/provider/index.aspx?1nkId=outcomesmanagement/outcomesfiles/Quality%20Alert%2010_%20Final.pdf

Maxfield, M., Achman, L., & Cook, A. (2004). *National estimates of mental health insurance benefits* (DHHS Publication No. SMA 04-3872). Rockville, MD: Center for Mental Health Services, Substance Abuse and Mental Health Services Administration.

Miller, W. R., & Rollnick, S. (2002). *Motivational interviewing: Preparing people for change* (2nd ed.). New York: Guilford Press.

Nathan, P. E., & Gorman, J. M. (Eds.). (1998). *A guide to treatments that work*. New York: Oxford University Press.

National Institute for Clinical Excellence. (2004). *Depression: Management of depression in primary and secondary care*. Retrieved January 12, 2005, from http://www.nice.org.uk/pdf/CG023quickrefguide.pdf

National Institutes of Health. (2004). *State implementation of evidence-based practices: Bridging science and service* (NIMH and SAMHSA Publication No. RFA MH-03-007). Retrieved November 19, 2004, from http://grants1.nih.gov/grants/guide/rfa-files/RFA-MH-03-007.html

Norcross, J. C., & Hill, C. E. (2004). Empirically supported therapy relationships. *The Clinical Psychologist, 57,* 19–24.

Olfson, M., Marcus, S. C., Druss, B., Elinson, L., Tanielian, T., & Pincus, H. A. (2002, January 9). National trends in the outpatient treatment of depression. *Journal of the American Medical Association, 287,* 203–209.

Oregon Office of Mental Health and Addiction Services. (2004). *Proposed operational definition for evidence-based practices: Final draft, June 1, 2004*. Retrieved November 19, 2004, from http://www.leg.state.or.us/orlaws/sess0600.dir/0669ses.htm

Reed, G. M., McLaughlin, C. J., & Newman, R. (2002). American Psychological Association policy in context: The development and evaluation of guidelines for professional practice. *American Psychologist, 57,* 1041–1047.

Sackett, D. L., Straus, S. E., Richardson, W. S., Rosenberg, W., & Haynes, R. B. (2000). *Evidence based medicine: How to practice and teach EBM* (2nd ed.). London: Churchill Livingstone.

Sapyta, J., Riemer, M., & Bickman, L. (2005). Feedback to clinicians: Theory, research, and practice. *Journal of Clinical Psychology, 61,* 145–153.

Sperry, L., Brill, P., Howard, K. I., & Grissom, G. (1996). *Treatment outcomes in psychotherapy and psychiatric interventions*. New York: Brunner/Mazel.

Stricker, G., Abrahamson, D. J., Bologna, N. C., Hollon, S. D., Robinson, E. A., & Reed, G. M. (1999). Treatment guidelines: The good, the bad, and the ugly. *Psychotherapy, 36,* 69–79.

Tanenbaum, S. J. (1999). Evidence and expertise: The challenge of the outcomes movement to medical professionalism. *Academic Medicine, 74,* 757–763.

Tanenbaum, S. J. (2003). Evidence-based practice in mental health: Practical weaknesses meet political strengths. *Journal of Evaluation in Clinical Practice, 9,* 287–301.

Tanenbaum, S. J. (2005). Evidence-based practice as mental health policy: Three controversies and a caveat. *Health Affairs, 24,* 163–173.

U.S. Census Bureau. (2004, August 26). *Income stable, poverty up, numbers of Americans with and without health insurance rise, Census Bureau reports.* Retrieved November 19, 2004, from http://www.census.gov/Press-Release/www/releases/archives/income_wealth/002484.html

U.S. Food and Drug Administration. (2005, January). *Antidepressant use in children, adolescents, and adults.* Retrieved January 17, 2005, from http://www.fda.gov/cder/drug/antidepressants/default.htm

Wampold, B. E., Lichtenberg, J. W., & Waehler, C. A. (2002). Principles of empirically supported interventions in counseling psychology. *The Counseling Psychologist, 30,* 197–217.

Wang, P. S., Berglund, P., Olfson, M., Pincus, H. A., Wells, K. B., & Kessler, R. C. (2005). Failure and delay in initial treatment contact after first onset of mental disorders in the National Comorbidity Survey Replication. *Archives of General Psychiatry, 62,* 603–613.

Wang, P. S., Lane, M., Olfson, M., Pincus, H. A., Wells, K. B., & Kessler, R. C. (2005). Twelve-month use of mental health services in the United States: Results from the National Comorbidity Replication Survey. *Archives of General Psychiatry, 62,* 629–640.

Wennberg, J. E. (1984). Dealing with medical practice variations: A proposal for action. *Health Affairs, 3,* 6–32.

Westen, D., Novotny, C., & Thompson-Brenner, H. (2004). The empirical status of empirically supported therapies: Assumptions, methods, and findings. *Psychological Bulletin, 130,* 631–663.

WHO World Mental Health Survey Consortium. (2004, June 2). Prevalence, severity, and unmet need for treatment of mental health disorders in the World Health Organization World Mental Health surveys. *Journal of the American Medical Association, 291,* 2581–2590.

World Health Organization. (2001). *The World Health Report 2000: Health systems: Improving performance.* Geneva, Switzerland: Author.

Zarin, D. A., Young, J. L., & West, J. C. (2005). Challenges to evidence-based medicine: A comparison of patients and treatments in randomized controlled trials with patients and treatments in a practice research network. *Social Psychiatry and Psychiatric Epidemiology, 40,* 27–35.

Zoellner, L. A., Feeny, N. C., Cochran, B., & Pruitt, L. (2003). Treatment choice for PTSD. *Behaviour Research and Therapy, 41,* 879–886.

2

EVIDENCE, ENDEAVOR, AND EXPERTISE IN PSYCHOLOGY PRACTICE

CAROL D. GOODHEART

There is a chronic gap between many clinical researchers and clinical practitioners on the topic of evidence-based practice in psychology. Researchers complain that clinicians are slow to adopt the high-quality treatments they have designed under rigorous and controlled scientific conditions. Clinicians complain that narrow treatments based on randomized controlled clinical trials for specific diagnostic categories are of limited use with the varied populations and problems of clients seen in general practice. However, the schism is not really between certain practitioners and researchers; it is between adherents of a medical drug model of psychotherapy (based on specific ingredients) and a contextual model of psychotherapy (based on common factors in well-established therapies). Both groups are delivering important messages to each other with implications for the future of health care practice.

Discussions about evidence-based practice take place within the larger framework of the evidence-based practice movement in the United States,

Part of this chapter is adapted from "Evidenced-Based Practice and the Endeavor of Psychotherapy," by C. D. Goodheart, 2004, *The Independent Practitioner*, 24, pp. 6–10. Phoenix, AZ: Psychologists in Independent Practice: A Division of the American Psychological Association. Adapted with permission.

which is a social and cultural phenomenon. The movement reflects an accelerating public policy trend related to accountability and costs that is occurring also in medicine, nursing, occupational and physical therapy, and education. In the midst of this movement, it is a challenge for practicing psychologists to balance their needs to develop and maintain a personally effective therapeutic voice, translate multiple streams of evidence into meaningful interventions, offer safe and confidential therapeutic relationships, and earn a living by practicing in the real world. Disparate voices carry conflicting messages about the need for psychotherapy and its costs, worth, components, allowable interventions, and effectiveness. These forces, both within the discipline of psychology and in the larger health care system, compete for supremacy.

It is hard to imagine how anyone could be against "evidence." However, there are fundamental and important philosophical differences about the proper balance between the positivistic empiricism of the medical drug model, on the one hand, and the contextual model's attention to the client's subjective experiences and needs, the therapist's characteristics and activities, and the therapeutic alliance and endeavor on the other.

These differences in worldview are represented by two differing sets of recommendations. On the basis of psychology's impressive advances in the treatment of numerous specific disorders, Barlow (2004) proposed a demarcation between the terms *psychological treatments* and *psychotherapy*. In this recommendation, manual-based interventions designed and targeted for specific forms of pathology or dysfunction would be named *psychological treatments* and be a part of the health care system; the term *psychotherapy* would be considered generic and perhaps dropped from the health care system, although it might then be reserved for adjustment and problems in living, as well as for personal growth. In an examination of the evidence-based treatment movement, Wampold and Bhati (2004) took a different point of view. They cautioned that the emphasis of the movement is increasingly on treatments, when the type of treatment accounts for little of the outcome, and the role of the psychologist and the subjective experience of the client are omitted. They recommended alternative conceptualizations that emphasize common factors and broader research perspectives, such as those proposed by two American Psychological Association (APA) divisions, the Society of Counseling Psychology (Division 17; Wampold, Lichtenberg, & Waehler, 2002) and Psychotherapy (Division 29; Norcross, 2001). In a similar vein, Ablon and Marci (2004) suggested that the focus of efficacy research be shifted from treatment packages to treatment change processes, because the level of abstraction of the packages is too far removed from the clinical encounter. Many practitioners adopt an integrative approach and incorporate some elements of both common factors and specific interventions, assimilating useful aspects of both models. No one yet has the final word on what achieves the greatest meaningful change for individuals with emotional and social problems.

I suggest that at the heart of disagreements about evidence-based practice in psychology are differences in how evidence is defined and how the endeavor of psychotherapy is viewed. The problem does not lie, for the most part, in antiscientific practice attitudes, substandard doctoral education, or poor clinical research. This chapter presents the perspective of a lifelong practitioner on psychological practice and its context, the endeavor of psychotherapy, the multiple streams of evidence needed for scientifically informed practice, and the role of clinical expertise. There is a continuing thread throughout the chapter: the importance of adapting approaches to the needs of the individuals, couples, families, and groups who seek psychological services.

CONTEXT FOR A PRACTITIONER PERSPECTIVE

The foundation of psychology is science. The practice of psychology is built on that base, although clinicians are faced also with problems that go beyond what the research has yet been able to describe, measure, or ameliorate. Its foundation in basic science and social science is what differentiates psychology from the other helping professions. Extensive training in the development of technical and interpersonal expertise also differentiates psychologists from other groups.

Definitions

What does one mean when one talks about evidence-based practice? The Institute of Medicine (2001) definition adapted from Sackett, Straus, Richardson, Rosenberg, and Haynes (2000) is widely accepted in health care: "Evidence-based practice is the integration of best research evidence with clinical expertise and patient values" (p. 147). This definition provides a broad perspective and does not imply that any one of the three components is weighted more than another. Nevertheless, many medical and psychological scientists consider research the most important component.

The American Psychological Association accepted the recommendations of its Presidential Task Force on Evidence Based Practice (2005a) and adopted a similar definition in its policy statement: "Evidence-based practice in psychology (EBPP) is the integration of the best available research with clinical expertise in the context of patient characteristics, culture, values, and preferences" (p. 1). The report of the Task Force provides an expanded discussion of the basis for the policy, including the rationale and references (2005b). The "Criteria for Evaluating Treatment Guidelines" (APA, 2002a) incorporate the three components as well. The APA "Ethical Principles of Psychologists and Code of Conduct," in Section 2.04, sets the standard that psychologists' work is based on established scientific and professional knowledge of the discipline (APA, 2002b).

Differences Between Practice and Research

Practice and research are different endeavors with distinct purposes. The professional interests, the cultures of work settings, and even the kinds of questions posed often differ for practitioners and researchers. Each group places different values on the kinds of evidence it uses to guide its work. All knowledge is socially constructed; hence, science is a social construction, and so is psychological practice, but the two rely on different subjective value frameworks (Tanenbaum, 2002). The presence of differing values affects the two groups' orientation toward treatment.

Practitioners and researchers differ in personality characteristics, such as the underlying dimension of egocentric–sociocentric views of the world, as well as in epistemic values (e.g., increasing knowledge vs. improving the human condition), theoretical orientations (e.g., learning theory vs. humanism), cognitive strengths, and developmental influences (Conway, 1988; Dana, 1987; Frank, 1984; Zachar & Leong, 1992). However, these differences reside on a continuum, and many psychologists combine characteristics of both groups.

Role demands for researchers and practitioners differ, too. Researchers must show that a treatment works under specified conditions; clinicians must do all they can to resolve the problem at hand. Researchers primarily seek efficacy, internal validity, and reliability based on clinical trials, whereas practitioners primarily seek effectiveness, external validity (utility), and feasibility (resources) for the particular client, couple, family, or group in the room at the moment. Researchers value knowledge based on hypothesis testing under controlled circumstances. Practitioners do, too, but many also value forms of knowledge based on discovery and give them precedence in the clinical encounter. Researchers usually link treatment and outcome, whereas practitioners usually link context and outcome. In a seminal article, Peterson (1991) presented a vibrant picture of practice activities as differentiated from science:

> Professional activity begins and ends in the condition of the client. Whether the client is an individual, a group, or an organization, the responsibility of the practitioner is to help improve the client's functional effectiveness. The practitioner does not choose the issue to examine; the client does. The simplifications and controls that are essential to science cannot be imposed in practice. Each problem must be addressed as it occurs in nature, as an open, living process in all its complexity, often in a political context that requires certain forms of action and prohibits others. All functionally important influences on the process under study must be considered. (p. 426)

Peterson (1991) expressed the view that "at its best practice runs ahead of research" (p. 426). However, as preparation for practice, he recommended that graduate programs teach procedures subjected to rigorous research and found useful and that they not teach procedures that have been tested repeatedly and failed to demonstrate utility, and he reiterated that claims of utility for useless procedures are unethical (Peterson, 1995). Thus, the strengths of both science and practice are needed to serve the public well. In recognizing the necessary differences between the goals of science and practice, the psychology profession must remember that the shared goal is to solve problems in society. Any signs of charlatanism on the part of practitioners and scientism on the part of scientists are a hindrance to that goal (Fox, 1996).

THE ENDEAVOR OF PSYCHOTHERAPY

Psychotherapy is first and foremost a human endeavor. It is messy. It is not solely a scientific endeavor, nor can it be reduced meaningfully to a technical mechanistic enterprise (Goodheart, 2004). The evidence-based treatment movement can disempower practitioners relative to researchers to the extent that clinical skill is equated solely with applied science and to the extent that science is restricted to randomized controlled clinical trials of treatment packages (Tanenbaum, 1999). Nevertheless, a sound basis for psychotherapy and guidance about its important elements exist. Psychology has a significant body of evidence for the treatment of specific kinds of distress and clusters of symptoms and a significant body of research concerning the importance of the therapeutic relationship and common factors. Practitioners need to rely on data from both nomothetic (attempts to discover general laws) and idiographic (attempts to understand a particular individual or event) processes, findings based on both quantitative and qualitative methods, and views based on both scientific and humanistic attitudes; these are psychology's dual heritage (Messer, 2004).

The triumvirate of factors that contribute to psychotherapy outcomes is the client's personal factors (e.g., motivation), the therapist's personal factors (e.g., capacity for empathy), and the interventions offered (e.g., stimulation of the client's curiosity about his or her problem). Sophisticated meta-analyses show that about 75% of people who enter psychotherapy benefit from the experience (Lambert & Ogles, 2004) and that there are few differences in outcome among therapeutic orientations (Lambert & Ogles, 2004; Wampold, 2001). Suffering is a part of the human experience, and psychotherapy is generally effective in easing that suffering.

Psychotherapy is a rich process. It encompasses efforts to reach understanding, ease pain, solve problems, facilitate adaptation, foster growth, prevent decline or dysfunction, and find meaning, all within the context of a trusting relationship. People seeking psychotherapy want to be heard and understood. They want respectful help in obtaining relief, making sense of their experience, and improving their lives. Each client wants to be treated as a whole person, not as a diagnosis or a case. Research findings are a necessary and vital part of psychotherapy, but they are not all of psychotherapy. Guiding principles are needed, too. The language of treatment manuals gives only a narrow and tightly structured view of the human condition. It is like looking at a landscape with a flashlight. The flashlight illuminates the dark, but it does not show the entire field. Practitioners need additional tools as well to function clinically. Scientific experiments are predicated on control and the ability to manipulate the variables under consideration or to vary them along selected dimensions. Real-world psychotherapy involves working in the face of a few variables one can control and with the knowledge that there are many others one cannot. This is where clinical knowledge, expertise, and the ability to use creative combinations and adaptations of interventions come into play. They widen the view from that illuminated by the flashlight to the broader field.

Psychotherapy draws on many theories. These theories include behavioral, cognitive–behavioral, psychodynamic, family systems, humanistic, feminist, integrative, and cultural competence orientations, among others. In diverse practices and clinical settings, underlying theories may differ somewhat, but most experienced clinicians are integrationists (Lambert, Bergin, & Garfield, 2004). They offer solid interventions, a confidential therapeutic relationship, and a shared expectation for a positive outcome. Good clinicians borrow from each other and borrow what works. Some psychotherapy-related theories contain constructs that are easy to isolate and measure; others do not. There are very few differences among bona fide therapies that have been widely practiced over time and that have a coherent theoretical structure and research underpinning (Wampold, 2001). Good clinicians also become aware of new and emerging approaches, such as cultural competence guidelines, that evolve as society and practices change.

Psychotherapy is an art as well as a science. In other words, psychotherapy is based on both clinical expertise and scientific knowledge. Art is a transformative human effort to mirror, alter, or counteract the work of nature; it is conception, form, and execution (American Heritage Dictionary, 1993). Psychotherapy is a fluid, mutual, interactive process. Each participant shapes and is shaped by the other. Good clinicians respond to the nuances of language, both verbal utterances and bodily expressions. They are masters of tact and timing, of when to push and when to be patient. They know the spectrum of disruptions that can occur in a working alliance and are versatile and empathic in their reparative responses. They are creative in finding paths to understanding, in matching an intervention to a need.

Psychotherapy is complex. Clients' biological predispositions, personalities, preferences, developmental level, and psychological functioning intertwine with their life circumstances and stressors. It is helpful to know that individually tailored and readiness stage-matched interventions and relationships can be much more effective than standardized ones (Prochaska &

Norcross, 2002). Most psychotherapy clients have cross-diagnostic issues and comorbid conditions. Dual diagnosis is common. Even within one diagnostic category, level of functioning varies widely. In my own practice, I had to tailor treatments individually for the following clients, all of whom met the criteria for major depression: the self-mutilating woman with a borderline personality disorder, the man lashing out at his work clients and on probation for a bad temper, the withdrawn and tearful mother and midlevel manager whose husband was a cocaine addict exhibiting bizarre behavior and frightening their children, and the elderly man with cancer who was suffering great losses.

RELEVANT STREAMS OF EVIDENCE AND INFORMATION FOR PSYCHOTHERAPY

Many appropriate and different kinds of evidence facilitate scientifically informed practice and are needed for clinical decision making. The more complex the case, the more resources one may have to call on. The information needs of practitioners are heterarchical in nature, rather than hierarchical, and mandate the consideration of a wide range of sources (Tickle-Degnen & Bedell, 2003).

Empirical Research

Several categories of research design offer useful information for practice. Each has its strengths and limitations. The categories are briefly summarized in the paragraphs that follow (see APA, 2005b, for a review of the relative value of evidence produced by different designs).

Randomized controlled trial (RCT) design is the research standard for drawing causal inferences about the effects of interventions. Efficacious interventions based on RCTs are considered solid for the situations in which they apply. The treatments based on RCTs are aimed at closely defined nonoverlapping disorders listed in the *Diagnostic and Statistical Manual of Mental Disorders* (4th ed., *DSM–IV*; American Psychiatric Association, 1994), such as panic disorder or sexual dysfunction, and are based on methods that lend themselves to quantification and the positivist empirical tradition (see Chambless, 2005, for a summary of empirically supported therapies, most of which, but not all, are based on RCTs done by cognitive–behaviorally oriented researchers). The RCT model of research is the medical drug research model. It is the predominant form of health care research funded by the National Institutes of Health and the National Institute of Mental Health, which explains why this method is driving much of the empirical research on psychotherapy. RCTs can evaluate existing treatments but cannot create new ones. RCT results offer probabilistic knowledge, but the practitioner still must make a subjective choice in how to treat each individual person based on a broad knowledge base and clinical skill (Tanenbaum, 2002).

Equally important to the practitioner are effectiveness research, which addresses the validity of interventions and approaches in real-world settings; process–outcome research, which investigates the mechanisms of change; meta-analysis research, which analyzes the size of effects based on syntheses of multiple studies; health service system research, which examines public health issues, utilization, acceptance, costs, and cost offsets; and qualitative research, which describes meaning and process and inductively builds hypotheses and theories. Psychotherapy also lends itself well to single-participant designs for tracking client progress.

Collaborative practitioner–researcher networks, such as the Pennsylvania Practice Research Network (Borkovec, Echemendia, Ragusea, & Ruiz, 2001), show promise for the further development of effectiveness research in natural settings. Also, there are interesting efforts under way to revisit the case-study method on a larger scale to provide quantitative and qualitative knowledge about psychotherapy process and outcomes. For example, the online journal *Pragmatic Case Studies in Psychotherapy* (at http:// pcsp.libraries.rutgers.edu) is a peer-reviewed, open-access journal and database (D. Fishman, personal communication, July 7, 2004; Fishman & Messer, 2005).

A Diverse Psychology Literature

Clinicians assemble knowledge from a varied literature related to psychology to inform their practices. The content of this body of knowledge is much larger than treatments for disorders. Some examples are observations of resilience and child development (Masten, 2001), the first new stress response and coping model in more than 70 years (Taylor et al., 2000), social epidemiology and the impact of psychosocial factors on the human immune system (Berkman & Kawachi, 2000), the genetics revolution and the psychological implications of genetics testing (Patenaude, 2005), and the literature on the likely impact of certain life events such as poverty or parental divorce on children (e.g., Belle & Dodson, 2006; Pedro-Carroll, 2001).

Professional consensus material, such as the "Ethical Principles of Psychologists and Code of Conduct" (APA, 2002b), is another category of information and is a living document that has been revised and updated regularly since the 1950s. In addition, the APA has published other practice guidelines that recommend professional conduct for psychologists, including the "Guidelines for Psychological Practice With Older Adults" (2004); the "Guidelines on Multicultural Education, Training, Research, Practice, and Organizational Change for Psychologists" (2003); the "Guidelines for Psychotherapy With Gay, Lesbian, and Bisexual Clients" (2002c); and the *Guidelines for Psychological Evaluations in Child Protection Matters* (1998). Practice guidelines represent an attempt to delineate best professional practices; they are different from treatment guidelines, which specify treatment interventions for disorders.

The literature includes many widely recognized theories of personality, psychopathology, and health, as well as theoretically based principles and aims for psychotherapy. The most frequently researched approach to psychotherapy is cognitive–behavioral therapy (CBT). It is interesting to note that as the pace of research on CBT quickens, the cross-fertilization of concepts is increasing, too. Important and useful constructs from other theories are being folded into the burgeoning literature on CBT. For example, the psychoanalytic concept of transference was described in an interview by Judith Beck, director of the Beck Institute for Cognitive Therapy and Research, as a client interrupting the process of therapy "by applying his or her dysfunctional beliefs to therapy itself" (Dingfelder, 2004). The therapeutic response to a negative transference or belief about the therapist or therapy is quite similar for both psychodynamically and cognitively oriented therapists: Help the client recognize the beliefs and test them for reality, responsiveness, and trustworthiness within the safety of the therapeutic relationship. Theoretical blending is also apparent in motivational interviewing for substance abuse, which combines cognitive–behavioral and nondirective Rogerian techniques (Burke, Arkowitz, & Mencola, 2003). There are similarly useful modifications to traditional behavioral-change-focused couples treatment (Jacobson, Christiansen, Prince, Cordova, & Eldridge, 2000); an emotional acceptance strategy has been added (based on empathic joining, unified detachment, and tolerance building), which mirrors the acceptance component found in existential approaches to psychotherapy.

Changes in practice over time seem to arise from a combination of research, theory, and consensus. In recent years, strengths-based approaches to practice have been on the rise, as opposed to a focus on deficits, with both children and adults (Goodheart, 2006).

Effectiveness Data

Conclusions about effectiveness are based on real-world outcomes in diverse communities. Information about effectiveness can be gained from numerous sources such as from an individual clinician's practice, from community trials, and from studies on special populations. Health system payers increasingly seek accountability and demonstrated services effectiveness from health care professionals. Pre- and posttreatment measures provide evidence of functional status, responsiveness, and outcome. Measurement can also improve clinical judgment by providing a feedback mechanism. However, it is important to remember that results depend on what questions are asked, and the selection of measures depends on what one wants to know (e.g., characteristics of the client or characteristics of the psychologist's practice across clients). Selection also depends on the focus of treatment, such as symptom reduction or quality-of-life issues, and the sensitivity of the measure in showing change.

The simplest way for a practitioner to track effectiveness is to do outcomes measurement. In principle, practitioners should have the option of using many kinds of interventions and combinations according to client needs if they have basic evaluation processes in place. However, apart from psychologists' scientific and professional interests in better understanding outcomes, there are cost-cutting factors associated with the health care marketplace's drive toward the demonstration of outcomes. The insurance industry may mishandle outcomes data or its collection process when cost containment is the primary goal. Managed care companies may not approve sufficient numbers of sessions for therapy to show improvements in clients whose problems call for a higher dose–response ratio. Practitioners are not likely to treat the most distressed and dysfunctional clients if the less positive short-term outcomes generated by a skewed population of clients will be used against them. Also, practitioners are not reimbursed by most systems for the time expended in measurement and outcomes tracking. Therefore, payment for the measurement services will need to be built into these systems in situations where outcome measurement is required.

Clinical Interview and Observation

Sensitive semistructured interviews and observation yield essential clinical information. Before making a treatment plan and selecting interventions, a practitioner must understand the unique person and situation, form a relationship of trust and confidence, and discover and frame the real problem, not just a few presenting symptoms. Very few clients reveal secrets in the first session, and none can tell the practitioner what is outside of their awareness. Sophisticated case formulation evolves over time as observation helps the clinician to build, modify, regroup, and strengthen the treatment.

Disciplined inquiry, anchored by a guiding conception, forms the basis for a coherent clinical assessment and practice (Peterson, 1991). In this process, the client's needs are paramount, rather than the need for general knowledge. One begins with the client and applies all useful knowledge, including qualitative or humanistic knowledge, if it helps to understand the client, rather than starting with a fixed set of strategies.

The term *local clinical scientist* describes practitioners with observational and scientific attitudes and skills (Stricker & Trierweiler, 1995). Observation, both in session and over time, is a powerful tool. It includes four types of observational skills (Shakow, 1976): objective (from the outside), participant (including awareness of the reciprocal effects on observer and observed), subjective (empathic and intuitive), and self (self-examination). An expert therapist functions as a finely tuned instrument and thinking person, not as a technician following a script. He or she asks, What do I see and hear, how do I understand it, and how am I reacting to it and to this person? Related to observation, there is a useful distinction between generalization and stereotyping (Galanti, 1997): A generalization is a starting point that indicates common trends, but further inquiry is needed to discover whether the hypothesis or conclusion is appropriate to a particular individual. A stereotype is an ending point, one in which no further attempts are made to discover if the person fits the hypothesis. Being observant, keeping an open mind, and maintaining an attitude of scientific inquiry are ways that clinicians use to keep a cautious eye on their own judgments. The scientific attitude allows practitioners to add knowledge and avoid blunders that can lead to breaks in the alliance, misunderstanding, and treatment failures. Problems in the generalizability of treatments based on the efficacy literature can be mitigated somewhat by using local observations and local solutions (Stricker & Trierweiler, 1995).

Patient Response to Intervention

Clients' responses guide practitioners to better tailor treatment to their preferences and needs. Even relatively standard interventions applied in unique circumstances may provide the therapist with another opportunity to receive feedback from clients about how well the therapist understands them and their needs. Client response is a critical source of information.

For example, I recently evaluated a client with major depression who left a previous treatment at a college counseling center after one session. According to the client's report, the therapist asked her to identify her goals for psychotherapy. She was unable to do so but wanted to talk about how badly her life was going. The therapist asked her a second and a third time about her goals, but the client did not know how to answer. The session ended unsatisfactorily. What was I to make of this event? After all, it is reasonable and customary to ask clients about what they hope to gain and what they hope can change. In fact, it is standard practice. However, this client's response and her inability to give a meaningful answer were clear indicators that another approach was needed. The client reported, in tears, "I am so depressed I can hardly get out of bed, and I don't know what my goals are." My intervention was to reassure her that she would know her goals when she felt better, and in the meantime we would sort out what was troubling her and what might be helpful. By the fourth session she was sufficiently improved to identify and start to pursue her goals.

A similar problem occurred in a training videotape that I reviewed shortly after seeing the client discussed in the preceding paragraph. In this example of a first meeting, the therapist was a young male graduate student in psychology, and the client was a depressed young woman. The session began well as he greeted her pleasantly and asked what brought her there. He seemed attentive and interested in learning about her. She began to talk about her life. In short order, he asked about her goals. She paused, looked down, and when she spoke, it was not about her goals. He listened for a few moments and gently brought her back to the topic of goals. She sighed, paused, and veered away again. He seemed to recognize her difficulty; he rephrased his question about goals and then tried to help her understand by giving her examples of goals. By the end of the session they produced a goal statement, in his words. What happened in this session? The graduate student was attempting to follow a protocol with instructions to identify a goal in the first session. He was not yet experienced enough to know how to respond when an intervention is not working in the way intended, although he did his best to follow the rules and still to be responsive to the client. I learned later that he did not know he was "allowed" to deviate from the planned sequence.

Clients are a primary source of information about how psychotherapy is progressing. An attuned clinician gains valuable feedback about improvements or setbacks that are taking place in the sessions or outside of the treatment room in the client's everyday life. Clients tell clinicians when things are going better or worse at work or in their relationships; they tell them they are sleeping or eating differently; they tell them they feel better or are not their old selves yet. But attuned clinicians also know that many clients have a tendency to be agreeable on the surface and tell them what they want to hear. Clinicians know it is important to be alert for signs of client disengagement or distance to address the issue being hidden. Clients often omit information, especially if it is associated with shame. It is not only the client who gives feedback to the clinician; it may be a spouse or parent who contributes observations about changes in the client. Under some circumstances, it may be the client's physician, attorney, or employer.

THE ROLE OF CLINICAL EXPERTISE

There is much less research on clinical expertise than on psychotherapy. However, as with the evolving evidence for specific treatments, common factors, therapeutic relationships, and client factors in psychotherapy, there is a sound basis on which to build further.

The APA Presidential Task Force on Evidence-Based Practice (APA, 2005b) identified competencies that foster positive therapeutic outcomes:

> a) assessment, diagnostic judgment, systematic case formulation, and treatment planning; b) clinical decision making, treatment implementation, and monitoring of patient progress; c) interpersonal expertise; d) continual self-reflection and acquisition of skills; e) appropriate evaluation and use of research evidence in both basic and applied psychological science; f) understanding the influence of individual and cultural differences on treatment; g) seeking available resources (e.g., consultation, adjunctive or alternative services) as needed; and h) having a cogent rationale for clinical strategies. (p. 10)

Psychotherapy requires clinical expertise because it is a complex interpersonal process that takes place in a context of uncertainty and ambiguity and under the press of clients' urgent needs. The relevance of the information obtained and the impact of decisions cannot be known in advance. Clinicians have to consider how best to achieve and maintain a working alliance. They have to consider not only the best treatment options but also the important consequences of those choices and the outcomes clients seek. Practitioners must attend to such client concerns as obtaining symptom relief, recovering from debilitating conditions, managing chronic conditions, adjusting to adversity, making important decisions, developing skills, resolving interpersonal conflicts, and improving quality of life. Often goals change over time. Clients' capacities and needs unfold as they progress and develop trust in the psychologist, sometimes seeming like the traditional nested Russian doll sets—when a doll is opened, it contains another version within, and another, and another. An adolescent female with an eating disorder may discuss a number of somatic symptoms but may hide her history of sexual exploitation by a family member until she decides how her story will be received. A depressed retired widower may reveal his social isolation with some embarrassment and only much later, in deep shame, may acknowledge a growing drinking problem.

Faced routinely with difficult or murky psychotherapy situations, clinicians call on their experiences and their expertise for a way to move the treatment forward to a good resolution and to preserve the client's dignity. What makes a master clinician? How do expert practitioners make decisions about what to do, how to relate, what to offer, when to reevaluate, when to change direction, and how to repair a ruptured alliance? Although psychology has not yet been able to answer these questions definitively, there are promising leads.

An Updated Model for Evidence-Based Clinical Decisions

Clinical expertise is appropriately recognized as one of the three components in evidence-based practice: research evidence, clinical expertise, and patient preferences (see Figure 2.1). Haynes, Devereaux, and Guyatt (2002) created an advanced model of evidence-based practice that reflects the expanded role of clinical expertise (see Figure 2.2). In the newer model, clinical expertise becomes a fourth element, one that is overlaid as the means to integrate all other components. *Clinical state and circumstances* is added as an essential element in clinical decisions, replacing clinical expertise in the original configuration; *patient preferences* is expanded to include patient actions and is reversed with research evidence to show its frequent precedence.

Clinical expertise lies in balancing the patient's state and circumstances, the relevant research, and the patient's preferences and actions to achieve a good outcome. The balancing process often involves tradeoffs, which should

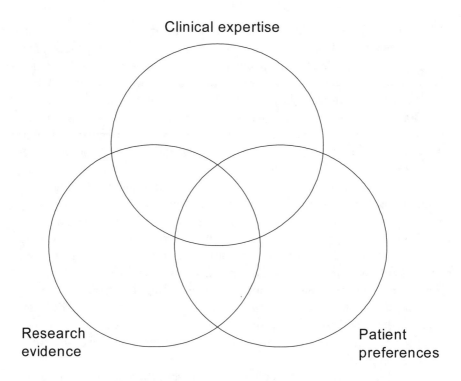

Clinical expertise

Research
evidence

Patient
preferences

Figure 2.1. Early model of the key elements for evidence-based clinical decisions.
From *Evidence-Based Medicine Notebook, Vol. 7* (p. 36), by R. B. Haynes, P. J.
Devereaux, and G. H. Guyatt, 2002, London: BMJ Publishing Group. Copyright
2002 by the BMJ Publishing Group. Reprinted with permission.

be made according to the patient's needs. Haynes et al. (2002) presented the
model as a recommendation for how decisions should be made, rather than
as a description of how they are made (health care systems often influence or
set the boundaries on treatment options). The recommendation gives precedence to patient preferences over clinician preferences, when feasible. In
individual clinical decisions, the role of the four components may vary according to the circumstances of care, which makes the model flexible and
responsive and seems to capture the role of clinical expertise in a more clinically sophisticated conceptualization. In addition, the model's focus on patients allows for inclusion of the central role of culture in patients' preferences and actions.

Novice–Expert Differences

The ability to reason and solve problems well is dependent on a system
of well-organized knowledge. It is not surprising that there are significant
differences between experts and novices. In an early influential study of ex-

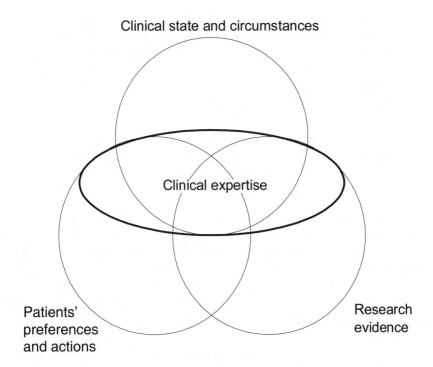

Clinical state and circumstances

Clinical expertise

Patients'
preferences
and actions

Research
evidence

Figure 2.2. An updated model for evidence-based clinical decisions. From
Evidence-Based Medicine Notebook, Vol. 7 (p. 37), by R. B. Haynes, P. J.
Devereaux, and G. H. Guyatt, 2002, London: BMJ Publishing Group. Copyright
2002 by the BMJ Publishing Group. Reprinted with permission.

pert chess players (Chase & Simon, 1973), results showed that experts chunk
information and are able to see many variations, many moves ahead. Since
then, expertise in many areas has been tested with such groups as historians,
physicians, social scientists, and sushi chefs. The factors involved in expertise, discussed in reviews by Bransford, Brown, and Cocking (1999) and
Gambrill (2005), are summarized below:

- *Pattern:* Experts recognize large patterns. They attend to features and meaningful patterns of information not noticed by
  novices.
- *Depth:* Experts know more. They have acquired extensive content knowledge and organize it in ways that reflect a deep understanding of their domain.
- *Content and access:* Experts' knowledge cannot be reduced to
  sets of isolated facts or propositions; instead, it is organized functionally rather than descriptively. The set of knowledge is
  "conditionalized" to specify the circumstances in which it will
  be useful.

- *Retrieval:* Experts are able to flexibly retrieve important aspects of their knowledge fluidly and automatically, with little focused effort. Their retrieval process is not always faster than novices, however, because they try to understand problems before moving to solutions. They approach problems in a different way and spend more time analyzing problems qualitatively than novices do.
- *Adaptive expertise:* Experts remain adaptive to new situations and continue to learn. They monitor their level of understanding and know when it is inadequate (a characteristic of metacognition).

Eells, Lombart, Kendjelic, Turner, and Lucas (2005) compared expert, experienced, and novice cognitive–behavioral and psychodynamic therapists on the quality of their case formulations, which is a core psychotherapy skill. The experts' formulations were more comprehensive, elaborated, and complex than those of novices or experienced therapists; their treatment plans were more elaborated and had a better fit with formulations; they showed more use of a systematic reasoning process; they elaborated more on diagnostic possibilities, problems in global functioning, inferred problems or symptoms, and psychological mechanisms; and they were superior in total quality ratings. Effect sizes for the quality ratings ranged from medium to large. It is interesting to note that novices were rated higher in total formulation quality than those in the experienced (but not expert) group. The authors hypothesized that experts keep themselves "calibrated" to a high standard of skill and novices are newly calibrated by graduate training, but experienced therapists are more distant from their training and case formulation experiences and may not be aware of the need to recalibrate. Eells et al. found few differences between therapists of differing orientations. These results are similar to those of Goldfried, Raue, and Castonguay (1988) and Wiser and Goldfried (1998), who found that peer-nominated expert cognitive–behavioral and psychodynamic therapists were similar in their explorations of emotionally significant events.

Judgment

All people are subject to errors in judgment and to biases in reasoning and problem solving; psychologists are no exception. Clinical expertise applied to this area diminishes these typical tendencies toward error. This section provides a brief synopsis of concepts and a few examples in judgment research that are relevant to practice but can only skim the surface (see Elstein & Schwartz, 2002; Gambrill, 2005; Griffin, Gonzales, & Varey, 2001, for more complete discussions). Heuristic processes for making judgments about probability fall on a continuum from purely impression-based processes (arising from automatic natural assessments) on one end, through a midpoint where one engages in monitoring and attention to particular questions (arising from conditionally automatic assessments), to purely argument-based processes (arising from purely controlled assessments) on the other end (Griffin et al., 2001).

Heuristics are simple rules that describe how judgments or predictions are made. For example, a judgment might vary by representativeness (the similarity of a sample case to a diagnostic category; error may lead to an over- or underrepresentation of the probability of a disorder), by availability (the vividness of an event or ease of retrieval from memory; error may lead to overestimation of vivid or easily recalled events or underestimation of ordinary or hard-to-recall events), and by anchoring and adjustment (final opinions are sensitive to the starting point; error may lead to insufficient revision of first impressions).

Cognitive biases describe errors. Examples are confirmatory bias (when one seeks or recalls only information that confirms but does not refute a hypothesis or support alternatives), hindsight (when the outcome is known, this increases the perceived likelihood of the outcome), and misestimation of covariance (the inaccurate estimation of a relationship between two events).

For prediction tasks, when formulas are available, statistical or actuarial aggregation outperforms informal subjective aggregation (often called *clinical prediction*); these differences are statistically significant but modest (Dawes, Faust, & Meehl, 2002). It is important to note that *clinical prediction* refers to a method of aggregating data, not to clinicians. For practice, one has to consider the context in which practitioners make judgments. Reed (2006) noted that behavioral prediction is not the emphasis in psychologists' training or work, except perhaps in the area of forensics. Clinicians provide reliable and valid data under research conditions most like their usual work: when their inferences are quantified using instruments designed for expert observers, when the responses require expertise with psychopathology, when the domain being assessed is apparent in behavior that can be decoded by expert observers, when the population being assessed is represented in clinical practice settings, and when the clinician knows the client relatively well (Westen, Novotny, & Thompson-Brenner, 2004).

Most practitioners are likely to be more interested in how to improve clinical judgment for everyday practice because they do not participate in research projects very often. Garb (1999) offered suggestions for improving clinical assessment and judgment and for heeding the lessons of the research on heuristics and biases. His recommendations were rooted specifically in cognitive–behavioral methods, but the principles can be adapted for practitioners with different orientations. These recommendations include the following:

1. Attend to empirical research.

2. Recognize and overcome cultural biases based on such categories as gender, ethnic minority status, disability, and social class.
3. Describe clients' strengths, and do not overweight deficits.
4. Be wary of judgment tasks that are known to be difficult, such as predicting violence or suicide or describing the traits of depressed people.
5. Be systematic and comprehensive when conducting interviews. For example, routinely ask whether clients in domestic abuse situations were abused as children or teens.
6. Use psychological tests and behavioral assessment methods.
7. Use cognitive debiasing strategies. For example, consider alternative diagnoses; attribute behavior to factors other than internal ones, such as factors in the environment; and do not rely on memory, but record observations and review progress notes regularly.
8. Follow ethical and legal principles, such as reporting child abuse or helping a client in danger establish a safety plan.
9. Follow scientific standards. For example, follow assessment standards to the degree supported by empirical research.
10. Use decision aids, such as *DSM–IV* diagnostic criteria.

Guiding Principles, Behaviors, and Commonalities

Clinical experts use broad principles for making decisions and implementing psychotherapy. Williams and Levitt (in press) and Levitt, Neimeyer, and Williams (2005) reported on a qualitative research study to identify implicit principles that are used by expert therapists across theoretical orientations to regulate values and interventions within their practice. The expert therapists were eminent psychologists from humanistic, feminist, constructionist, cognitive–behavioral, and psychodynamic traditions. Analysis led to the following principle concerning their handling of clients' values in the service of therapeutic change: Expert therapists use clients' values to guide the therapeutic process unless those values actively impede client progress, in which case (e.g., disregard for life or safety) therapists would directly engage clients in evaluating that value. These experts used five identified components of the psychotherapy process to facilitate change:

> Therapists act to (1) *stimulate* clients' curiosity about their own experience to assist them to (2) *sustain* the exploration of distressing experiential states for the purpose of (3) generating *experiences* of difference. These experiences, in turn, can lead to (4) a process of reflexive *symbolization*, during which therapists provide the structure to allow for (5) the *integration* of these differences. (Levitt et al., 2005, p. 126)

Meichenbaum (2002) isolated core tasks that expert therapists pursue and engage in, also regardless of therapeutic orientation. Some of the identified tasks are directed toward victims of violence because a high percentage of clients fit that profile, but the tasks are quite broad based. His approach is a strengths-based model and creates a positive context for change. The basic expert skills Meichenbaum identified include developing a therapeutic alliance, offering psychoeducation and stimulating curiosity, nurturing hope, teaching psychological skills and the ability to generalize them, fostering self-attributions about change, and providing for relapse prevention. For victims of violence, additional expert tasks include assessing for comorbidity and risk for further victimization, helping clients to cognitively reconstruct and find meaning in the event, and promoting healthy social connections. Of course, part of clinical expertise lies in knowing which strategies to pursue and in which order or combination. Such decision making is a part of the process of tailoring treatment to individual needs.

Because of the importance of the therapeutic alliance to outcomes (see the meta-analytic review by Martin, Garske, & Davis, 2000), it is useful to understand the personal attributes and interventions of therapists that strengthen the alliance, which is an expert skill. Ackerman and Hilsenroth (2003) provided a comprehensive review and identified important practitioner attributes across a range of psychotherapy orientations, including being flexible, honest, respectful, trustworthy, confident, warm, interested, and open. They also identified the interventions that contribute to alliance: exploration, reflection, review of past therapy success, accurate interpretation, facilitation of the expression of affect, and attending to the client's experience.

Clinical Expertise: Putting It All Together

There are recurring themes and overlapping concepts in the descriptions of expert therapists' competencies, value principles, and tasks, despite differing theoretical orientations and research designs. It seems fair to conclude that expert practitioners are client focused and alliance centered. They stimulate curiosity about psychological functioning, explore subjective experience, and foster the expression of affect. They teach new psychological skills (behavioral, cognitive–representational, affective, interpersonal) and ways of understanding subjective experience (personal meanings of objects, events, and relationships). Clinical experts encourage hope, integration, and change.

I propose that clinical expertise, as described in Exhibit 2.1, is an indispensable part of the foundation of EBP. Clinical activities and best practices that lead to positive outcomes are built on this foundation. Because clinical expertise is such a vital part of EBP, it merits further research to identify the conditions that increase expertise and to identify the skill constellations of clinicians who obtain good outcomes in the community.

EXHIBIT 2.1
Foundation of Clinical Expertise in Psychology

1. Knowledge of the scientific literature on psychology, psychotherapy processes and interventions, and their applicability for specific patients and local circumstances.
2. Incorporation of sound therapeutic principles based on psychological theory and research.
3. Breadth and depth of therapeutic and interpersonal skills.
4. A genuine therapeutic alliance and a respectful understanding of the person, problem, context, and circumstances.
5. Consultation, when appropriate, with peers and experts, especially when the clinical picture is not clear or there are problems in the treatment process.
6. Critical thinking about the psychotherapy process and fine-tuning of interventions based on patients' response patterns, progress, and outcomes.
7. Lifelong learning.

CONCLUSION

The purposes of practice and science necessarily differ. Practitioners learn over time to use evidence without subscribing to specific hierarchies of which type of evidence is most important because usefulness varies widely depending on context. The discussion of evidence focuses on practitioners' need to seek information from a broad range of research; from the literature of reasoned theories and consensus and diverse forms of knowledge; from the fruits of clinical observation and inquiry; and from clients' contributions, responses, and progress. This chapter has presented the endeavor of psychotherapy as a complex multilayered interpersonal enterprise with both scientific and humanistic foundations. It has described the important role of clinical expertise and discussed competencies, recurring concepts across theoretical orientations, overlapping themes, and identified variables related to expertise. Psychologists use a combination of tools and approaches to do meaningful and effective psychotherapy. They use research evidence where it exists, modify it where necessary, and create new interventions in the field on a case-by-case basis, often by combining accepted techniques from different areas in novel ways. Most practitioners use guiding principles, rather than fixed rules, to assess and treat people who seek their help.

Psychotherapy is a rewarding but very challenging enterprise. It can be exciting, maddening, boring, pleasant, confusing, agitating, frustrating, frightening, or discouraging at times. But when clients heal, the therapeutic process is a deeply satisfying and transformative experience. It is a humbling experience to make psychotherapy one's life work.

REFERENCES

Ablon, J. S., & Marci, C. (2004). Psychotherapy process: The missing link: Comment on Westen, Novotny, & Thompson-Brenner. *Psychological Bulletin, 130,* 664–668.

Ackerman, S. J., & Hilsenroth, M. J. (2003). A review of therapist characteristics and techniques positively impacting the therapeutic alliance. *Clinical Psychology Review, 23,* 1–33.

American heritage dictionary (3rd ed.). (1993). Boston: Houghton Mifflin.

American Psychiatric Association. (1994). *Diagnostic and statistical manual of mental disorders* (4th ed.). Washington, DC: Author.

American Psychological Association. (1998). *Guidelines for psychological evaluations in child protection matters.* Washington, DC: Author.

American Psychological Association. (2002a). Criteria for evaluating treatment guidelines. *American Psychologist, 57,* 1052–1059.

American Psychological Association. (2002b). Ethical principles of psychologists and code of conduct. *American Psychologist, 57,* 1060–1073.

American Psychological Association. (2002c). Guidelines for psychotherapy with gay, lesbian, and bisexual clients. *American Psychologist, 55,* 1440–1451.

American Psychological Association. (2003). Guidelines on multicultural education, training, research, practice, and organizational change for psychologists. *American Psychologist, 58,* 377–402.

American Psychological Association. (2004). Guidelines for psychological practice with older adults. *American Psychologist, 59,* 236–260.

American Psychological Association. (2005a). *Policy statement on evidence-based practice in psychology.* Retrieved October 24, 2005, from http://www.apa.org/practice/ebpstatement.pdf

American Psychological Association. (2005b). *Report of the 2005 Presidential Task Force on Evidence-Based Practice.* Retrieved October 24, 2005, from http://www.apa.org/practice/ebpstatement.pdf

Barlow, D. H. (2004). Psychological treatments. *American Psychologist, 59,* 869–878.

Belle, D., & Dodson, L. (2006). Poor women and girls in a wealthy nation. In J. Worell & C. D. Goodheart (Eds.), *Handbook of girls' and women's psychological health* (pp. 122–128). New York: Oxford University Press.

Berkman, L., & Kawachi, I. (2000). A historical framework for social epidemiology. In L. Berkman & I. Kawachi (Eds.), *Social epidemiology* (pp. 3–12). New York: Oxford University Press.

Borkovec, T. D., Echemendia, R. J., Ragusea, S. A., & Ruiz, M. (2001). The Pennsylvania Practice Research Network and future possibilities for clinically meaningful and scientifically rigorous psychotherapy effectiveness research. *Clinical Psychology: Research and Practice, 8,* 155–167.

Bransford, J. D., Brown, A. L., & Cocking, R. R. (Eds.). (1999). *How people learn: Brain, mind, experience, and school.* Washington, DC: National Academy of Sciences. Retrieved April 12, 2004, from http://www.nap.edu/html/howpeople1/ch2.html

Burke, B. L., Arkowitz, H., & Mencola, M. (2003). The efficacy of motivational interviewing: A meta-analysis of controlled clinical trials. *Journal of Consulting and Clinical Psychology, 71,* 843–861.

Chambless, D. L. (2005). Compendium of empirically supported therapies. In G. P. Koocher, J. C. Norcross, & S. S. Hill (Eds.), *Psychologists' desk reference* (2nd ed., pp. 183–192). New York: Oxford University Press.

Chase, W. G., & Simon, H. A. (1973). Perception in chess. *Cognitive Psychology, 1,* 33–81.

Conway, J. B. (1988). Differences among clinical psychologists: Scientists, practitioners, and scientist–practitioners. *Professional Psychology: Research and Practice, 19,* 642–655.

Dana, R. H. (1987). Training for professional psychology: Science, practice, and identity. *Professional Psychology: Research and Practice, 18,* 9–16.

Dawes, R. M., Faust, D., & Meehl, P. E. (2002). Clinical versus actual judgment. In T. Gilovich & D. Griffin (Eds.), *Heuristics and biases: The psychology of intuitive judgment* (pp. 716–729). New York: Cambridge University Press.

Dingfelder, S. F. (2004, March). Treatment for the "untreatable." *Monitor on Psychology, 35,* 46.

Eells, T. D., Lombart, K. G., Kendjelic, E. M., Turner, L. C., & Lucas, C. (2005). The quality of case formulations: A comparison of expert, experienced, and novice cognitive–behavioral and psychodynamic therapists. *Journal of Consulting and Clinical Psychology, 73,* 579–589.

Elstein, A. S., & Schwartz, A. (2002). Clinical problem solving and diagnostic decision-making: A selective review of the cognitive research literature. In J. S. Knottenerus (Ed.), *The evidence base of clinical diagnosis* (pp. 179–195). London: BMJ Publishing.

Fishman, D. B., & Messer, S. B. (2005). Case-based studies as a source of unity in applied psychology. In R. J. Sternberg (Ed.), *The unification of psychology: Prospect or pipedream?* (pp. 37–60). Washington, DC: American Psychological Association.

Fox, R. E. (1996). Charlatanism, scientism, and psychology's social contract. *American Psychologist, 51,* 777–784.

Frank, G. (1984). The Boulder model: History, rationale, and critique. *Professional Psychology: Research and Practice, 1,* 417–435.

Galanti, G.-A. (1997). *Caring for patients from different cultures: Case studies from American hospitals* (2nd ed.). Philadelphia: University of Pennsylvania Press.

Gambrill, E. (2005). *Critical thinking in clinical practice: Improving the accuracy of judgments and decisions about clients.* New York: Wiley.

Garb, H. N. (1999). *Studying the clinician: Judgment research and psychological assessment.* Washington, DC: American Psychological Association.

Goldfried, M. R., Raue, P. J., & Castonguay, L. G. (1998). The therapeutic focus in significant sessions of master therapists: A comparison of cognitive–behavioral and psychodynamic interpersonal interventions. *Journal of Consulting and Clinical Psychology, 66,* 803–810.

Goodheart, C. D. (2004). Evidence-based practice and the endeavor of psychotherapy. *Independent Practitioner, 24,* 6–10.

Goodheart, C. D. (2006). An integrated view of girls' and women's psychological health: Psychology, physiology, and society. In J. Worell & C. D. Goodheart (Eds.), *Handbook of girls' and women's psychological health* (pp. 3–14). New York: Oxford University Press.

Griffin, D., Gonzales, R., & Varey, C. (2001). The heuristics and biases approach of judgment under uncertainty. In A. Tesser & N. Schwartz (Eds.), *Blackwell handbook of social psychology: Intraindividual processes* (pp. 207–235). Malden, MA: Blackwell.

Haynes, R. B., Devereaux, P. J., & Guyatt, G. H. (2002). Clinical expertise in the era of evidence-based medicine and patient choice. *Evidence-Based Medicine Notebook, 7,* 1–3.

Institute of Medicine. (2001). *Crossing the quality chasm: A new health system for the 21st century.* Washington, DC: National Academy of Sciences.

Jacobson, N. S., Christiansen, A., Prince, S. E., Cordova, J., & Eldridge, K. (2000). Integrative behavioral couple therapy: An acceptance-based, promising new treatment for couple discord. *Journal of Consulting and Clinical Psychology, 68,* 351–355.

Lambert, M. J., Bergin, A. E., & Garfield, S. L. (2004). Introduction and historical overview. In M. J. Lambert (Ed.), *Bergin and Garfield's handbook of psychotherapy and behavior change* (5th ed., pp. 3–15). New York: Wiley.

Lambert, M. J., & Ogles, B. M. (2004). The efficacy and effectiveness of psychotherapy. In M. J. Lambert (Ed.), *Bergin and Garfield's handbook of psychotherapy and behavior change* (5th ed., pp. 139–193). New York: Wiley.

Levitt, H. M., Neimeyer, R. A., & Williams, D. C. (2005). Rules versus principles in psychotherapy: Implications of the quest for universal guidelines in the movement for empirically supported treatments. *Journal of Contemporary Psychotherapy, 35,* 117–129.

Martin, D. J., Garske, J. P., & Davis, M. K. (2000). Relation of the therapeutic alliance with outcome and other variables: A meta-analytic review. *Journal of Consulting and Clinical Psychology, 68,* 438–450.

Masten, A. S. (2001). Ordinary magic: Resilience processes in development. *American Psychologist, 56,* 227–238.

Meichenbaum, D. (2002, December). *Core tasks of psychotherapy: What "expert" therapists do.* Keynote address presented at the Milton Erickson Foundation Brief Therapy Conference, Orlando, FL.

Messer, S. B. (2004). Evidence-based practice: Beyond empirically supported treatments. *Professional Psychology, 35,* 580–588.

Norcross, J. C. (2001). Purposes, processes, and products of the task force on empirically supported therapy relationships. *Psychotherapy: Theory, Research, Practice, Training, 38,* 345–356.

Patenaude, A. F. (2005). *Genetic testing for cancer: Psychological approaches for helping patients and families.* Washington, DC: American Psychological Association.

Pedro-Carroll, J. (2001). The promotion of wellness in children and families: Challenges and opportunities. *American Psychologist, 56,* 993–1004.

Peterson, D. R. (1991). Connection and disconnection of research and practice in the education of professional psychologists. *American Psychologist, 46,* 422–429.

Peterson, D. R. (1995). The reflective educator. *American Psychologist, 50,* 975–983.

Prochaska, J. O., & Norcross, J. C. (2002). Stages of change. In J. C. Norcross (Ed.), *Psychotherapy relationships that work* (pp. 303–313). New York: Oxford University Press.

Reed, G. M. (2006). Clinical expertise. In J. C. Norcross, L. E. Beutler, & R. F. Levant (Eds.), *Evidence-based practices in mental health: Debate and dialogue on the fundamental questions* (pp. 13–23). Washington, DC: American Psychological Association.

Sackett, D. L., Straus, S. E., Richardson, W. S., Rosenberg, W., & Haynes, R. B. (2000). *Evidence-based medicine: How to practice and teach EBM.* New York: Churchill Livingstone.

Shakow, D. (1976). What is clinical psychology? *American Psychologist, 31,* 553–560.

Stricker, G., & Trierweiler, S. J. (1995). The local clinical scientist. *American Psychologist, 50,* 995–1002.

Tanenbaum, S. J. (1999). Evidence and expertise: The challenge of the outcomes movement to medical professionalism. *Academic Medicine, 74,* 757–763.

Tanenbaum, S. J. (2002). Evidence-based practice in mental health: Practical weaknesses meet political strengths. *Journal of Evaluation in Clinical Practice, 9,* 287–301.

Taylor, S. E., Klein, L. C., Lewis, B. P., Gruenewald, T. L., Gurung, R. A. R., & Updegraff, J. A. (2000). Biobehavioral responses to stress in females: Tend-and-befriend, not fight-or-flight. *Psychological Review, 107,* 411–429.

Tickle-Degnen, L., & Bedell, G. (2003). Heterarchy and hierarchy: A critical appraisal of the "levels of evidence" as a tool for clinical decision-making. *American Journal of Occupational Therapy, 57,* 234–237.

Wampold, B. E. (2001). *The great psychotherapy debate: Models, methods, and findings.* Mahwah, NJ: Erlbaum.

Wampold, B. E., & Bhati, K. S. (2004). Attending to the omissions: A historical examination of evidence based practice movements. *Professional Psychology: Research and Practice, 35,* 563–570.

Wampold, B. E., Lichtenberg, J. W., & Waehler, C. A. (2002). Principles of empirically supported interventions in counseling psychology. *The Counseling Psychologist, 30,* 197–207.

Westen, D., Novotny, C. M., & Thompson-Brenner, H. (2004). The empirical status of empirically supported psychotherapies: Assumptions, findings, and reporting in controlled clinical trials. *Psychological Bulletin, 130,* 631–663.

Williams, D. C., & Levitt, H. M. (in press). A question of values: Developing principles for change. *Journal of Psychotherapy Integration.*

Wiser, S., & Goldfried, M. R. (1998). Therapist interventions and client emotional experiencing in expert psychodynamic–interpersonal and cognitive–behavioral therapies. *Journal of Consulting and Clinical Psychology, 66*, 634–640.

Zachar, P., & Leong, F. T. (1992). A problem of personality: Scientist and practitioner differences in psychology. *Journal of Personality, 60*, 665–677.

3

THEORETICAL PLURALISM AND TECHNICAL ECLECTICISM

JEAN A. CARTER

The real world of psychotherapy practice is complex, requiring moment-by-moment decisions about the treatment plan, the techniques being used, the working diagnosis, and even the goals. Patients rarely can be put into neat diagnostic boxes, and there is a great deal about their lives that psychotherapists cannot control. Clinicians know that psychotherapy occurs within a relationship that is personal and interpersonal, deeply textured, and responsive to the patient. Psychologists are trained in both the science and the practice of psychology, and they firmly believe in the value of evidence and the science base for their practice. The integration of these factors in recent calls for greater accountability and quality improvement in health care practice creates important challenges for both the scientists and the practitioners within psychology. Although the two groups share the goals of improving the effectiveness of psychotherapy and enhancing outcomes for patients, the tools and methods each uses to approach these goals may reflect quite different viewpoints. Like the blind men exploring an elephant, the part of psychotherapy one touches shapes how one understands the nature of the endeavor.

Although psychology has been committed to the integration of science and practice throughout its history, current initiatives to articulate and implement evidence-based practice principles highlight both that commitment and the difficulties inherent in integrating disparate views (American Psychological Association [APA], 2005). From a scientific perspective, psychologists seek greater control of variables, clarity of questions and methods, and general principles that are valid and reliable. From a practice perspective, they are committed to enhancing the lives of patients, drawing on general psychological principles, treatment-oriented research, and their experience in the multilayered world of practice.

Inevitably, divergent perspectives result in conflicts as psychologists attempt to bring together different approaches to the same shared goal of more effective practice. The significance of these conflicts, and the tension surrounding them, rises as funding and policy implications are increasingly based on demonstrable effectiveness and its evidence base. Practitioners are concerned about the limitations required by scientific methodologies and the direct application of research findings to any particular individual or treatment, as well as funding and treatment constraints arising out of misapplications of methodologies and results. Following various initiatives by groups within APA to address this difficulty, the APA Presidential Task Force on Evidence-Based Practice, appointed by 2005 President Ronald Levant, undertook the development of a statement that values the contributions of multiple perspectives on these issues and offers guidance to scientists, practitioners, policymakers, and funders (APA, 2005).

Clinicians know the impact of psychotherapy; they experience it as they sit with their patients hour after hour, struggling with the anguish and difficulties patients bring into their offices. A long history of evidence supports the effectiveness and durability of psychotherapy (Ahn & Wampold, 2001; Barlow, 2004; Elkin et al., 1989; Lambert & Barley, 2002; Lambert & Bergin, 1994; Lipsey & Wilson, 1993; Roth & Fonagy, 1996; Sloane, Staples, Cristol, Yorkston, & Whipple, 1975; Smith, Glass, & Miller, 1980; Wampold et al., 1997). These reports include psychotherapy studies, literature reviews, and meta-analyses and represent many theoretical perspectives, patient and treatment types, and a variety of outcome measures. The picture is clear—psychotherapy works, and works well, much of the time.

At the same time, no particular form or model of therapy has been found to consistently work better than others (Wampold, 2001). In recent research designed to evaluate psychological interventions to relieve specific target problems in well-defined treatment populations using controlled treatment protocols (Barlow, 2004), the data support the efficacy of specific treatments but do not clearly support differential treatment effects (Wampold, 2001; Westen, Novotny, & Thompson-Brenner, 2004). In addition, questions about the applicability of the results of these studies to the general treatment population and therapeutic realities abound. One cannot conclude that particular treatments are clearly better than other treatments or clearly better than treatment as usual in the community. The research literature thus supports clinicians' experiential knowledge that psychotherapy works but does not offer them specific information about what to do when or with whom to provide effective psychotherapy.

Practitioners value the grounding of practice within evidence, including the evidence that they collect and draw on as they engage in a version of science within the hour (Carter, 2002; Stricker & Trierweiler, 1995). They continually ask questions about what is or is not working and why, and they attempt to understand how to enhance the multilayered practice that occurs within a specific interpersonal context (Samstag, 2002) and with its own unique demands. This chapter is based on the daily experience of a practitioner–scholar and the contextual model of psychotherapy (Wampold, 2001), which is adapted to the particular patient and practitioner and offers a good match to the clinical world. Within this continually changing world of practice, clinicians rely on the therapeutic relationship; a broad knowledge of individual differences, psychological principles, and change processes; a theoretical grounding that offers cogent explanations; and techniques that provide the necessary tools for change.

This chapter offers a perspective on the importance of maintaining multiple theoretical formulations for effective psychological practice and on the role of related techniques in the psychotherapy process. Evidence-based practice in psychology has as its background the complex factors that affect the psychotherapy process and the history of research demonstrating the effectiveness of psychotherapy. It reflects an understanding of the contextual model of psychotherapy with its emphasis on common factors. I propose the essential integration of theoretical pluralism and technical eclecticism as significant components of real-world applications of evidence-based practice in psychology.

THE MULTILAYERED REAL WORLD OF PSYCHOTHERAPY

Psychotherapy is complex and requires continual responsiveness. Many factors operate at any given moment, all of which may call for the clinician's attention, and many of which are not within his or her control. Clinicians look for ways to understand psychological distress and to effect change in a way that takes into account this complexity. Although this chapter does not primarily address the wide range of presentations and problem types or specific treatments designed to be effective with the variety of clients clinicians face, it is important that the reader understand the psychotherapy process as an ongoing complex interplay of factors in which the clinician makes frequent decisions within an uncertain context, using their own clinical expertise and probabilistic research evidence to guide them in the moment. To set the stage, I offer a sample of the myriad ways clients can present and note a few of the factors that operate within the therapeutic hour:

- Roberta is 41, White, single, and successful at work but limited by the anxiety that keeps her up at night, worrying about decisions she made the day before and the ramifications she will face the following day. Although she has close women friends, she has no partner. She is nearing menopause and has no children. She is depressed and anxious.
- Another patient, Michael, is 27, also White, also single, but with no work life, love life, or friendships. He is frequently suicidal and eventually reveals a history of physical abuse by his father and emotional abandonment by his mother. He has had several psychiatric hospitalizations and does not expect to survive his 30s, assuming he will die by his own hand if he cannot keep a job that pays for his medical care. He, too, is depressed and anxious.
- Mary is 64, African American, and bisexual and has an adult child who moves in and out of her apartment at will. She spent some time in jail for petty theft she committed during a time when she was homeless. She is now working but is deeply in debt, and her life is chaotic. Her few friends are men and women who use her sexually and then disappear for months at a time. She, too, is depressed and anxious.
- Rhonda is 19, White, a student, a binge drinker, and a self-mutilator. She lives with her mother and her mother's boyfriend, who both drink heavily; her alcoholic father lives nearby and takes her out for drinks after he gets off work. She has great difficulty being alone and often goes to a nearby bar to pick up men for casual sex, which she remembers only in brief images after the encounter. She is failing classes, and her mother will allow her to live at home only if she is a student. She, too, is depressed and anxious.

As is evident in these examples, patients present dramatically different pictures, even those who meet the same diagnostic criteria from the *Diagnostic and Statistical Manual of Mental Disorders* (American Psychiatric Association, 1994). Clinicians attend to disorder-related issues, including presenting problem, level of distress, level of function, co-occurring problems, and attachment style (see Norcross, 2002). They attend to life circumstances (e.g., available resources and support systems, medical concerns, social skills), individual and group characteristics (APA, 2002, 2003; Sue, 2003; Sue & Lam, 2002), and values. These factors are what patients bring into treatment and what influences their lives outside of treatment as well as the treatment itself (see Miller, Duncan, & Hubble, 1997). In addition, these patient factors do not remain static and do not follow neat lines of development or change and may be affected by happenstance, or things that occur in people's lives that may not be under their control but that significantly affect their lives and the treatment.

In addition to patient factors, there are a number of factors related specifically to the therapist that operate throughout treatment (see Norcross, 2002, for a discussion of clinician factors). Clinicians vary in interpersonal skills and abilities, experience, training, values, personal characteristics, knowledge base, and worldview, as well as other factors. Just as no two patients are exactly the same, clinicians are not interchangeable.

Structural aspects of the clinical situation affect what can or does occur within treatment. These factors may include the resources available and costs related to engaging in treatment (Yates, 1994, 1995, 2000). The payer or agency may impose session or treatment limits. Moves, job changes, and other life events may affect the length or nature of treatment independent of patient preference or clinician recommendation.

Theoretical models also play a significant role in psychotherapy. Clinicians may rely on theory to explain change processes, and in the contextual model (Wampold, 2001) theories are valuable because they provide rationales for treatment, help organize it, and guide appropriate therapeutic goals for the particular clinical context. Clinicians also rely on a range of techniques drawn from multiple theoretical perspectives that research has found to be effective for particular symptom pictures or particular patient types and that the clinicians have found to be effective through their own experience and expertise (e.g., Arnkoff, Glass, & Shapiro, 2002; Beutler, Alomohamed, Moleiro, & Romanelli, 2002; Norcross, 2002).

THE CONTEXTUAL MODEL OF PSYCHOTHERAPY

Psychotherapy practice is inextricable from the context in which it occurs. Psychotherapy is an interpersonal experience, with a patient who is in distress and a treatment based on psychological principles and offered by a therapist. Wampold (2001), in *The Great Psychotherapy Debate*, presented a compelling differentiation between the medical model of psychotherapy and the contextual model of psychotherapy and described the research foundation on which the contextual model rests. Although not all clinicians or researchers see this model as a more accurate fit for psychotherapy process and outcomes data, the presentation closely matches the lived experience of many clinicians. It also provides the foundation for the remainder of this chapter.

History of the Contextual Model

Rosenzweig's early insightful article (1936/2002) laid out four factors that he believed were essential to effective psychotherapy; in this chapter I focus on the first three. As described by Weinberger (2002), Rosenzweig's four factors common to all psychotherapy include

- the therapeutic relationship,
- the provision of an ideology or rationale,
- the integration of the subsystems of personality, and
- the personality of the therapist.

This was the first presentation of what has come to be called a *common factors approach* and was the first articulation of the Dodo bird conclusion: Everybody has won, and all must have prizes. Obviously, Rosenzweig did not have access to the thousands of research reports in the current literature or to the rapid expansion of theoretical models, but his writing was strikingly prescient (Jorgensen, 2004).

Rosenzweig (1936/2002), offering early support for theoretical pluralism, believed that the particular doctrine, ideology, or rationale offered is unimportant but that the formal consistency and the extent to which it provides the patient with a schema for reorganization of personality are essential. By *integration of the subsystems of personality*, Rosenzweig was referring to his belief that all of the factors of personality are dynamically related and that changing one affects the others. From this perspective, he believed in the importance of a "repertoire of methods to be drawn upon as needed for the individual case" (p. 8). This is a clear statement of the need for technical eclecticism.

Frank (1973; Frank & Frank, 1991), in *Persuasion and Healing*, built on Rosenzweig's cogent statement of the components or factors common to all forms of psychotherapy. According to Frank, the three common components are as follows:

1. Psychotherapy occurs within an emotionally charged and confiding relationship with a therapist.
2. It occurs within a healing setting, in which the patient believes that the therapist can provide help and is trustworthy in doing so.
3. There is a rationale, conceptual schema, or myth that provides a plausible explanation for the distress and a procedure or ritual for helping to resolve the distress.

For Frank, as for Rozenzweig, the therapeutic relationship (Items 1 and 2) is essential, as is an ideology or rationale that offers a cogent explanation for the treatment (Item 3). Neither Frank nor Rosenzweig focused on the truth value or scientifically derived foundation for the rationale; their concern was the coherence of the explanation and the extent to which patient and therapist can use the explanation to understand the patient's distress, to develop goals, and to implement procedures. The importance of both the explanation (theory) and the procedures or rituals (techniques) that derive from the explanation is noteworthy, although both Rosenzweig and Frank recognized the importance of flexible techniques to adapt the treatment to the specific patient. The contextual model of psychotherapy, following Frank, relies on a strong therapeutic relationship and the development of a coherent and cogent treatment approach, including techniques, that the therapist believes in and that is convincing to patients (Wampold, 2001).

How do these factors—the relationship, the cogent rationale, and the techniques that arise from that rationale—relate to a discussion of evidence-based practice and to the scientific literature on which evidence-based practice rests? What does this mean for the role of theory and technique in the practice application of evidence-based practice?

The Therapeutic Relationship

The therapeutic relationship is foundational to the psychotherapy endeavor. Just as psychotherapy cannot proceed without patients, it cannot proceed without a clinician,[1] and the therapeutic relationship is built by the two participants. The therapeutic relationship accounts for 30% of the variance in outcome in psychotherapy, second only to patient factors, which represent 40% of the variance (Assay & Lambert, 1999; Lambert, 1992; Lambert & Barley, 2002). The therapeutic relationship is considered by many psychotherapy researchers and clinicians to be so central that the APA Division of Psychotherapy (Division 29) created a task force to review the literature on effective psychotherapy relationships and published their report both in a special issue of *Psychotherapy: Theory, Research, Practice, Training* (Norcross, 2001) and as a part of the book *Psychotherapy Relationships That Work* (Norcross, 2002).

The Working Alliance

The *therapeutic relationship* and the *working alliance* are often referred to synonymously, particularly in the research literature. The working alliance (originally conceptualized by Bordin, 1975) includes a bond between patient and therapist, agreement on goals, and consensus on therapeutic tasks. The alliance has repeatedly been found to be significantly related to outcome; Wampold (2001) and Horvath and Bedi (2002) provided summaries of this research. Given the large proportion of variance in outcome accounted for by the alliance, it is clearly important for clinicians and researchers to be continually attentive to the role and impact of the alliance and to the ways in which the alliance as a relationship can be enhanced.

The agreement on tasks and consensus on goals that are components of the alliance are significant in any consideration of the role of theory in evi-

---

[1]Some computer models of intervention do not require the active participation of a clinician. However, psychotherapy is commonly understood to be an interpersonal process between a patient and a therapist.

dence-based practice in psychology. Although well-designed research supports the effectiveness of psychotherapy, it does not offer clear support for relative effectiveness—that is, of one form of treatment over another, including treatment as usual in the community (Westen et al., 2004). The Dodo bird appears to have been right. If none of the treatment approaches arising out of any particular theoretical model is clearly superior to another, what does that mean in terms of the alliance?

The working alliance includes clinician and patient agreement on goals and tasks as major components of a successful alliance, and positive working alliance is related to better outcomes. The question may arise, however, about which goals and tasks the clinician and patient may agree on and how they come to the definition and the agreement. There are many possible goals and expected or desirable outcomes from psychotherapy, and it sometimes appears that there are as many measures of goals and outcomes as there are possible outcomes. Some examples included in studies of outcomes are self-esteem, premature termination, global change, symptom severity, interpersonal functioning, addiction severity, change in distress, drug use, alleviation of depressive symptoms, social adjustment, specific symptoms, social relationships, indecision, personal growth, relations with others, social or sexual adjustment, interpersonal problems, defense style, employment status, legal status, self-concept, anxiety symptoms, medication compliance, quality of life, hospitalization, productivity, and satisfaction with treatment (Horvath & Bedi, 2002). It is clear that the range of possible outcomes is huge. At the same time, the clinician and patient must identify outcomes they believe to be desirable and goals to be achieved and must reach agreement on these goals as an essential part of the alliance. The definition of outcomes arises from a shared perspective held by the clinician and patient.

Typically, the desirable goals for any particular psychotherapy are derived from patient need and problem type and patient and clinician worldviews. They are consistent with the theoretical framework from which the treatment was developed. Thus, agreement on goals implies agreement (whether implicit or explicit) on the theoretical framework (cogent and coherent explanation or rationale) from which the clinician operates. Therefore, the theoretical framework provides an important structure within which psychotherapy occurs and is significantly related to one of the components of psychotherapy outcome (agreement on goals as part of the alliance).

Patient Belief in the Treatment

According to Frank (1973; Frank & Frank, 1991) and Wampold (2001), the patient's belief in the treatment, its context, and the clinician is a component shared by all psychotherapy approaches. Indeed, it is hard to imagine how a patient without some belief and hope in the effectiveness of treatment could be an active participant in psychotherapy or could share an agreement on goals or outcome with the clinician. The participation of patients is essential, of course. Duncan (2002) described patients as the heroes of the treatment; it is the patient's therapy, and he or she makes whatever changes are to be made. Successful collaboration between clinician and patient (Tryon & Winograd, 2002) and lower levels of resistance (Beutler, Moleiro, & Talebi, 2002) are related to positive outcomes. Patient factors such as positive expectation, motivation, and openness to treatment (Grencavage & Norcross, 1990) account for 40% of the variance (Assay & Lambert, 1999). These factors, which are central to the patient's belief in the treatment, make patient characteristics and values the most potent component of successful treatment. These findings support the importance of agreement on goals and consensus on tasks, which are part of the alliance and part of the patient's belief in the healing benefit of psychotherapy. When there are difficulties in collaboration and resistance to the treatment is high (both reflect difficulties in the alliance), existing evidence suggests that acknowledging the patient's concerns, attending to the relationship, and renegotiating goals and roles may be effective in ameliorating problems in the alliance (Beutler & Harwood, 2002; Beutler, Moleiro, et al., 2002; Safran & Muran, 2002).

The Value of Flexible Theoretical Frameworks

Effective treatment clearly needs a cogent rationale, and clinician and patient need to agree on goals and tasks based on that rationale. At the same time, the complexity of psychotherapy may require renegotiating goals and roles to better align patient and clinician and to better match patient characteristics and worldview. Renegotiation and realignment call for flexibility in the theoretical framework guiding the treatment designed for the specific patient and his or her situation, as well as flexibility in the use of techniques derived from various theoretical approaches. The clinician needs to be adaptive and conversant with multiple theoretical perspectives that may guide his or her ability to integrate clinician worldview and patient worldview to match the particular patient. The clinician must be prepared to incorporate additional or different theoretical components to achieve better fit for the patient. In other words, the clinician's effectiveness rests in part on maintaining theoretical pluralism and the ability to be integrative in those theories.

A CONCEPTUAL SCHEME

Rosenzweig (1936/2002) and Frank (Frank & Frank, 1991) supported the importance of an ideology or rationale provided by the clinician that presents a cogent, coherent, and plausible explanation for both the patient's distress and the approach the clinician will take to help the patient. This ideology engages the patient. It offers the patient hope and expectation (remoralization through positive expectation) in the treatment, as well as a way to understand the goals and tasks of treatment, which in turn enhance outcomes. Ideology, rationale, and coherent and cogent explanation are all different words for the *theoretical formulation* that guides the clinician in the treatment.

Patient Expectancy

Patient expectancy and hope are potent contributors to positive outcomes. Assay and Lambert (1999) suggested that the accumulation of research puts the contribution of patient expectancy for outcomes at about 15% of the variance. Expectation is typically cast as a placebo effect in medical model approaches, but the contextual model includes it as a central component of effective treatment. Placebo effects are essentially psychological effects and thus are undesirable in a model that attempts to minimize extrinsic factors through tight control and adherence to the treatment as defined. However, increased psychological effects as a result of psychological treatments seem desirable—not undesirable—outcomes and should be supported, and factors that increase positive expectations should be promoted. For example, a patient who moves into a hopeful state and no longer exhibits hopelessness (one of the primary symptoms of depression) because of his or her belief in the treatment demonstrates the effectiveness of nonspecific psychological factors in the treatment. The clinician wants to enhance the patient's belief in what he or she is offering to enhance expectancy effects. Therefore, the clinician would promote the importance of the theoretical framework to engage and encourage patients and heighten expectancy effects, as well as to take advantage of the positive contribution theory makes to agreement on goals and tasks.

Allegiance

Trust is a significant part of therapy; patient belief in and openness to treatment and the patient–clinician bond component of the alliance rely on trust (Horvath & Bedi, 2002). Clinicians' belief in their therapeutic models or theories is related to outcomes through its impact on clinician–patient agreement on goals and desirable outcomes and the extent to which it engages the patient. Therefore, the clinician must believe in his or her own treatment model, just as the patient does. The theoretical framework must therefore be cogent, coherent, and explanatory for the clinician as well as for the patient. Theory also provides the clinician with an underlying organization for the large amounts of information that are relevant to psychotherapy and that must be available for the clinician's use in the treatment.

To the extent that the clinician believes the theory to be explanatory for the patient's distress and to provide a rationale for the treatment plan and its implementation, one would expect the clinician to have considerable allegiance to the theoretical model he or she is using. Wampold (2001) offered extensive evidence regarding clinician allegiance to an espoused theoretical model and its strong positive relationship to outcomes.

It is important to note that the relationship between allegiance and outcomes appears to hold regardless of the truth value of the theory. One might think that this would lead to rampant development of a vast array of untested and untestable theoretical models. Despite frequent counts of theoretical models that number several hundred (e.g., Bergin & Garfield, 1994), the major models remain largely consistent categories.[2] At the same time, consistent with the importance of the theoretical model to both clinician and patient, clinicians would be expected to do one of two things: either endorse one of the existing general theoretical models or endorse an approach that draws from more than one model. Both seem to occur simultaneously, however. Clinicians choose one model as primary (often with a secondary choice when that is an alternative) and may also espouse an integrative perspective (drawing on multiple models) or eclecticism as their theoretical perspective (Garfield & Bergin, 1994; Jensen & Bergin, 1990; Norcross, Prochaska, & Farber, 1993; Wampold, 2001). Typically, *eclectic* draws the largest endorsement as a single category. Norcross et al. (1993) found that 40% of the members of the Division of Psychotherapy of the APA who responded to a survey of theoretical orientation chose *eclectic*, reflecting individualized versions based on experience, training in multiple models, and alterations in response to patient need. Clinicians' choice of eclectic as a theoretical perspective needs attention to understand its meaning, impact, and role as an explanatory system and the extent to which it is a well-developed individualized model versus a process for integrating multiple models (Carter, 2002).

Currently, theoretical integration, technical eclecticism, and common factors are receiving considerable attention, reflecting dissatisfaction with individual theoretical approaches and attempts to develop more flexible approaches. Theoretical integration is problematic if it becomes its own model, because it then has all of the problems that are associated with a single theoretical model (Feixas & Botella, 2004; O'Brien, 2004). However, it provides a useful framework if it provides procedures for integrating diverse perspectives into a system that is applicable for the particular clinician–patient pair, to the particular patient problems, and in the particular context (Feixas & Botella, 2004).

Technical eclecticism alone as a response to the poor fit of theoretical models is limited, because it takes only interventions into account and ignores the relevance and role of theoretical models. From an integrative or

---

[2]The major models are behavioral and cognitive–behavioral, psychodynamic, humanistic or experiential, systems theory, and feminist theory. All of them have multiple variants that reflect shifts in perspective or incorporation of new knowledge drawn from general psychological principles or research on the treatment model itself.

theoretically eclectic perspective, however, it is important for clinicians to be skilled in techniques drawn from the multiple theories from which their own theoretical perspective is derived. Because allegiance to a cogent rationale is important and clinicians and patients rely on theories to organize and guide their work, clinicians are expected to modify models as needed to be responsive to patients. Thus, psychologists must continue to develop and teach multiple models, to understand the components of the theories as explanatory tools, and to understand and effectively implement the techniques derived from the models.

Rituals and Procedures (Otherwise Known as *Techniques*)

Frank and Frank (1991), drawing on Rosenzweig's formulation (1936/ 2002), focused on the importance of rituals and procedures that are consistent with the rationale given for the treatment. The rituals and procedures that Frank and Frank suggested may best be understood as the interventions or techniques that are logically derived from the theoretical formulation of the causes of the patient's distress and the approach to ameliorating the dysfunction. Clinicians design techniques, then, to have a specific impact on symptoms, behaviors, or other components as defined by the theory from which they arise and with which they are consistent. Rosenzweig believed that an impact on any subsystem (or aspect) of personality affects all of the personality, suggesting that effective treatment may occur with any one of multiple symptoms as the target of interventions. If Rosenzweig was correct, techniques should have a positive impact on outcomes, but the impact should account for a relatively small portion of the variance. According to Assay and Lambert (1999), techniques overall account for only 15% of the variance, and specific techniques appear to make little additive difference in outcome (Wampold, 2001). Valuable research using designs that offer well-controlled and targeted interventions for specific symptom pictures demonstrates their effectiveness in both absolute and relative terms (Barlow, 2004). Although application of these results may call for adaptation to the particular treatment picture, these are useful tools for the clinician to have readily available. It is interesting to note that Westen et al. (2004), in a review of the current status of what have been known as empirically supported treatments, offered a hypothesis on the role of negative diatheses as an underlying principle that may be common to all psychological disorders and explanatory for varied presentations and comorbidity. The relationship between specific techniques for specific symptoms and the complex symptom picture in a typical clinical practice offers great opportunities for collaboration between research and practice.

Nevertheless, techniques do matter. Interventions are the tools through which psychotherapy occurs within the context previously described. They are the expression of the belief system arising from theoretical models. They operationalize the therapeutic tasks that are part of the alliance. They are the medium by which the relationship is developed and maintained. They build hope in the patient through active engagement in the tasks of therapy. They effectively alter specific symptoms. Hence, it is essential for clinicians to be technically eclectic and prepared with a wide range of tools to address the needs of patients in the continually changing world of psychotherapy. The contextual model, which reflects the deeply complex interpersonal world of psychotherapy, supports the importance of techniques as tools in trade (Wampold, 2001), with clinicians having the ability to apply multiple techniques in the service of an individually tailored psychotherapy.

CONCLUSION

Most clinicians strongly support models of psychotherapy that are context centered, that place a strong value on the relationship and alliance, and that are embedded in theoretical models. At the same time, clinicians rely on eclectic or integrative models, and their work reflects theoretical pluralism. In addition, experienced clinicians from different theoretical perspectives are more similar than different within the psychotherapy hour, using techniques drawn from a variety of theoretical approaches and reflecting technical eclecticism in the application of psychotherapy.

Psychological scientists and psychological practitioners have a number of areas of agreement about the evidence base underlying practice. The therapeutic relationship, a central component to practice, has strong evidentiary support as an essential factor in successful outcomes. Therefore, clinicians should devote considerable attention to building and maintaining a strong therapeutic relationship in the implementation of evidence-based practice. Evidence drawn from research on psychotherapy supports the importance of coherent and cogent explanations for distress, dysfunction, and treatment to positive outcomes. Therefore, clinicians who engage in evidence-based practice should devote time, energy, and attention to strengthening the cogency and clarity of their theoretical formulations, including both the major theoretical perspectives and the variants that are consistent with their own worldviews and psychology's scientific base. Theoretical pluralism is an important part of evidence-based practice.

The therapeutic alliance (which is part of the relationship) rests on agreement on goals and tasks and is positively related to outcomes. Agreement on goals and tasks is drawn from agreement on and belief in the explanations for and implementation of the treatment (the theoretical model the clinician uses and the techniques drawn from that model). The alliance necessarily takes into account the therapist's role, the patient's role, and the relationship between them. Clinicians who integrate principles of evidence-based practice devote energy to learning techniques that emanate from their own theoretical model. In addition, they should maintain openness to techniques that may complement or supplement those derived from their model, that may enhance the relationship, and that may fit the patient's desired goals, problems, and characteristics.

Placebo or expectancy effects are essentially belief in or hope for the treatment that rests on the patient's and the therapist's belief that the explanation is valid and that it will work—again, the important role of theory. Clinicians demonstrating evidence-based practice should support patients' hopes and beliefs, as well as their own, which requires a somewhat different approach to the evidence foundation for psychotherapy that draws on a context of discovery rather than a context of justification for the scientific thinking occurring within the hour.

Skill with a range of techniques is important as an expression of the theory (agreement on tasks), as a way to effectively manage the alliance and relationship, as rituals, and as ways to accommodate multiple problems, worldviews, and expected outcomes. Technical eclecticism is an important component of evidence-based practice in psychology.

Psychological research underlying evidence-based practice in psychology

- supports the use of theoretical pluralism and technical eclecticism to enhance the alliance and strengthen the therapeutic relationship;
- supports a coherent, cogent, and organized explanation for patient distress and its amelioration;
- fosters patient hope; and
- uses a range of techniques to maximize effectiveness.

Evidence-based practice in psychology has at its core an effort to enhance patient involvement and choice, as well as participation in his or her own health care. Implementing evidence-based practice requires the continuous and deliberate incorporation of both a scientific attitude and empirical research into an understanding and appreciation for the unique demands of psychotherapy practice. Commitment to evidence-based practice continues a strong belief in the integration of science and practice in psychology. Embracing it reflects psychology's past and supports its future.

REFERENCES

Ahn, H., & Wampold, B. E. (2001). Where oh where are the specific ingredients? A meta-analysis of component studies in counseling and psychotherapy. *Journal of Counseling Psychology, 48,* 251–257.

American Psychiatric Association. (1994). *Diagnostic and statistical manual of mental disorders* (4th ed.). Washington, DC: Author.

American Psychological Association. (2002). Guidelines for psychotherapy with gay, lesbian, and bisexual clients. *American Psychologist, 55*, 1440–1451.

American Psychological Association. (2003). Guidelines on multicultural education, training, research, practice, and organizational change for psychologists. *American Psychologist, 58*, 377–402.

American Psychological Association. (2005). *Report of the 2005 Presidential Task Force on Evidence-Based Practice.* Retrieved October 24, 2005, from http://www.apa.org/practice/ebpstatement.pdf

Arnkoff, C. B., Glass, C. R., & Shapiro, S. J. (2002). Expectations and preferences. In J. C. Norcross (Ed.), *Psychotherapy relationships that work: Therapist contributions and responsiveness to patients* (pp. 335–356). New York: Oxford University Press.

Assay, T. P., & Lambert, M. J. (1999). The empirical case for the common factors in therapy: Quantitative findings. In M. A. Hubble, B. Duncan, & S. D. Miller (Eds.), *The heart and soul of change: What works in therapy* (pp. 33–56). Washington, DC: American Psychological Association.

Barlow, D. H. (2004). Psychological treatments. *American Psychologist, 59*, 869–878.

Bergin, A. E., & Garfield, S. L. (Eds.). (1994). *Handbook of psychotherapy and behavior change* (4th ed.). New York: Wiley.

Beutler, L. E., Alomohamed, S., Moleiro, C., & Romanelli, R. K. (2002). Systematic treatment selection and prescriptive therapy. In F. W. Kaslow (Ed.), *Comprehensive handbook of psychotherapy: Integrative/eclectic* (Vol. 4, pp. 255–271). New York: Wiley.

Beutler, L. E., & Harwood, T. M. (2002). *Prescriptive psychotherapy: A practical guide to systematic treatment selection.* New York: Oxford University Press.

Beutler, L. E., Moleiro, C., & Talebi, H. (2002). Resistance in psychotherapy: What conclusions are supported by research? *Journal of Clinical Psychology, 58*, 207–217.

Bordin, E. S. (1975). The generalizability of the psychoanalytic concept of the working alliance. *Psychotherapy: Theory, Research and Practice, 16*, 252–260.

Carter, J. A. (2002). Integrating science and practice: Reclaiming the science in practice. *Journal of Clinical Psychology, 58*, 1285–1290.

Duncan, B. L. (2002). The legacy of Saul Rosenzweig: The profundity of the Dodo bird. *Journal of Psychotherapy Integration, 12*, 32–57.

Elkin, I., Shea, T., Watkins, J. T., Imber, S. D., Sotsky, S. M., Collins, J. F., et al. (1989). National Institute of Mental Health treatment of depression collaborative research program: General effectiveness of treatments. *Archives of General Psychiatry, 46*, 971–982.

Feixas, G., & Botella, L. (2004). Psychotherapy integration: Reflections and contributions from a constructivist epistemology. *Journal of Psychotherapy Integration, 14*, 192–222.

Frank, J. (1973). *Persuasion and healing: A comparative study of psychotherapy* (2nd ed.). Baltimore: Johns Hopkins University Press.

Frank, J. D., & Frank, J. B. (1991). *Persuasion and healing: A comparative study of psychotherapy* (3rd ed.). Baltimore: Johns Hopkins University Press.

Garfield, S. L., & Bergin, A. E. (1994). Introduction and historical review. In A. E. Bergin & S. L. Garfield (Eds.), *Handbook of psychotherapy and behavior change* (4th ed., pp. 3–18). New York: Wiley.

Grencavage, L. M., & Norcross, J. C. (1990). Where are the commonalities among the therapeutic common factors? *Professional Psychology: Research and Practice, 21*, 372–378.

Horvath, A. O., & Bedi, R. P. (2002). The alliance. In J. C. Norcross (Ed.), *Psychotherapy relationships that work: Therapist contributions and responsiveness to patients* (pp. 37–70). New York: Oxford University Press.

Jensen, J. P., & Bergin, A. E. (1990). The meaning of eclecticism: New survey and analysis of components. *Professional Psychology: Research and Practice, 21*, 124–130.

Jorgensen, C. R. (2004). Active ingredients in individual psychotherapy: Searching for common factors. *Psychoanalytic Psychology, 21*, 516–540.

Lambert, M. J. (1992). Psychotherapy outcome research: Implications for eclectic and integrative psychotherapists. In J. C. Norcross & M. R. Goldfried (Eds.), *Handbook of psychotherapy integration* (pp. 94–129). New York: Basic Books.

Lambert, M. J., & Barley, D. E. (2002). Research on the therapeutic relationship and psychotherapy outcome. In J. C. Norcross (Ed.), *Psychotherapy relationships that work: Therapist contributions and responsiveness to patients* (pp. 17–32). New York: Oxford University Press.

Lambert, M. J., & Bergin, A. E. (1994). The effectiveness of psychotherapy. In A. E. Bergin & S. L. Garfield (Eds.), *Handbook of psychotherapy and behavior change* (4th ed., pp. 143–189). New York: Wiley.

Lipsey, M. W., & Wilson, D. B. (1993). The efficacy of psychological, educational and behavioral treatment: Confirmation from meta-analysis. *American Psychologist, 48*, 1181–1209.

Miller, S. D., Duncan, B. L., & Hubble, M. A. (1997). *Escape from Babel*. New York: Norton.

Norcross, J. C. (Ed.). (2001). Empirically supported therapy relationships: Summary report of the Division 29 Task Force [Special issue]. *Psychotherapy: Theory, Research, Practice, Training, 38*.

Norcross, J. C. (Ed.). (2002). *Psychotherapy relationships that work: Therapist contributions and responsiveness to patients*. New York: Oxford University Press.

Norcross, J. C., Prochaska, J. O., & Farber, J. A. (1993). Psychologists conducting psychotherapy: New findings and historical comparisons on the psychotherapy division membership. *Psychotherapy, 30*, 692–697.

O'Brien, M. (2004). An integrative therapy framework: Research and practice. *Journal of Psychotherapy Integration, 14*, 21–37.

Rosenzweig, S. (2002). Some implicit common factors in diverse methods of psychotherapy: "At last the Dodo said, 'Everybody has won and all must have prizes.'"

Journal of Psychotherapy Integration, 12, 32–57. (Reprinted from *American Journal of Orthopsychiatry, 6,* 412–415, 1936)

Roth, A., & Fonagy, P. (1996). *What works for whom? A critical review of psychotherapy research.* New York: Guilford Press.

Safran, J. D., & Muran, J. C. (2002). A relational approach to psychotherapy. In F. W. Kaslow & J. J. Magnavita (Eds.), *Comprehensive handbook of psychotherapy* (Vol. 1, pp. 253–281). New York: Wiley.

Samstag, L. W. (2002). The common versus unique factors hypothesis in psychotherapy research: Did we misinterpret Rosenzweig? *Journal of Psychotherapy Integration, 12,* 58–66.

Sloane, R. B., Staples, F. R., Cristol, A. H., Yorkston, N. J., & Whipple, K. (1975). *Psychotherapy vs. behavior therapy.* Cambridge, MA: Harvard University Press.

Smith, M. L., Glass, G. V., & Miller, T. I. (1980). *The benefits of psychotherapy.* Baltimore: Johns Hopkins University Press.

Stricker, G., & Trierweiler, S. J. (1995). The local clinical scientist. *American Psychologist, 50,* 995–1002.

Sue, S. (2003). In defense of cultural competency in psychotherapy and treatment. *American Psychologist, 58,* 964–970.

Sue, S., & Lam, A. G. (2002). Cultural and demographic diversity. In J. C. Norcross (Ed.), *Psychotherapy relationships that work: Therapist contributions and responsiveness to patients* (pp. 401–421). New York: Oxford University Press.

Tryon, G. S., & Winograd, G. (2002). Goal consensus and collaboration. In J. C. Norcross (Ed.), *Psychotherapy relationships that work: Therapist contributions and responsiveness to patients* (pp. 109–125). New York: Oxford University Press.

Wampold, B. E. (2001). *The great psychotherapy debate: Models, methods and findings.* Mahwah, NJ: Erlbaum.

Wampold, B. E., Mondin, G. W., Moody, M., Stich, F., Benson, K., & Ahn, H. (1997). A meta-analysis of outcome studies comparing bona-fide psychotherapies: Empirically "All must have prizes." *Psychological Bulletin, 122,* 203–215.

Weinberger, J. (2002). Short paper, large impact: Rosenzweig's influence on the common factors movement. *Journal of Psychotherapy Integration, 12,* 67–76.

Westen, D., Novotny, C. M., & Thompson-Brenner, H. (2004). The empirical status of empirically supportive psychotherapies: Assumptions, findings and reporting in controlled clinical trials. *Psychological Bulletin, 130,* 631–663.

Yates, B. T. (1994). Toward the incorporation of costs, cost-effectiveness analysis, and cost–benefit analysis into clinical research. *Journal of Consulting and Clinical Psychology, 62,* 729–736.

Yates, B. T. (1995). Cost-effectiveness analysis, cost–benefit analysis, and beyond: Evolving models for the scientist–manager–practitioner. *Clinical Psychology: Science and Practice, 2,* 385–398.

Yates, B. T. (2000). Cost–benefit analysis and cost-effectiveness analysis. In A. Kazdin (Ed.), *Encyclopedia of psychology* (Vol. 3, pp. 311–312). Washington, DC: American Psychological Association.

4

CULTURAL VARIATION IN THE THERAPEUTIC RELATIONSHIP

LILLIAN COMAS-DÍAZ

Different schools of psychotherapy recognize the therapeutic relationship as a core factor in treatment. Psychotherapy research highlights the healing relationship and the working alliance as important variables for predicting psychotherapeutic change (Marmar, Horowitz, Weiss, & Marziali, 1986). In his extensive literature review on this topic, Norcross (2002) concluded, "Both clinical experience and research findings underscore that the therapy relationship accounts for as much of the outcome variance as specific treatments" (p. 5).

A challenge in delivering effective psychotherapy to clients from other cultures is balancing clinical expertise and cultural relevance with the use of treatments that are informed by science. Unfortunately, the dearth of significant psychotherapy research studies with ethnic minorities makes it difficult to assess the efficacy of interventions for these populations (Roselló & Bernal, 1999). Several multicultural scholars have identified dominant psychotherapy in the United States as Eurocentric and insensitive to the cultural and spiritual experiences of people of color (G. C. N. Hall, 2001; D. W. Sue, Bingham, Porche-Burke, & Vasquez, 1999). Mainstream psychotherapy is predominantly informed by Western White middle-class cultural values such as individualism, independence, future orientation, and linear thinking (among others), in contrast to sociocentric values such as collectivism, interdependence, holism, and circular thinking (Ho, 1987; Sato, 1998; Tamura & Lau, 1992). Dominant psychotherapy's monocultural bias is seldom addressed and thus is difficult to manage, particularly in the therapeutic relationship. This bias is critically significant, however, because all clinical relationships can be considered to be cross-cultural (Comas-Díaz, 1988).

The therapeutic alliance is of utmost importance in the multicultural therapeutic relationship. Indeed, clinicians of most orientations agree that a positive alliance increases psychotherapy's effectiveness with all clients. This chapter explores the role of culture within the therapeutic relationship and examines the relevant literature, including that on evidence-based treatment of individuals from other cultures. Moreover, it offers recommendations for addressing the cultural components of the client–therapist relationship to increase psychotherapy's effectiveness.

For the purposes of this chapter, I use the term *culture* in a broad sense to include ethnicity, race, gender, age, sexual orientation, social class, physical ability, religion and spirituality, nationality, language, immigration and refugee status, and generational level and the interactions among these characteristics. Culture is layered and complex—consider ethnicity, for example. At a global level, there are hundreds of ethnicities. According to data from Infoplease (Information Please Database, n.d.), in Afghanistan there are Pashtun (4%), Tajik (27%), Uzbek (9%), Hazara (9%), and other smaller ethnic groups; in Bhutan there are Bhote (50%), ethnic Nepalese (35%), and migrant tribes (15%). In Cambodia, the population is 90% Khmer, 5% Vietnamese, and 1% Chinese, whereas France is home to Celtic and Latin Teutonic, Slavic, North African, Southeast Asian, and Basque minorities. In Guatemala, the Ladino (also called *mestizo*, or mixed Amerindian-Spanish ancestry) population is 55%, the Mayan (Amerindian) population is 43%, and Whites and others constitute 2%. The population of the United States is 75.1% White, 12.5% Hispanic/Latino, 12.3% Black, 3.6% Asian, 0.9% Native Indian and Alaska Native, 0.1% Native Hawaiian and other Pacific Islander, and 5.5% other ethnicities.

ADAPTATION OF MAINSTREAM PSYCHOTHERAPY TO CULTURALLY DIVERSE POPULATIONS

Clients who enter a consulting room for the first time often wonder whether psychotherapy will be responsive to their life experiences. However, individuals from other cultures seldom see their faces reflected in the therapeutic mirror, and many speculate about their practitioner's cultural attunement. According to Ramirez (1991), many people of color suspect the techniques and goals of psychotherapy to be acculturation instruments used by the dominant Western culture. The history of people of color receiving inappropriate psychotropic treatment may be partly responsible for this suspicion.

The field of ethnopsychopharmacology has described the cultural insensitivity of mainstream medical treatment and the need for ethnocultural specificity. The absence of people of color in drug clinical trials mirrors the absence of ethnic minorities in psychotherapy research, and both result in inappropriate care for persons of ethnic minorities. Psychopharmacological treatment can be unsuitable and even harmful when gender, race, and ethnicity are not taken into consideration. For example, extensive literature documents that African Americans with affective disorders are often undertreated or treated inappropriately with antipsychotic medications (Lawson, 1996; Strickland, Ranganeth, & Lin, 1991). As a group, Hispanics or Latinos—a widely diverse population—have been treated inappropriately with psychopharmacology, partly because their rate of drug metabolization is variable (Jacobsen & Comas-Díaz, 1999; Mendoza & Smith, 2000). In a similar way, Asian patients require lower doses of haloperidol than do White patients to produce similar clinical effects because of differences in drug metabolization between Asians and non-Asians (Pi & Gray, 2000). The lack of recognition of racial differences in drug responses has resulted in the psychopharmacological mistreatment of many people of color (Melfi, Croghan, Hanna, & Robinson, 2000). When membership in a cultural group correlates with health-related genetic traits, clinicians can increase their effectiveness by becoming culturally competent (Bamshad & Olson, 2003).

There is growing empirical evidence that ethnicity is a central variable in an individual's response to psychotropic medications (Ruiz, 2000). Although ethnopsychopharmacologists acknowledge the significant racial variability among individuals, they often divide racial populations on the basis of genetic differences for pragmatic reasons. Differences in the genetic structure of drug-metabolizing enzymes can explain most of the ethnic variations in psychopharmacological responses (Ruiz, 2000). Smith and Mendoza (1996) stated that the cytochrome P450 (CYP) enzyme system is the main pathway of drug metabolism and that these enzymes are responsible for the metabolism of most psychopharmacological agents. Ethnic differences in drug metabolism appear to be related to polymorphic variation of the same enzyme, attributable to evolutionary pressures on the CYP system. Ruiz (2000) stated that body size and composition often vary across ethnic groups, and therefore the volume of distribution of drugs can vary, particularly with drugs that are absorbed by fatty tissue. Culturally infused behaviors such as diet, response to placebo (Lin, Anderson, & Poland, 1995), health beliefs, and lifestyle choices also influence drug metabolization. Furthermore, culture influences how people take their medication. Many Latinos appear "noncompliant" because they self-prescribe and share medication among family members (Comas-Díaz & Jacobsen, 1995). Cultural beliefs can add to practitioner–patient miscommunication. For example, a common belief, the hot–cold theory of illness, indicates that one maintains health by taking a "cold" medication for a "hot" illness and vice versa (Harwood, 1971). Thus, if psychopharmacologists prescribe a hot drug for a hot condition, the patient may not comply.

As with psychopharmacology, psychotherapists can benefit from understanding the role of ethnicity and culture in treatment. Practitioners and patients negotiate their relationship not only in terms of their worldviews but also in terms of cultural variables that are permeated by subjective and contextual meanings. For instance, clinicians need to recognize that all individuals, including themselves, are influenced by their contexts, which in turn are influenced by historical, ecological, and sociopolitical forces (American Psychological Association [APA], 2003). Culture profoundly affects clinical practice. As an illustration, mainstream psychotherapy often promotes a Western ideal of selfhood, viewing the normative behaviors of patients of different cultures as resistance to treatment (Chin, 1993). When insensitive to culture, Eurocentric practitioners can violate personal and family norms by asking clients to reveal intimate personal information (including family history), soliciting the expression of emotion and affect, and asking individuals to air family disputes before achieving credibility and earning their patients' trust (Varma, 1988).

Cross-cultural encounters are frequently rife with missed empathetic opportunities. *Missed empathetic opportunities* are moments when a client reports emotional issues, and the clinician suddenly changes the topic without addressing the client's feelings (Suchman, Markakis, Beckman, & Frankel, 1997). Missed empathetic opportunities are usually subtle in cross-cultural interactions, because the signs are not as visible as in the monocultural dyad. Clients from other cultures frequently communicate in an indirect manner; they raise racial, ethnic, gender, sexual orientation, socioeconomic, ideological, and political issues, among others, as a means of evaluating the therapist.

The APA's "Guidelines on Multicultural Education, Training, Research, Practice, and Organizational Change" (APA, 2003; hereafter referred to as "Multicultural Guidelines") and *Guidelines for Providers of Psychological Services to Ethnic, Linguistic, and Culturally Diverse Clients* (APA, 1990) highlight the importance of psychologists' commitment to cultural awareness and knowledge of self and others. Although all multicultural guidelines provide a context to inform the client–practitioner dyad, there are two guidelines of particular relevance to multicultural practice. Multicultural Guideline 1 encourages psychologists to recognize that they may hold detrimental attitudes and beliefs that can influence their perceptions of and interactions with individuals who differ from them culturally, racially, and ethnically (APA, 2003). The YAVIS–HOUND dichotomy illustrates the need for clinicians to recognize their misperceptions of their clients. The YAVIS person—young, attractive, verbal, intelligent, and successful—has been considered an ideal client for exploratory and problem-solving talk psychotherapy. The HOUND client—humble, old, unattractive, nonverbal, and dumb—has been perceived as more suitable for nonverbal and supportive psychotherapy. Clinicians often perceive clients from other cultures as HOUND when they are unable to understand these clients.

Multicultural Guideline 5 states that psychologists must strive to apply culturally appropriate skills in clinical and other applied psychological practices (APA, 2003). Effective psychotherapy with individuals from other cultures focuses on the client's life experience, uses culturally appropriate assessment tools, and endorses a plurality of interventions (Hays, 1995). Practitioners of mainstream therapeutic orientations are revising their basic tenets with respect to their application to clients from other cultures. Some psychoanalysts, for instance, are incorporating patients' diverse social, communal, and spiritual orientations into their practices (Foster, Moskowitz, & Javier, 1996). In a similar manner, Altman (1995) used a modified object relations framework in examining his clients' progress on the basis of their ability to use relationships to grow rather than the insights they gained. Because object relations theory focuses on how significant interpersonal relationships are internalized and become central to the person's interactions with the world (Horner, 1984), such adaptation is highly consistent with the relational orientation of people from other cultures.

These are a few examples of *culturally sensitive psychotherapy*, or the modification of therapeutic interventions to specific cultural contexts (G. C. N. Hall, 2001). As a clinician who began her practitioner–scientist career with a cognitive–behavioral and interpersonal psychotherapy research orientation, I confronted the dilemma common to many multicultural practitioners: how to deliver effective psychotherapy grounded simultaneously in clinical skill, science, and culture. There is a definite need for treatments that are both empirically supported and culturally sensitive (G. C. N. Hall, 2001; Zane, Hall, Sue, Young, & Nunez, 2004). Unfortunately, many empirically supported treatments seem to miss the important role diversity variables have on the process and outcome of psychotherapy (Howard, Moras, Brill, Martinovich, & Lutz, 1996).

Some multicultural scholars have questioned the efficacy of empirically supported treatments with people of color (Matt & Navarro, 1997; S. Sue, 1998). When these approaches are assessed, treatment groups are often compared with control groups, usually no-treatment groups. Some studies, however, have focused on treatment approaches with people of color. Inspired by the effectiveness of empirically supported treatments for the majority culture population (Chambless et al., 1996), researchers of color found that cognitive–behavioral approaches are also effective in treating depression among Latinos (Comas-Díaz, 1981; Organista, Munoz, & Gonzales, 1994). Moreover, Roselló and Bernal (1999) found cognitive–behavioral therapy (CBT) and interpersonal therapy (IPT) to be beneficial in alleviating depression among Latino adolescents. CBT was shown to reduce Latinos' panic symptoms in a community medical center setting (Sanderson, Rue, & Wetzler, 1998). Interpersonal therapy has been found to be effective in reducing depression in African Americans (Brown, Schulberg, Sacco, Perel, & Houck, 1999). Although another study found that CBT reduced depression in African Americans, it was not as effective as with their European American counterparts (Organista et al., 1994). This finding may be explained by G. C. N. Hall's (2001) assertion that individuals of one cultural group may require a form of psychotherapy different from that required by members of another cultural group. It is clear that more studies are needed comparing diverse treatment orientations, including culturally sensitive psychotherapy.

Indeed, multicultural research has identified the need for culturally sensitive approaches in the delivery of evidence-based psychotherapy to people of color. For example, examining the validity of empirically supported treatments for persons of ethnic minorities, Bernal and Scharron del Rio (2001) recommended the addition of multicultural awareness and culture-specific strategies to cognitive–behavioral, person-centered, and psychodynamic forms of psychotherapy. Similarly, Lewis (1994) considered not only the culture of women of color in her application of CBT to these populations but also the systemic and historical influences in their lives. More specifically, CBT clinicians need to assess the role of racism and oppression in their clients' ability to achieve mastery and agency.

CBT can be useful in addressing societal oppression by offering techniques to alleviate ethnic and racial victimization, such as racial stress inoculation (a derivative of stress inoculation described by Foa, Rothbaum, Riggs, & Murdock, 1991) and racial stress management (Comas-Díaz, in press). Tools such as relaxation techniques, imagery, visualization, systematic desensitization, and stress management are consistent with a holistic healing perspective, an orientation endorsed by many collectivist cultures. Moreover, these tools have the potential to help disempowered individuals develop a personal sense of agency and mastery when they are used within a systemic perspective.

Cane (2000) successfully used holistic techniques combined with an empowerment framework with traumatized Central American Indians, abused women, violence victims, and other marginalized individuals. The self-healing practices included Tai Chi, Pal Dan Gum, acupressure, visualization, breath work, ritual, polarity, massage, labyrinth, body movement, and intuition work. The research methods involved quantitative and qualitative methods such as questionnaires, focus groups, and in-depth interviews. The study's findings showed a reduction of symptoms related to traumatic stress and posttraumatic stress disorder (PTSD). Cane concluded that the empowerment component was an effective way to promote the inherent healing capacity of the person and the community.

Clinicians can modify CBT to accommodate non-Western cultures by emphasizing its teaching component. For instance, the CBT technique of challenging negative cognitions is consistent with the collectivistic cultural value of viewing life as a spiritual learning experience where karma (law of cause and effect) and dharma (code of proper conduct conforming to duty) are mediated by achieving wisdom (Comas-Díaz, 1992). CBT can help clients who deal with losses and trauma to perceive life setbacks as learning experiences with opportunities for growth and improvement. If modified through the addition of a cultural component, CBT can be used to address special needs of underserved populations. There is a long history of loss, violence, abuse, and coercion leading to learned helplessness and PTSD among many women of color (Vasquez, 1994). Indeed, the incidence of PTSD among young urban Latinas is reported to be significantly higher than among other populations (Lipschitz, Rasmusson, Anyan, Cromwell, & Southwick, 2000). Culturally sensitive CBT can help promulgate an educational approach that facilitates women's abilities to assume credit for their gains and success.

Feminist perspectives can empower women from diverse cultural backgrounds (Worell & Remer, 2003). In my clinical experience, the empowerment of disenfranchised clients requires assertiveness training. However, the expression of assertiveness is context specific. For example, the direct expression of assertiveness among Puerto Rican women is culturally discouraged, leaving room for the indirect expression of assertiveness through "guerrilla tactics" or strategies characteristic of the socially powerless. Moreover, the cultural taboo against the direct expression of anger and the colonial status of the island contribute to the development of unassertiveness as a coping mechanism. My colleague and I (Comas-Díaz & Duncan, 1985) developed and applied a more direct assertiveness training program encased in a cultural context relevant to Latinas. Our findings indicated that assertiveness training was effective; it helped women to freely and directly express their assertiveness in a culturally relevant manner while exploring the cultural consequences of their actions (Comas-Díaz & Duncan, 1985).

The therapeutic relationship is crucial for working within a CBT framework. For example, Kala, a 40-year-old Indian immigrant who had been in the United States for 20 years, came to see me after a failed trial of systematic desensitization for social phobia. When I asked her about her previous psychotherapeutic experience, Kala replied, "That Western approach did not work with me." Upon exploration, I uncovered that Kala perceived her previous therapist—a White woman—as "too technical, following a treatment manual, and being more interested in having me fit her notions." Kala raised her voice when she relayed the information. She continued, "When I told her I was not used to measuring discomfort with a numeric scale, the psychologist asked me to keep trying it, that it was the way it was supposed to work." I asked Kala how she felt, and she replied, "I was furious, but my culture tells me to be respectful to authority figures, so I did not express my anger." Kala concluded, "I stopped seeing her."

I worked on developing a therapeutic alliance with Kala by obtaining family data after securing her trust. I did not interpret her refusal to use a rating scale as resistance to treatment. Although rating scales may be helpful in diagnosis and treatment, they may contain bias and ambiguity; thus, a clinician needs to question their use with individuals from other cultures. Moreover, self-report scales are susceptible to response bias and may contain terms that are not clearly defined, causing clients to be uncertain of what they are being asked (Beere, 1990). As an illustration, East Asian students are more likely than U.S. students to use the midpoint on scales, whereas U.S. students are more likely than other groups to use the extreme values (Chen, Lee, & Stevenson, 1995).

I discussed the cross-cultural research findings on rating scales with Kala. She stated that my approach was consistent with her cultural belief that healers teach. APA Multicultural Guideline 4 (APA, 2003) states, "Culturally sensitive psychological researchers are encouraged to recognize the importance of conducting culture-centered and ethical psychological research among persons from ethnic, linguistic, and racial minority backgrounds" (p. 388), and to comply with this guideline I asked Kala to collaborate with me in designing a way to measure her level of discomfort in a nonnumerical way. Then I taught her relaxation techniques and how to visualize a safe place. Kala found both techniques very useful. Afterward, I introduced the healing light-stream technique (Shapiro, 1995) and informed her that this technique was borrowed from yoga. Kala commented that as an Indian, she believed in the healing effects of yoga. This exchange helped to solidify the therapeutic alliance, and she agreed to try systematic desensitization a second time. Kala's trust in me, her clinician, helped her successfully complete her treatment. She stated that she was "doing fine" at a 6-month telephone follow-up.

Interpersonal psychotherapy can be culturally sensitive for clients with a strong relational orientation. Based on the legacies of relational theorists Harry Stack Sullivan and John Bowlby, IPT focuses on interpersonal and attachment factors in mental distress. Initially developed as a therapy for depression, IPT targets four problem areas—grief, interpersonal disputes, role transitions, and interpersonal deficits (Klerman, Weissman, Rounsanville, & Chevron, 1984). Most of these areas are particularly relevant to individuals who experience losses, relational difficulties, and cultural role transitions.

Roselló and Bernal (1999) found both CBT and IPT beneficial in alleviating depression among Latinos. Participants in the IPT condition, however, had an added advantage: Their self-concept and social adaptation also improved. The researchers suggested that IPT is culturally congruent with the Latino values of *familismo* and *personalismo*, the latter representing the preference for personal contact in interactions. The study's finding that IPT enhances self-esteem seems congruent with many collectivistic clients' relational orientation. However, caution is required in the generalization of these findings; Roselló and Bernal's sample consisted of Puerto Rican adolescents living in Puerto Rico. There is wide variation among the Latino groups and great individual differences within cultures. Gender, age, acculturation to mainstream U.S. culture, nationality, generational status, foreign birth, language use, skin color, socioeconomic class, and residence area, among many other factors, can influence Latinos' adherence to traditional cultural values. It is clear that more research is needed.

SOCIOPOLITICAL CONTEXT

In addition to the confluence of therapist and client worldviews, therapists in multicultural psychotherapy need to acknowledge the ecological reality of historical and sociopolitical factors. Sociopolitical behaviors and attitudes such as discrimination and oppression, racism, ethnocentrism, sexism, heterosexism, and other "isms" permeate the lives of many individuals from diverse cultures. Furthermore, the post-September 11th climate has created fertile ground for xenophobia and hate crimes in the United States. For instance, many Latinos were attacked because they looked Arab (Dudley-Grant, Comas-Díaz, Todd-Bazemore, & Hueston, 2004). These sociopolitical and historical realities affect the therapeutic relationship.

The best empirically supported treatment is going to fail if the client feels that the therapist is unconsciously racist, sexist, homophobic, elitist, or the like. The recognition of ecological and political factors in the cross-cultural encounter is of particular importance given the salience of race, ethnicity, gender, and other highly visible cultural diversity variables. For example, the contexts of race, class, and gender and their interaction permeate the therapeutic hour. The televised beating of Rodney King by the police, for instance, galvanized the African American community and was a popular topic among African Americans in psychotherapy. The O. J. Simpson trial became a nationwide Rorschach test on race relations. Some African Americans saw O. J. as a successful Black person who was framed by the racist White establishment; he became a symbol of the historic racial oppression of the "uppity" Black man. Moreover, they perceived his acquittal as an example of righting a historical wrong within race relations. From a contrary viewpoint, many Whites believed that the African American ex-football player and actor murdered his White ex-wife and her White male friend and then got away with it. This national event reminded us that mental health issues extend beyond the consulting room (Shorter-Gooden, 1996).

CULTURAL VARIATION IN THE CLINICIAN'S ROLE

Culture affects not only the process and outcome of psychotherapy but also how clients perceive their clinicians. A therapist's personal qualities are a contributing factor to psychotherapy outcome (Shahar, Blatt, Zuroff, Krupnick, & Sotsky, 2004), and this finding is particularly relevant to multicultural therapeutic relationships.

The ideal psychotherapist–client relationship varies from culture to culture (Portela, 1971). Many Asian immigrants, for instance, tend to expect their clinician to conform to a cultural hierarchy (Sakauye, 1996). Attitudes toward authority figures are likely to inform clients' expectations about their practitioners. If not recognized, these expectations may interfere with the establishment of a therapeutic alliance within a multicultural therapeutic dyad. More specifically, there are different cultural responses to authority figures inside the family (nuclear and extended), authorities in the social hierarchy such as clergy and community leaders, and outside authorities such as health care providers, teachers, and lawyers, in addition to general members of the mainstream community such as police and politicians. When interacting with clinicians, clients from traditional collectivistic societies may be overly deferential, inhibited, and ashamed to reveal personal information, or they may alternatively be suspicious, defensive, or hostile (Sakauye, 1996).

In addition, some Asian cultural values may not be congruent with Eurocentric and Western expectations of the therapeutic relationship. For instance, humility and modesty are expected in social interactions and are often expressed in deferential behavior (Leong, 1996). Asians who have been influenced by Confucian thought may expect the therapeutic relationship to follow a hierarchical mode between the self and other, with relatively well-defined roles, reciprocal obligations, rules, and rituals (Yi, 1995). Such hierarchies are clearly delineated for parent and child, husband and wife, teacher and student, and older and younger sibling relationships (Shon & Ja, 1982).

Feelings of affection and closeness are different from obligation and affiliation within an Eastern relational framework. Yi (1995) posited that patients may develop a positive, idealized feeling toward practitioners as authority figures. If clients perceive their clinician as a wise teacher, they will assume the role of a student. Clients may expect the clinician to provide warmth, benevolence, and knowledge that will help them. Southeast Asian refugees seem to prefer relatively structured, hierarchical relationships in treatment (Westermeyer, Williams, & Nguyen, 1991). In addition, expectations, roles, and rules guiding the therapeutic relationship are frequently informed by clients' need to save face (Paniagua, 1994).

To develop a working alliance, clinicians need to understand culturally diverse expectations, because the interaction style of egalitarian and nondirective therapists can unsettle clients who are more comfortable with hierarchical and directive professional interactions (Koss-Chioino & Vargas, 1992). For example, during my first session with May, a highly educated Thai woman, I said, "I'll do my best to help you." May replied, "No, I don't want you to say you will do your best." She continued, "As my doctor, I want you to say that you *will* heal my depression." Upon exploration, May stated that in her culture doctors are experts and do not say they will try. With a smile, May continued, "Of course I understand what you meant, but you can use the technique of suggestion to help me heal myself."

Another cultural variation is the perception of the psychologist as the expert of the heart (Chao, 1992). The Chinese characters for the word *psychologist* translate as *expert of the inner heart;* in Vietnamese, *psychologist* translates as *expert of the heart* or *expert of the soul.* In other words, the psychologist is the expert who understands the metaphorical seat of the emotions—the heart. This perception highlights the mind–body and mind–soul connection present among many Asian groups. As the expert of the soul, the psychologist appreciates spiritual matters and thus endorses a holistic approach.

The complex expectations of practitioners are also reflected among some American Indian patients. Trimble and his associates (1996) asserted that in many American Indian communities, mental health providers are expected to exemplify empathy, genuineness, availability, respect, warmth, congruence, and connectedness. These characteristics need to be present in all therapeutic relationships, regardless of cultural background. It is interesting to note that Messer and Wampold (2002) advised prospective clients to evaluate clinicians' reputations within a local community of practitioners and to select a well-regarded clinician whose theoretical orientation is compatible with their own outlook, instead of choosing a practitioner on the basis of expertise in empirically supported treatments.

Clinicians' interpersonal style is of vital importance for Latino clients. Many Latinos expect their therapist to become part of their families, or at least part of their extended supportive network, an expectation that can be attributed to the cultural value of *familismo.* Some Latinos may appear initially resistant to address serious topics and to waste time making small talk. This cultural behavior is *plática,* or the informal small talk that breaks the ice before discussing serious topics. The initial *plática* additionally serves Latinos as means of evaluating the practitioner. For example, they may ask their clinician personal information during a *plática* to develop trust. As a Latina clinician, I register it differently when clients of color, particularly Latinos, ask me personal questions. Of course, I use clinical judgment about appropriate boundaries, but I also balance it with sensitivity to cultural expectations. As a consequence, I selectively self-disclose, balancing clinical skill with cultural norms.

On the basis of cultural variation in clients' expectations of their providers, Atkinson, Thompson, and Grant (1993) identified eight intersecting roles. They divided clients into low and high acculturation to the dominant U.S. culture as follows: Less acculturated clients may expect the practitioner to act as the following:

1. *Advisor:* The problem is external in nature, and prevention is the treatment goal.

2. *Advocate:* The problem is external in nature, and remediation is the treatment goal.
3. *Facilitator of indigenous support systems:* The problem is internal in nature, and prevention is the treatment goal.
4. *Facilitator of indigenous healing systems:* The problem is internal in nature, and remediation is the treatment goal.

More acculturated clients may expect the therapist to act as the following:

5. *Consultant:* The problem is external in nature, and prevention is the treatment goal.
6. *Change agent:* The problem is external in nature, and remediation is the treatment goal.
7. *Counselor:* The problem is internal in nature, and prevention is the treatment goal.
8. *Psychotherapist:* The problem is internal in nature, and remediation is the treatment goal.

In my clinical experience, the main difference between less acculturated and more acculturated clients is that the therapist needs to educate the former about psychotherapy. Nonetheless, the diverse expectations of the practitioner's role can develop in a circular fashion, in which clinicians move from one role to another, or engage in several roles simultaneously, regardless of the client's level of acculturation. For instance, a highly acculturated client may require the psychologist's involvement as an advisor, advocate, and consultant, as well as a psychotherapist. In a converse situation, I have worked with recent immigrants who have responded well to my role as a psychotherapist without any need for me to act as an advocate, consultant, or change agent. Acculturation is not the only determining factor. Clients' relational needs, psychological developmental stages, and ethnic identity development are also important in determining their expectations of a clinician.

It is interesting to note that some mainstream psychotherapeutic orientations may benefit from the complex set of practitioner and psychotherapy expectations predominant among collectivist individuals. For instance, in rational-emotive therapies, the therapist is a combination of philosopher, teacher, and scientist (Prochaska & Norcross, 1994). In coaching practices, the coach's directive role is similar to the practitioner's role as an advisor, counselor, consultant, and change agent. Similarly, active and directive approaches can be particularly helpful during the initial stages of treatment, and they reduce the client's presenting symptoms. A directive therapeutic style can facilitate the clinician's credibility, earning clients' trust at the beginning of treatment.

Some research has examined the complex expectations of people of color regarding clinicians and therapy. My colleagues and I (Comas-Díaz, Geller, Melgoza, & Baker, 1982) studied the expectations of clients of color regarding their therapists. The results of the empirical investigation showed that people of color expected their practitioner to be active by giving advice, teaching, and guiding. These expectations were accompanied by the clients' belief that their clinicians would help them grow emotionally in a process that at times would be painful. We concluded that people of color have a complex set of expectations related to the cultural variation in clinician roles. We also studied ethnic minority clients' pretherapy expectations. The results suggested that although clients of color expected to get relief from their symptoms, they also expected to work to overcome their contribution to their distress. In addition, the clients perceived psychotherapy as a process that would take time to achieve their therapeutic goals. These empirical findings suggest that clients do not need to be YAVIS to be psychologically minded.

INDIVIDUAL AND COLLECTIVE: CULTURAL VARIATIONS IN THE SELF–OTHER RELATIONSHIP

Most cultural variations in healing encounters relate to the value attributed to the relationship between self and other or to how individuals define the self and how they relate to others. According to Triandis (1995), Eurocentric and Western cultures tend to endorse individuation and separation, where self is clearly demarcated and separate from other. Within this worldview, identity development is based on affirmation of the self in contrast to the other. "I am not you" is an individualistic developmental task. In a converse manner, indigenous and Eastern cultures tend to value connectedness between self and other, where the boundary between them is fluid: "I am part of you," and "I am we." In summary, the individualistic, separate sense of self is at odds with the interdependent communal identity. Moreover, among some collectivist cultures, illness is considered a family affair, requiring a communal intervention (Canino & Canino, 1982).

Differences in communication styles between members of collectivist and individualist cultures further complicate the multicultural psychotherapeutic relationship. Collectivists tend to be implicit and indirect, because in maintaining harmonious relationships they rely substantially on nonverbal communication and pay great attention to context (Triandis, 1995). By contrast, individualists prefer to communicate in a direct, explicit, and specific manner, paying less attention to context. E. T. Hall (1983) labeled these two styles as *context rich*, where communication adheres to a rich web of cultural nuances and meaning, and *context poor*, where communication relies on the literal meaning of words. As a consequence, the multicultural practitioner needs to pay more attention to context-rich communication, that is, indirect messages and nonverbal language.

Indeed, effective multicultural practice requires the inclusion and recognition of nonverbal communication as well as sensitivity to the subjective aspects of the client's life (Kinzie, 1978). I use the term *cultural resonance* to identify this process. Cultural resonance involves the ability to understand clients through clinical skill, cultural competence, and intuition. Cultural resonance acknowledges intuition as an important variable in the multicultural encounter. *Intuition* is a collectivistic nonverbal communication that relies on internal cues, hunches, and vibes as a means of problem solving (Butler, 1985). Given the diverse worldviews that the clinician must examine, cultural resonance becomes a guide for understanding the cross-cultural divide. The ability to resonate culturally with clients offers information about their internal emotional state based on nonverbal communication and can be used to supplement knowledge regarding their behavior. Cultural resonance helps the clinician decipher the client's inner processes and provides information beyond messages that the client communicates verbally.

MANAGEMENT OF THE MULTICULTURAL THERAPEUTIC RELATIONSHIP

The therapeutic relationship requires special attention in multicultural dyads. Like clinical practice, the therapeutic relationship needs to be modified to the client's culture. In addition to tailoring the relationship to the client's interpersonal and developmental needs, clinicians need to acknowledge cultural variations in the relationship. Moreover, they need to add additional flexibility to the clinician role (Seeley, 2000). For example, Nikelly (1996) recommended that clinicians use modeling, selective self-disclosure, and didactic approaches when working with immigrant clients. He asserted that these relational styles are less threatening to the client's ego than explorations into psychological and personality realms that may be unfamiliar. In a similar manner, Kakar (1985) modified his psychoanalytic approach for working with East Indians by being active and didactic and by feeling and expressing empathy, interest, and warmth. Regardless of theoretical orientation, the common elements in the process of psychotherapy include a shared worldview, the healing qualities of the therapist, the client's expectations, and an emerging sense of mastery (Torrey, 1986). However, in multicultural healing encounters, these conditions may be perceived and experienced differently. For instance, clinician and client may not necessarily share worldviews, even if they are from the same culture. The feeling of being understood by another person can be intrinsically therapeutic, because it bridges the isolation of the distress and helps restore a sense of connectedness (Suchman et al., 1997).

Practitioners need to understand their clients' voices. Like a psycholinguist, the multicultural clinician's role is to echo, resonate, translate, and recreate the client's voice and language. To fully accomplish this, the psychologist needs to learn the client's use of words to facilitate and guide the learning of a new common language. Therefore, part of the therapeutic task is to incorporate the client's vocabulary into the therapeutic dialogue to promote change. The translation of psychotherapeutic concepts into the client's language is a central aspect in healing. I have found the explanatory model to be extremely helpful in beginning the therapeutic dialogue. The explanatory model is a socioanthropological method advanced by Kleinman (1980) to elicit clients' perspectives of their illness and experience. This brief ethnographic approach solicits clients' views and beliefs regarding their distress and healing through the following questions:

- What do you call your problem (illness)?
- What do you think your illness (problem) does?
- What do you think the natural course of your illness is?
- What do you fear?
- Why do you think this illness or problem has occurred?
- How do you think the sickness should be treated?
- How do want me to help you?
- Whom do you turn to for help?
- Who should be involved in decision making?

These questions not only initiate the therapeutic dialogue but also unfold clients' expectations of both treatment and clinician (Callan & Littlewood, 1998). Moreover, the explanatory model enlists the patient's support systems in the healing process. Research on a short interview to elicit explanatory models showed differences between the explanatory models of White, African Caribbean, and Asian clients in London and in Harare, Zimbabwe (Lloyd et al., 1998).

Most clinicians agree that a psychotherapeutic alliance increases treatment effectiveness. However, how can clinicians enter the life of a client from a different culture? Effective treatment for clients from other cultures requires therapists' credibility and giving (S. Sue & Zane, 1987). *Credibility* refers to the client's perception of the practitioner as a trustworthy and effective helper. For some people of color, the clinician's role can be initially associated with a traditional role of a healer, to whom wisdom and respect are awarded because of his or her esoteric knowledge (Koss-Chioino, 1992). The archetype of the healer is present in many societies. Traditional healers reach deep-feeling states such as benevolent love, empathy, and compassion to provide life-enriching experiences to their clients. Many people of color expect these qualities from their healers–psychotherapists. Nonetheless, client familiarity with this role does not mean that he or she will automatically award this credibility to the therapist.

Psychotherapists need to give to their clients in addition to earn credibility (S. Sue & Zane, 1987). *Giving* refers to the client's perception that he or she gained something from the encounter. There are several examples of giving, including acknowledging, and at times addressing, realistic issues in the therapeutic hour. To illustrate, in their work with African American clients of low socioeconomic status, Thomas and Dansby (1985) asserted that helping their clients solve concrete problems or difficulties with significant others was a significant building block in gaining trust within the therapeutic relationship. These authors cited involvement in day-to-day living as another building block in the development of trust.

I try to earn credibility by being active during the initial stages of treatment. An active, focused style consistent with cognitive–behavioral approaches seems responsive to many of my clients' explanatory models of illness and treatment. I give to my clients by summarizing insights and connections learned at the end of each session. Such an approach can also be an indication of a therapist's sense of caring. However, I always keep a dynamic and systemic understanding of my clients' circumstances. In addition, I try to meet them where they are. Depending on their cultural and spiritual beliefs, I often use mind–body approaches within a holistic framework.

CULTURAL EMPATHY

One fundamental task in the management of multicultural encounters is the development and enhancement of empathy. *Empathy* involves recognition of the self in the other. Such recognition is critical because of the human tendency to like people who remind them of themselves, which in turn can inhibit empathy toward individuals who are different. People, including therapists, tend to have difficulty empathizing with those they dislike or disrespect or whose cultures, values, experiences, customs, beliefs, or ideals are different from their own.

The interpersonal construct of empathy includes affective and cognitive components (Jordan & Surrey, 1986). The emotive and moral components of empathy pertain to a clinician's intrinsic capacity and motivation to attend to the emotional experience of others and are prerequisites to empathic communication. In addition, empathy has perceptual, aperceptual, kinesthetic, and somatic elements. The affective component involves emotional connectedness, or a capacity to take in and contain the feelings of the client, similar to a subjective and phenomenological experience of being like the other. The cognitive component involves an intellectual understanding of the client, similar to witnessing the other's experience (Kleinman, 1988). Kaplan (1991) observed that the cognitive component follows a different and contradictory course from the affective component. She argued that although there may be an interpretation of affect, identity tends to remain differentiated in cognitive empathy.

The development of empathy in a multicultural context facilitates an understanding of the client's experience (Stewart, 1981). Within the multicultural encounter, clinicians may be able to empathize at a cognitive level but not necessarily at an affective level. In cognitive empathy, therapists can study the client's culture and confer with colleagues who share the client's cultural background. Kleinman (1988) termed this concept *empathic witnessing*; the therapist recognizes his or her cultural ignorance of the client's reality and reaffirms, through empathic witnessing, the client's experience and reality. The emergence of empathy with the emotional experience of clients from other cultures may be difficult. Accepting this difference is a useful component in managing the therapeutic relationship within the multicultural framework. For example, a European American female clinician began working with a Vietnamese refugee woman who was raped by pirates before her arrival in the United States. The therapist, a social worker, felt qualified to work with this client because she was trained as a sexual assault counselor and was fluent in French, the client's second language. The counselor believed that she had both cognitive and affective empathy because she too had been a victim of sexual abuse. However, she was unprepared for the devastating effects of the client's story about her ordeal in Vietnam, her refugee trauma, and her experiences of repeated rape victimization. The therapist did not differentiate between cognitive and affective empathy and could not relate to the client's combined sexual and refugee trauma. Unable to deal with her strong reactions (and countertransferential feelings), the psychotherapist decided to transfer the client to another clinician. After consulting with a clinical consultant, she decided that her patient needed a therapist who spoke French, was familiar with Vietnamese culture, and had expertise in treating trauma. She then contacted national mental health associations and organizations working with war trauma for referrals. This decision illustrates the importance of referral when clinicians are not adequately prepared to address their clients' therapeutic needs.

The multicultural therapeutic relationship requires more than cognitive and affective empathy. It needs to be grounded in cultural empathy. Ridley and Lingle (1996) identified the concept of *cultural empathy* as "a learned ability of counselors to accurately gain an understanding of the self-experience of clients from other cultures—an understanding informed by counselors' interpretations of cultural data" (p. 32). These authors proposed a cultural empathy model that integrates a variety of perceptual, cognitive, affective, and communication skills and places empathic understanding and cultural responsiveness at the center. The model proposes perspective taking—using a cultural framework as a guide for understanding the client from the outside in—as well as the recognition of cultural differences between self and other. The affective processes of cultural empathy include vicarious affect and expressive concern. In *vicarious affect*, psychotherapists understand clients by comparing vicarious or similar experiences in their own lives with the client's reality. *Expressive concern* involves clinicians' manifestation of genuine concern for the clients' challenges and conflicts, as well as the expression of affirmation of the client's achievements. The communicative processes involve the clinicians' exploration for insight into the clients' whole experience using sensitivity and asking clarifying questions, in addition to conveying accurate understanding.

Psychotherapists can facilitate change through clinical collaboration. Research suggests that clients working with clinicians of similar ethnic backgrounds and languages tend to remain in treatment longer than do clients whose therapists are not ethnically nor linguistically matched (S. Sue, 1998). However, ethnic and linguistic match does not imply cultural identification (G. C. N. Hall, 2001). As an illustration, Karlsson (2005) reviewed the research on ethnic matching between psychotherapists and clients and found inconclusive results and low validity for ethnic matching. Nonetheless, research indicated that patients of color in race-concordant clinical dyads participate more in their care than do those in race-dissimilar dyads (Cooper-Patrick et al., 1999). The empirical results on the effects of ethnic matching on treatment satisfaction among Mediterranean migrants showed that these patients did not value ethnic matching as important to the clinical relationship (Knipscheer & Kleber, 2004). Research also indicates that patients of color in race-concordant clinical dyads participate more in their care than do those in race-dissimilar dyads (Cooper-Patrick et al., 1999). Regardless of their ethnicity, race, gender, sexual orientation, class, physical ability, or other diversity variables, therapists who are proficient in cultural communication enhance their clients' satisfaction with treatment. An effective basis for communication is collaboration. The explanatory model can lay the foundation for collaboration; the therapist's cultural adaptation helps to cement the alliance.

CONCLUSION

Culture mediates psychotherapy. Clinicians need to adapt their interventions to culturally diverse clients. Effective multicultural psychotherapy requires a balance of clinical expertise with treatments that are both informed by science and grounded in culture. Such a balance is solidified in the development of a psychotherapeutic alliance. Clinicians who endorse evidence-supported treatments need to acknowledge the cultural variation within the psychotherapeutic relationship. For instance, clinicians can expand their therapeutic style to include the roles of advisor, consultant, teacher, and change agent, among others. Treatment expectations of individuals from other cultures are often complex and even paradoxical. Although many people of color expect their practitioner to give advice, teach, and guide, they also believe that their clinician will help them grow emotionally in a process that at times will be painful.

A positive multicultural therapeutic relationship requires more than cognitive and affective empathy; it needs to be grounded in cultural empathy. Cultural empathy involves a process of perspective taking using a cultural framework as a guide for understanding the client from the outside in and the recognition of cultural differences between self and other (Ridley & Lingle, 1996). Practitioners communicate with their clients through resonance, affinity, and identification. Therapists' need to identify with clients from other cultures offers a challenge as well as a growth opportunity. The explanatory model of distress and treatment can help multicultural clinicians act as psycholinguists to echo, resonate, translate, and recreate their clients' voice and language. The explanatory model, a socioanthropological method advanced by Kleinman (1980), helps clients articulate their perspectives on their own illness and healing. The explanatory model can help address multicultural clients' complex treatment expectations. As an illustration, although many clients of color expect to obtain relief from their symptoms, they also expect to work to overcome their own contribution to their distress to develop agency and mastery. The recognition of extratherapy variables such as history, ecology, and sociopolitical factors is required for the solidification of a multicultural psychotherapeutic relationship. Finally, the cultural examination of both client and practitioner circumstances, the expansion of the clinician's role, increased flexibility in therapeutic style, and the development of cultural empathy and resonance are strategies that psychologists of all orientations can implement to improve the effectiveness of their interventions.

REFERENCES

Altman, N. (1995). *The analyst in the inner city: Race, class and culture through a psychoanalytic lens*. New York: Analytic Press.

American Psychological Association. (1990). *Guidelines for providers of psychological services to ethnic, linguistic, and culturally diverse populations*. Washington, DC: Author.

American Psychological Association. (2003). Guidelines on multicultural education, training, research, practice, and organizational change for psychologists. *American Psychologist, 58*, 377–402.

Atkinson, D. R., Thompson, C. E., & Grant, S. K. (1993). A three-dimensional model for counseling racial/ethnic minorities. *The Counseling Psychologist, 21*, 257–277.

Bamshad, M. J., & Olson, S. E. (2003). Does race exist? *Scientific American, 289*(6), 78–85.

Beere, C. A. (1990). *Gender roles: A handbook of tests and measures*. New York: Greenwood Press.

Bernal, G., & Scharron del Rio, M. R. (2001). Are empirically supported treatments valid for ethnic minorities? Toward an alternative approach for treatment research. *Cultural Diversity and Ethnic Minority Psychology, 7*, 328–342.

Brown, C., Schulberg, H. C., Sacco, D., Perel, J. M., & Houck, P. R. (1999). Effectiveness of treatment for major depression in primary medical care practice: A post hoc analysis of outcomes for African American and White patients. *Journal of Affective Disorders, 53,* 185–192.

Butler, L. (1985). Of kindred minds: The ties that bind. In M. A. Orlandi (Ed.), *Cultural competence for evaluators: A guide for alcohol and other drug abuse prevention practitioners working with ethnic/racial communities* (pp. 23–54). Rockville, MD: U.S. Department of Health and Human Services.

Callan, A., & Littlewood, R. (1998). Patient satisfaction: Ethnic origin or explanatory model? *International Journal of Social Psychiatry, 44,* 1–11.

Cane, P. (2000). *Trauma, healing and transformation: Awakening a new heart with body mind spirit practices.* Watsonville, CA: Capacitar.

Canino, G., & Canino, I. (1982). Culturally syntonic family therapy for migrant Puerto Ricans. *Hospital and Community Psychiatry, 33,* 299–303.

Chambless, D. L., Sanderson, W. C., Shoham, V., Johnson, S. B., Pope, K. S., Crits-Christoph, P., et al. (1996). An update on empirically validated therapies. *The Clinical Psychologist, 49,* 5–18.

Chao, C. (1992). The inner heart: Therapy with Southeast Asian families. In L. A. Vargas & J. Koss-Chioino (Eds.), *Working with culture: Psychotherapeutic interventions with ethnic minority children and adolescents* (pp. 157–181). San Francisco: Jossey-Bass.

Chen, C., Lee, S., & Stevenson, H. W. (1995). Response style and cross-cultural comparisons of rating scales among East Asian and North American students. *Psychological Science, 6,* 170–175.

Chin, J. L. (1993). Toward a psychology of difference: Psychotherapy for a culturally diverse population. In J. L. Chin, V. De La Cancela, & Y. Jenkins (Eds.), *Diversity in psychotherapy* (pp. 69–91). Wesport, CT: Praeger.

Comas-Díaz, L. (1981). Effects of cognitive and behavioral group treatment in the depressive symptomatology of Puerto Rican women. *Journal of Consulting and Clinical Psychology, 49,* 627–632.

Comas-Díaz, L. (1988). Cross cultural mental health treatment. In L. Comas-Díaz & E. E. H. Griffith (Eds.), *Clinical guidelines in cross cultural mental health* (pp. 337–361). New York: Wiley.

Comas-Díaz, L. (1992). The future of psychotherapy with ethnic minorities. *Psychotherapy, 29,* 88–94.

Comas-Díaz, L. (in press). Ethnopolitical psychology. In E. Aldarondo (Ed.), *Promoting social justice in mental health practice.* Mahwah, NJ: Erlbaum.

Comas-Díaz, L., & Duncan, J. W. (1985). The cultural context: A factor in assertiveness training with mainland Puerto Rican women. *Psychology of Women Quarterly, 9,* 463–475.

Comas-Díaz, L., Geller, J., Melgoza, B., & Baker, R. (1982, August). *Ethnic minority patients' expectations of treatment and of their therapists.* Paper presented at the 90th Annual Convention of the American Psychological Association, Washington, DC.

Comas-Díaz, L., & Jacobsen, F. M. (1995). Women of color and psychopharmacology: An empowering perspective. *Women & Therapy, 16*, 85–112.

Cooper-Patrick, L., Gallo, J., Gonzales, J. J., Vu, H. T., Powe, N. E., Nelson, C., & Ford, D. (1999, August 11). Race, gender and partnership in the patient–physician relationship. *Journal of the American Medical Association, 282*, 583–589.

Dudley-Grant, R., Comas-Díaz, L., Todd-Bazemore, B., & Hueston, J. D. (2004). *Fostering resilience in response to terrorism: For psychologists working with people of color.* Retrieved November 4, 2005, from the American Psychological Association Practice Directorate's Online Help Center Web site: http://www.apahelpcenter.org/featuredtopics/feature.php?id=6

Foa, E. B., Rothbaum, B. O., Riggs, D. S., & Murdock, T. B. (1991). Treatment of posttraumatic stress disorder in rape victims: A comparison between cognitive–behavioral procedures and counseling. *Journal of Consulting and Clinical Psychology, 59*, 715–723.

Foster, R. F., Moskowitz, M., & Javier, R. (Eds.). (1996). *Reaching across the boundaries of culture and class: Widening the scope of psychotherapy.* New York: Jason Aronson.

Hall, E. T. (1983). *The dance of life: The other dimension of time.* Garden City, NY: Anchor Press/Doubleday.

Hall, G. C. N. (2001). Psychotherapy research with ethnic minorities: Empirical, ethical, and conceptual issues. *Journal of Consulting and Clinical Psychology, 69*, 502–510.

Harwood, A. (1971, May 17). The hot–cold theory of disease: Implications for treatment of Puerto Rican patients. *Journal of the American Medical Association, 216*, 1153–1158.

Hays, P. (1995). Multicultural applications of cognitive behavioral therapy. *Professional Psychology: Research and Practice, 26*, 306–315.

Ho, M. H. (1987). *Family therapy with ethnic minorities.* Newbury Park, CA: Sage.

Horner, A. J. (1984). *Object relations and the developing ego in therapy.* New York: Jason Aronson.

Howard, K. I., Moras, K., Brill, P. L., Martinovich, Z., & Lutz, W. (1996). Evaluation of psychotherapy: Efficacy, effectiveness, and patient progress. *American Psychologist, 51*, 1059–1064.

Information Please Database. (n.d.). *Ethnicity and race by counties.* Retrieved November 4, 2005, from http://www.infoplease.com/ipa/A0855617

Jacobsen, F. M., & Comas-Díaz, L. (1999). Psychopharmacological treatment of Latinas. *Essential Psychopharmacology, 3*, 29–42.

Jordan, J. V., & Surrey, J. L. (1986). The self-in-relation: Empathy and the mother–daughter relationship. In T. Bernay & D. W. Cantor (Eds.), *The psychology of today's woman: New psychoanalytic visions.* Hillsdale, NJ: Analytic Press.

Kakar, S. (1985). Psychoanalysis and non-Western cultures. *International Review of Psychoanalysis, 12*, 441–448.

Kaplan, A. (1991). The self in relation: Implications for depression in women. In J. V. Jordan, A. G. Kaplan, J. B. Miller, I. P. Stiver, & J. I. Surrey (Eds.), *Women's growth in connection: Writings from the Stone Center* (pp. 206–222). New York: Guilford Press.

Karlsson, R. (2005). Ethnic matching between therapist and patient in psychotherapy: An overview of findings, together with methodological and conceptual issues. *Cultural Diversity and Ethnic Minority Psychology, 11*, 113–129.

Kinzie, J. D. (1978). Lessons from cross-cultural psychotherapy. *American Journal of Psychotherapy, 32*, 510–520.

Kleinman, A. (1980). *Patients and healers in the context of culture: An exploration of the borderland between anthropology, medicine, and psychiatry.* Berkeley: University of California Press.

Kleinman, A. (1988). *Rethinking psychiatry: From cultural category to personal experience.* New York: Free Press.

Klerman, G. L., Weissman, M. M., Rounsanville, B., & Chevron, E. (1984). *Interpersonal psychotherapy of depression.* New York: Basic Books.

Knipscheer, J. W., & Kleber, R. J. (2004). A need for ethnic similarity in the therapist–patient interaction? Mediterranean migrants in Dutch mental health care. *Journal of Clinical Psychology, 60*, 543–554.

Koss-Chioino, J. (1992). *Women as healers, women as patients: Mental health care and traditional healing in Puerto Rico.* Boulder, CO: Westview Press.

Koss-Chioino, J., & Vargas, L. (1992). Through the cultural looking glass: A model for understanding culturally responsive psychotherapies. In L. A. Vargas & J. D. Koss-Chioino (Eds.), *Working with culture: Psychotherapeutic interventions with ethnic minority children and adolescents* (pp. 1–22). San Francisco: Jossey-Bass.

Lawson, W. B. (1996). Clinical issues in pharmacotherapy of African Americans. *Psychopharmacological Bulletin, 32*, 275–281.

Leong, F. T. (1996). MCT theory and Asian American populations. In D. W. Sue, A. E. Ivey, & P. B. Pedersen (Eds.), *A theory of multicultural counseling and therapy* (pp. 204–216). Pacific Grove, CA: Brooks/Cole.

Lewis, S. Y. (1994). Cognitive–behavioral therapy. In L. Comas-Díaz & B. Greene (Eds.), *Women of color: Integrating ethnic and gender identities in psychotherapy* (pp. 223–238). New York: Guilford Press.

Lin, K.-L., Anderson, D., & Poland, R. E. (1995). Ethnicity and psychopharmacology: Bridging the gap. *Psychiatric Clinics of North America, 18*, 635–647.

Lipschitz, D. S., Rasmusson, A. M., Anyan, W., Cromwell, P., & Southwick, S. M. (2000). Clinical and functional correlates of posttraumatic stress disorder in urban adolescent girls at a primary care clinic. *Journal of the American Academy of Child and Adolescent Psychiatry, 39*, 1104–1111.

Lloyd, K. R., Jakob, K. S., Patel, V., St. Louis, L., Bhugra, D., & Mann, A. H. (1998). The development of the short explanatory interview (SEMI) and its use among primary-care attenders with common mental disorders. *Psychological Medicine, 28*, 1231–1237.

Marmar, C. R., Horowitz, M. J., Weiss, D. S., & Marziali, E. (1986). The development of the therapeutic alliance rating system. In L. S. Grenber & W. M. Pinsof (Eds.), *The psychotherapeutic process: A research handbook* (pp. 367–390). New York: Guilford Press.

Matt, G. E., & Navarro, A. M. (1997). What meta-analyses have and have not taught us about psychotherapy effects: A review and future directions. *Clinical Psychology Review, 17*, 1–32.

Melfi, C. A., Croghan, T. W., Hanna, M. P., & Robinson, R. (2000). Racial variation in antidepressant treatment in a medication population. *The Journal of Clinical Psychiatry, 61*, 16–21.

Mendoza, R., & Smith, M. W. (2000). The Hispanic response to psychotropic medications. In P. Ruiz (Ed.), *Ethnicity and psychopharmacology* (pp. 55–89). Washington, DC: American Psychiatric Press.

Messer, S. B., & Wampold, B. E. (2002). Let's face facts: Common factors are more potent than specific therapy ingredients. *Clinical Psychology: Science and Practice, 9*, 21–25.

Nikelly, A. G. (1996). Cultural Babel: The challenge of immigrants to the helping professions. *Cultural Diversity and Mental Health, 3*, 221–233.

Norcross, J. C. (Ed.). (2002). *Psychotherapy relationships that work: Therapist contributions and responsiveness to patients.* New York: Oxford University Press.

Organista, K. C., Munoz, R. F., & Gonzales, G. (1994). Cognitive behavioral therapy for depression in low income and minority medical outpatients: Description of a program and exploratory analyses. *Cognitive Therapy and Research, 18*, 241–259.

Paniagua, F. (1994). *Assessing and treating culturally different clients.* Newbury Park, CA: Sage.

Pi, E. H., & Gray, G. E. (2000). Ethnopharmacology for Asians. In P. Ruiz (Ed.), *Ethnicity and psychopharmacology* (pp. 91–113). Washington, DC: American Psychiatric Press.

Portela, J. M. (1971). Social aspects of transference and countertransference in the patient–psychiatrist relationship in an underdeveloped country: Brazil. *International Journal of Social Psychiatry, 17*, 177–188.

Prochaska, J. O., & Norcross, J. C. (1994). *Systems of psychotherapy: A transtheoretical analysis* (3rd ed.). Pacific Grove, CA: Brooks/Cole.

Ramirez, M. (1991). *Psychotherapy and counseling with minorities: A cognitive approach to individual and cultural differences.* New York: Pergamon Press.

Ridley, C., & Lingle, D. W. (1996). Cultural empathy in multicultural counseling: A multidimensional process model. In P. B. Pedersen, J. G. Draguns, W. J. Lonner, & J. E. Trimble (Eds.), *Counseling across cultures* (4th ed., pp. 21–46). Thousand Oaks, CA: Sage.

Roselló, J., & Bernal, G. (1999). The efficacy of cognitive–behavioral and interpersonal treatments for depression in Puerto Rican adolescents. *Journal of Consulting and Clinical Psychology, 67*, 734–745.

Ruiz, P. (Ed). (2000). *Ethnicity and psychopharmacology*. Washington, DC: American Psychiatric Press.

Sakauye, K. (1996). Ethnocultural aspects. In J. Sadavoy, L. W. Lazarus, L. F. Jarvik, & G. T. Grossberg (Eds.), *Comprehensive review of geriatric psychiatry* (2nd ed., pp. 197–221). Washington, DC: American Psychiatric Press.

Sanderson, W. C., Rue, P. J., & Wetzler, S. (1998). The generalization of cognitive behavior therapy for panic disorder. *Journal of Cognitive Psychotherapy, 12,* 323–330.

Sato, T. (1998). Agency and communion: The relationship between therapy and culture. *Cultural Diversity and Mental Health, 4,* 278–290.

Seeley, K. M. (2000). *Cultural psychotherapy: Working with culture in the clinical encounter.* Northvale, NJ: Jason Aronson.

Shahar, G., Blatt, S. J., Zuroff, D. C., Krupnick, J. L., & Sotsky, S. M. (2004). Perfectionism impedes social relations and response to brief treatment for depression. *Journal of Social and Clinical Psychology, 23,* 140–154.

Shapiro, F. (1995). *Eye movement desensitization and reprocessing: Basic principles, protocols, and procedures.* New York: Guilford.

Shon, S., & Ja, D. Y. (1982). Asian families. In M. McGoldrick, J. K. Pearce, & J. Giordano (Eds.), *Ethnicity and family therapy* (pp. 208–228). New York: Guilford Press.

Shorter-Gooden, K. (1996). The Simpson trial: Lessons for mental health practitioners. *Cultural Diversity and Mental Health, 2,* 65–68.

Smith, M., & Mendoza, R. (1996). Ethnicity and psychopharmacogenetics. *Mt. Sinai Journal of Medicine, 63,* 285–290.

Stewart, E. C. (1981). Cultural sensitivities in counseling. In P. B. Pedersen, J. G. Draguns, W. J. Lonner, & J. E. Trimble (Eds.), *Counseling across cultures* (pp. 61–68). Honolulu: University Press of Hawaii.

Strickland, T. L., Ranganeth, V., & Lin, K.-M. (1991). Psychopharmacologic considerations in the treatment of Black American populations. *Psychopharmacology Bulletin, 27,* 441–448.

Suchman, A. L., Markakis, K., Beckman, H. B., & Frankel, R. (1997, February 26). A model of empathic communication in the medical interview. *Journal of the American Medical Association, 277,* 678–682.

Sue, D. W., Bingham, R. P., Porche-Burke, L., & Vasquez, M. (1999). The diversification of psychology: A multicultural revolution. *American Psychologist, 54,* 1061–1069.

Sue, S. (1998). In search of cultural competence in psychotherapy and counseling. *American Psychologist, 53,* 440–448.

Sue, S., & Zane, N. (1987). The role of culture and cultural techniques in psychotherapy: A critique and reformulation. *American Psychologist, 55,* 37–45.

Tamura, T., & Lau, A. (1992). Connectedness versus separateness: Applicability of family therapy to Japanese families. *Family Process, 31,* 319–340.

Thomas, M. B., & Dansby, P. G. (1985). Black clients: Family structures, therapeutic issues, and strengths. *Psychotherapy, 22*(Suppl.), 398–407.

Torrey, E. F. (1986). *With doctors and psychiatrists: The common roots of psychotherapy and its future*. New York: Harper & Row.

Triandis, H. (1995). *Individualism and collectivism*. Boulder, CO: Westview Press.

Trimble, J. E., Fleming, C. M., Beauvais, F., & Jumper-Thurman, P. (1996). Essential cultural and social strategies for counseling Native American Indians. In P. B. Pedersen, G. G. Draguns, P. B. Lonner, & J. E. Trimble (Eds.), *Counseling across cultures* (4th ed., pp. 177–209). Thousand Oaks, CA: Sage.

Varma, V. K. (1988). Culture personality and psychotherapy. *International Journal of Social Psychiatry, 43*, 142–149.

Vasquez, M. (1994). Latinas. In L. Comas-Díaz & B. Greene (Eds.), *Women of color: Integrating ethnic and gender identities in psychotherapy* (pp. 114–138). New York: Guilford Press.

Westermeyer, J., Williams, C. L., & Nguyen, A. N. (Eds.). (1991). *Mental health services for refugees* (DHHS Publication No. ADM 91–1824).Washington, DC: U.S. Government Printing Office.

Worell, J., & Remer, P. (2003). *Feminist perspectives in therapy* (2nd ed.). New York: Wiley.

Yi, K. (1995). Psychoanalytic psychotherapy with Asian clients: Transference and therapeutic considerations. *Psychotherapy, 32*, 308–316.

Zane, N., Hall, G. C. N., Sue, S., Young, K., & Nunez, J. (2004). Research on psychotherapy with culturally diverse populations. In M. J. Lambert (Ed.), *Handbook of psychotherapy and behavior change* (5th ed., pp. 767–804). New York: Wiley.

EDITORS' COMMENTS

Part I introduced both large systems and solo or small-practice clinically based contexts for evidence-based practice (EBP). Contributors challenged the restrictive aspects of EBP but supported a framework of EBP rooted in the findings of science and necessities of practice. Implicit across these chapters has been respect for a broad range of useful research and theory; for the autonomy and expertise of well-trained clinicians; and for the individuality, culture, preferences, and characteristics of clients. There were repeated themes, such as the look and feel of daily EBP considerations with clients, the overall efficacy of psychotherapy, the importance of starting with the patient rather than the disorder, the predominance of common factors and the therapeutic relationship as the prism through which interventions are integrated and applied, and the implementation of outcomes measurement as the wave of the future.

In Part II, contributors present the fruits of their research and that of others as it applies to the scientific knowledge base of EBP and clinical care. These areas include treatments, effects of treatments, evaluation of treatments, and extension of treatments into practice settings. Most of the clinical research contributors also do clinical work, and it shows in their sensitivity to clinical implications and practices. They share the themes of the overall efficacy of psychotherapy and an emphasis on outcomes measurement with the practice section authors, as well as some of the reservations about the restrictive elements of the EBP movement that have been misapplied. Most do not share an emphasis on common factors and the therapeutic relationship. The research section also spans large issues beyond treatments, from the proposal that patient-oriented research provides a way to bridge the distance between research and practice, to the idea that the methods (as differentiated from the results) of randomized controlled trials (RCTs) are not generalizable to practice, to the possibilities for researcher–clinician collaboration to improve clinical care. Differences in the fundamental purposes of research and practice are discussed in both Parts I and II. These distinctions are helpful to keep in mind as the reader transitions between perspectives.

II

THE RESEARCH
PERSPECTIVE

5

RESEARCH FINDINGS ON THE EFFECTS OF PSYCHOTHERAPY AND THEIR IMPLICATIONS FOR PRACTICE

MICHAEL J. LAMBERT AND ANDREA ARCHER

The findings of empirical research on the effects of treatment, by definition, do not necessarily respect the intuitive conceptions of clinicians, the pursuit of standardized treatments, or the economic goals of managed care companies. Instead, they form a matrix of data that is as likely to challenge as to support the assumptions of various perspectives on psychotherapy. It is therefore prudent to allow professional conclusions and rules to remain as dynamic as the data as they become accepted principles in the field of psychotherapy. Studies from the last decade show trends that are at times counterintuitive regarding principles of efficacy in psychotherapy outcomes. For example, historically psychologists have sought scientific legitimacy by imitating the field of medicine, leading to a search for specific treatments for specific diagnoses. Instead, the field of psychology is achieving scientific legitimacy through a proliferation of empirical data showing that psychotherapy is generally efficacious for a broad range of psychopathology, regardless of the therapeutic approach of the clinician.

Because the number of interventions that are applied in a variety of contexts (e.g., medical, internet, educational) with patients who have diverse problems continues to grow, as does the number of researchers and journals showing interest in studying treatment efficacy, a discussion of all studies and reviews in the area of behavior change is not possible. We limited our study population of interest mainly to adult outpatients in individual therapy as we considered an integration and comparison of results on issues of central importance to the effectiveness of all therapies. In this chapter, we review the status of empirically supported evidence on the effectiveness of psychotherapy, assessing the results of specific studies and the implications of these studies for the practice, further research, and funding of psychotherapy. We address the following important questions: Is psychotherapy effective? Do clients make clinically meaningful changes? Does therapy show greater benefits than placebo? Do clients maintain their gains? How many sessions of therapy are necessary? and Do some clients deteriorate during or following therapy?

EFFICACY OF PSYCHOTHERAPY

Overall, psychotherapy is efficacious. Hundreds of studies, both qualitative and quantitative, have now been conducted on the effects of psychotherapy, including research on psychodynamic, humanistic, behavioral, and cognitive approaches and variations and combinations of these approaches. Reviews of this research have shown that about 75% of clients who enter treatment show some benefit (Lambert & Ogles, 2004). This finding generalizes across a wide range of disorders, with the exception of severe biologically based disturbances, such as bipolar disorder and the schizophrenias, in which the impact of psychological treatments is secondary to psychoactive medications.

Quantitative reviews (meta-analyses) of psychotherapy efficacy support these conclusions and provide a numerical index for treatment effects. Early applications of meta-analysis to psychotherapy efficacy (e.g., Smith, Glass, & Miller, 1980) addressed the broad question of the extent of benefit associated with psychotherapy. For example, an average effect size of 0.85 standard deviation units was found over 475 studies comparing treated and untreated groups. This finding indicates that at the end of treatment, the average person was better off than 80% of the untreated control sample. A second round of meta-analytic findings (e.g., Shapiro & Shapiro, 1982) supported the consistent benefit of treatment over control. More recent analyses (e.g., Lipsey & Wilson, 1993; Shadish et al., 1997) also reported the broad finding of therapy benefit across a range of treatments for a variety of disorders. Variability is found within disorders, such that some disorders (e.g., phobias, panic disorder) yield to treatment more easily than others (e.g., obsessive–compulsive disorder), and some require longer and more intense interventions.

COMPARATIVE OUTCOMES

Whether or not there are uniquely effective psychotherapies is a salient question in the minds of many researchers. More narrow analyses that have focused on specific treatments and specific disorders have attempted to illuminate comparative effects. When all available meta-analytic reviews comparing different psychotherapies were collected, these studies usually showed little difference between treatments (Lambert & Ogles, 2004). For example, meta-analyses focused on behavioral, cognitive–behavioral, and general verbal therapies supported the finding that a range of therapeutic interventions resulted in improvement in mood and other symptoms for patients with depression.

An extensive meta-analysis comparing treatments is representative of findings from contemporary meta-analytic reviews (Wampold et al., 1997). This review examined studies that directly compared two or more treatments, eliminating the potential confounds associated with comparing treatments administered in different (i.e., across) studies (Shadish & Sweeney, 1991). The authors did not divide treatments into general types or categories, and they included only "bona fide" treatments—that is, studies in which the treatments were delivered "by trained therapists and were based on psychological principles, were offered to the psychotherapy community as viable treatments . . . , or contained specified components" (Wampold et al., 1997, p. 205). Thus, they excluded studies in which a viable treatment was compared with an alternative therapy that was "credible to participants in the study but not intended to be therapeutic" (p. 205).

To test whether one treatment was superior to another, Wampold et al. (1997) randomly gave effect sizes calculated comparing two treatments a positive or negative sign. They then tested the distribution of effects to see whether variability in effects was homogeneously centered on 0. Using several databases with different numbers of effect sizes, "none of the databases yielded effects that vaguely approached the heterogeneity expected if there were true differences among bona fide psychotherapies" (p. 205). Further analyses also indicated that more sophisticated methods associated with more recent studies were not related to increased differences between treatments, and theoretically dissimilar treatments did not produce larger effect sizes. Both of these findings provide evidence for the substantial equivalence of bona fide treatments.

In addition to studies comparing various orientations or methods of treatment, some studies examined the comparative benefit of differing modes of therapy (e.g., family vs. individual treatment). Some of the earliest meta-analyses compared the various modalities of therapy using between-group comparisons (Robinson, Berman, & Neimeyer, 1990; Smith et al., 1980). The potential confounding variables of between-study comparisons, however, led to several meta-analyses that eliminated this confound. Although the number of studies was typically small and the detailed results varied somewhat, these studies generally found no difference between group and individual therapy (McRoberts, Burlingame, & Hoag, 1998; Tillitski, 1990) or between marital or family therapies and individual therapy (Shadish et al., 1993).

The foregoing meta-analyses examining the comparative effectiveness of differing theories or modes of psychotherapy reveal a mixed picture. A strong trend toward no differences between techniques or modes in amount of change produced is counterbalanced by indications that under some limited circumstances, certain methods (e.g., applying behavioral techniques that rely on systematic exposure to fear-provoking situations with anxiety-based disorders) proved to be superior (Emmelkamp, 2004). The potential confounds of cross-study comparisons, differences in measurement and samples, and investigator allegiance complicate the process of making general conclusions. An examination of selected exemplary studies allowed us to explore this matter further. But even this research, carried out with the intent of contrasting two or more bona fide treatments, shows surprisingly small differences between the outcomes for patients who underwent a treatment that was fully intended to be therapeutic.

Similar results have been found in comparative studies that examined the effects of medication and psychotherapy. Two early meta-analyses supported the notion that psychotherapy is at a minimum equivalent to antidepressant medication (Robinson et al., 1990; Steinbrueck, Maxwell, & Howard, 1983). A third early meta-analysis suggested that antidepressant medications surpass psychotherapy only in the treatment of endogenous depression (Andrews, 1983). This finding was supported by the National Institute of Mental Health (NIMH) Treatment for Depression Collaborative Research Program (TDCRP) data (Elkin, 1994), which showed that medication (in this case, imipramine) surpassed psychotherapy only for more severe cases of depression.

Therapy plus medication was found to be more effective than therapy alone (Thase & Jindal, 2004), but other comparisons (e.g., Gloaguen, Cottraux, Cucherat, & Blackburn, 1998) found that cognitive–behavioral therapy (CBT) was more effective than medication alone (newer antidepressant medications may have been underrepresented in Gloaguen et al.'s study).

The consistent finding that the benefits of psychotherapy are equal to or surpass a variety of antidepressant medications is of great interest to practicing clinicians. The medical community has long considered antidepressant medication to be the treatment of choice for depression. With the advent of the selective serotonin reuptake inhibitors, such as fluoxetine and other newer drugs, medication for depression as the first line of treatment has been emphasized even more heavily. Indeed, the Agency for Health Care Policy and Research guidelines for the treatment of depression in primary care settings suggest medication as the first line of treatment (Munoz et al., 1994). However, for the most part, psychological interventions have been found to be equal to or to surpass the effects of medication for psychological disorders and should be offered before medications (except with the most severely disturbed patients) because they are less dangerous and less intrusive, or at the very least they should be offered in addition to medications, because they reduce the likelihood of relapse once medications are withdrawn (Elkin, 1994; Thase & Jindal, 2004). Findings that psychotherapies produce comparable or superior effects to medications are an important contribution of psychotherapy research.

Of course, one should never rely on a single study of psychotherapy, or even a single meta-analysis of psychotherapy, to draw firm conclusions about efficacy. For example, Sharpe (1997) described three notable criticisms of meta-analyses: (a) they mix dissimilar studies, (b) publication bias cannot be ruled out, and (c) they may also include poor-quality studies. Many meta-analysis reviewers have addressed these potential problems in one or more of four ways:

- by focusing on a narrow group of studies that investigate a specific treatment or a particular disorder (addressing the dissimilarity criticism),
- by testing effect size homogeneity to empirically investigate the similarity of the study results and to search for moderators when sufficient variability exists within the data,
- by calculating a "failsafe N" or including both published and unpublished studies (to address the publication bias), and
- by examining the methodological integrity of the studies in relation to effect sizes.

Standard criticisms must therefore be tempered by recent improvements in meta-analytic methodology.

Although research in the past 15 years has placed great emphasis on comparative outcome studies as a means of identifying causative mechanisms of patient improvement, a great deal of evidence suggests that factors common to many psychotherapies are highly important in determining patient outcome. Unlike interventions such as surgery and medication, where best practices are more likely to be specific and technical, psychological health depends far more on a human encounter in which the clinician's understanding attitude, warmth, acceptance, and respect play a significant role. Research evidence is clear in implicating the therapist and therapist attitudes as significantly related, important determinants of psychotherapy outcome (Norcross, 2002; Watson & Geller, 2005).

Regardless of the weight that can be accorded to the causes of client improvement, the consistent finding across thousands of studies and hundreds of meta-analyses leaves no room for debate—psychotherapy is beneficial. Having established this foundation, researchers have turned to other important questions, such as the clinical significance of the changes that occur.

CLINICALLY MEANINGFUL CHANGE

The outcomes of psychotherapy are substantial. Those who have studied psychotherapy have been rigorous in defining and measuring important factors of individual functioning. In a survey of outcome practices, Froyd, Lambert, and Froyd (1996) reviewed articles from 20 scientific journals published over a 5-year period. They found that measures of outcomes included patient reports; physiological changes; expert judge ratings; ratings by family members, friends, and coworkers; and employment, medical, and legal status (e.g., arrest, incarceration). These rating sources tapped a variety of areas of functioning, mainly psychiatric symptoms (e.g., anxiety, depression, anger, stress), interpersonal functioning (e.g., family conflict, loneliness, intimacy), and social role performance (e.g., conflict at work, absenteeism, employment status). These factors are of considerable importance to the patient, the family, and society at large. In addition, much recent effort has been expended to define what a "normal" state of functioning is and how to assess the degree to which patients have attained this state at the end of treatment. In current parlance, changes of this substantial kind are referred to as being clinically significant (Jacobson & Traux, 1991).

Clinical significance takes a somewhat narrow view of meaningful change by identifying methods defined by clinician–researchers (Ogles, Lunnen, & Bonesteel, 2001). The two most prominent definitions of clinically significant change are (a) treated clients make statistically reliable improvements as a result of treatment (Jacobson, Roberts, Berns, & McGlinchey, 1999) and (b) treated clients are empirically indistinguishable from normal or nondeviant peers following treatment recovery (Kendall, Marrs-Garcia, Nath, & Sheldrick, 1999). The question is, What do researchers find when they use these methods to evaluate the clinical importance of client change occurring during psychotherapy? Do clients make changes that are clinically meaningful? Several examples of typical findings provide initial evidence of the clinical benefits of therapy.

In a large-scale, comprehensive meta-analysis, Lipsey and Wilson (1993) addressed the issue of practical versus statistical effects of treatment. They suggested that "the practical significance of an effect, of course, is very much dependent on the nature of the outcome at issue and its importance to patients or clients" (p. 1198). They illustrated this point by presenting the effect sizes for a variety of medical interventions, some of which have small effects but serious ramifications in life-and-death situations. Obviously, small effects in critical situations can be extremely important, especially in the context of examining the health of large populations. Although the nature of outcomes resulting from therapy is highly variable, effect sizes generally exceed or equal many medical interventions.

Two early meta-analytic studies addressed the issue of clinically meaningful change by examining the pre- and posttreatment scores of clients on specific measures of outcome (Nietzel, Russell, Hemmings, & Gretter, 1987; Trull, Nietzel, & Main, 1988). In both studies, clients moved within 1.0 standard deviation of the normative mean, suggesting that many individuals receiving treatment might be considered meaningfully improved. A more recent meta-analysis examined the clinical significance of treatment for obsessive–compulsive disorder (Abramowitz, 1996). The average patient with the disorder started 2.0 standard deviations away from the general population mean but moved to 0.7 standard deviations away from the general population mean and below the cutoff (1.0 standard deviation) following treatment, suggesting that treated patients made clinically meaningful changes, although many had some remaining symptoms.

Not only are psychological interventions producing outcomes that are statistically superior to control conditions but many clients also are shown to improve to levels that are clinically meaningful in both primary studies and meta-analytic reviews. The study of clinical significance will remain a promising field for investigation in the years to come. Especially in this age of accountability, the ability of behavioral health professionals to demonstrate that their interventions are not merely statistically significant is a critical task. The establishment of clinical relevance has helped to verify that psychosocial interventions are meaningful not only to clients and therapists but to society as a whole.

SUPPORT SYSTEMS AND PLACEBO COMPARISON

The effects of psychotherapy are more substantial than those of informal support systems and placebo controls. In medical research, the effects of an active pharmacological agent are tested against the effects of a *placebo*, or pharmacologically inert or nontherapeutic substance. With psychological mechanisms, defining and using a placebo is more complex and has taken on a variety of meanings. For example, Rosenthal and Frank (1956) defined a placebo as being theoretically inert. As Critelli and Neumann (1984) pointed out, "Virtually every currently established psychotherapy would be considered inert, and therefore a placebo, from the viewpoint of other established theories of cure" (p. 33). Others have suggested that placebo effects in psychological treatments should most appropriately be labeled "nonspecific" factors (e.g., Oei & Shuttlewood, 1996). This conceptualization, however, becomes problematic when *nonspecific* includes factors like "therapist warmth," which studies have shown to be a specific and substantial factor in client change (see Herbert & Gaudiano, 2005, for similar discussions).

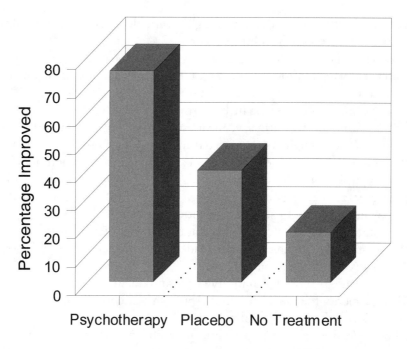

Figure 5.1. Estimates of percentages of patients improving as a function of treatment condition based on meta-analytic literature reviews.

Others have suggested the term *common factors* for referring to elements of therapy that are not unique (such as the expectation for improvement, persuasion, warmth, attention, feedback, exposure, understanding, encouragement, a confidential relationship, and the like). Research on placebo effects is more functionally conceptualized as research on common factors versus the specific effects of a particular technique. Such common factors should not be viewed as theoretically inert or as trivial. Indeed, these factors are central to psychological interventions in both theory and practice because they play an active role in patient improvement (cf. Critelli & Neumann, 1984; Parloff, 1986).

Figure 5.1 provides an illustration drawn from numerous studies and reviews of the literature in which researchers designed experiments that randomly assigned patients to a no-treatment control group, a placebo control group, or a psychotherapy treatment group (Lambert, 2005). These experimental designs allowed researchers to narrow down the causes of improvement while isolating and ruling out competing factors that might have accounted for improvements that were observed. As evident in the figure, patients who did not get psychotherapy improved, probably as a result of homeostatic mechanisms such as support from friends, family, clergy, and the like. Patients who entered a placebo control group fared even better than untreated patients, probably as a result of contact with a therapist, the expectation that they would be helped, and the reassurance and support they received during the study. In contrast, patients who entered psychotherapy had the best outcomes, suggesting that the active ingredients of bona fide treatments contain additional elements that facilitate improvements.

MAINTENANCE

The outcomes of therapy tend to be maintained. Many recent outcomes research and meta-analytic reviews considered the maintenance of treatment gains, rather than simply the immediate posttreatment status of patients. Results show that many patients who underwent therapy, including those with a long history of recurrent problems, achieved healthy adjustment for long periods of time. At the same time, substantial evidence shows that a portion of patients who had improved at termination relapsed and continued to seek help from a variety of mental health providers, including their former therapists. Several problems, such as alcohol and drug dependence, smoking, obesity, and possibly depression, are so likely to recur that they are not considered properly studied without data collection at least 1 year after treatment.

Numerous follow-up studies have tracked patients after they left treatment for periods ranging from 6 months to over 5 years. These studies are fairly consistent in demonstrating that treatment effects are enduring. For example, reviews of depression (Nicholson & Berman, 1983; Robinson et al., 1990), social phobia (Feske & Chambless, 1995), substance abuse (Stanton & Shadish, 1997), agoraphobia and panic disorder (Bakker, van Balkom, Spinhoven, Blaauw, & van Dyck, 1998), pain (Flor, Fydrich, & Turk, 1992), generalized anxiety disorder (Gould, Otto, Pollack, & Yap, 1997), and many other disorders (Carlson & Hoyle, 1993; Murtagh & Greenwood, 1995; Sherman, 1998; Taylor, 1996) all demonstrated maintenance of gains, on average, for at least 1 year after treatment.

In the earliest and most influential meta-analysis to determine whether follow-up is necessary in evaluating psychotherapy, Nicholson and Berman (1983) concluded that posttherapy status correlated with follow-up status, and differences between treatments apparent at the end of therapy were virtually the same at follow-up. Many of the meta-analyses conducted in the past decade have also considered the outcome of treatment at both the end of treatment and at a follow-up assessment. For example, an analysis of 21 studies of cognitive–behavioral and exposure-only treatment for social phobia showed that both treatments produced significant pre- to posttreatment gains that were maintained at follow-up 1 to 12 months later (Feske & Chambless, 1995; see also Stanton & Shadish, 1997).

Other findings show a remarkable endurance of treatment benefits for agoraphobia, including continuing gains between the end of treatment and follow-up (Bakker et al., 1998). Despite these positive findings, two methodological problems limit conclusions: Attrition between the end of treatment and follow-up data collection is a significant problem in many studies, and follow-up findings are "naturalistic" in most cases because most studies do not continue to follow control groups after treatment ends (Bakker et al., 1998). Given these limitations, greater selection in the application of follow-up designs is recommended. For example, continuing use of follow-up studies on depression outcomes is recommended, but only if the length of the follow-up is extended to at least 1 year. Short-term follow-up studies are no longer needed to establish the durability of effects, unless such studies help identify risk factors for relapse or patterns of deterioration.

Many high-quality studies have followed clients for several years after treatment. In these studies, researchers generally found that treatment effects were maintained for clients who continued to participate in data collection. Demonstrating that treatments are beneficial for long periods of time, identifying clients who are at risk of relapse, and developing methods of improving treatments that have acute benefits will be important future projects. Presently, it appears that treatment does offer a long-term benefit for many clients. Definitive conclusions are difficult because of the many methodological difficulties of longitudinal research with therapy participants (e.g., dropout, uncontrolled designs, clients seeking extrastudy treatment). Thus, the maintenance of treatment gains remains a rich, yet difficult, area of study.

Efficiency of Psychotherapy

Psychotherapy is relatively efficient. Researchers of psychotherapy have examined the speed with which patients improve over the course of treatment using numerous research designs. Treatment efficiency has important practical as well as social policy implications, with the number of sessions needed for improvement being front and center in the management of mental health services. Historically, the issue of treatment length was associated with psychoanalysis and its derivatives, especially in contrast with planned, brief psychotherapies. Howard, Kopta, Krause, and Orlinsky (1986) were the first to address the question of treatment length with a medication metaphor—the "dose–response" statistic—that examined the relationship of amount of therapy to patient improvement. They concluded that the relationship between the number of sessions and client improvement took a form similar to that evidenced by many medications, a positive relationship characterized by a negatively accelerated curve; the more psychotherapy, the greater the probability of improvement, with diminishing returns at higher doses. Their analysis of the data indicated that 14% of clients improved before attending the initial session, 53% improved following 8 weekly sessions, 75% by 26 sessions, and 83% by 52 sessions.

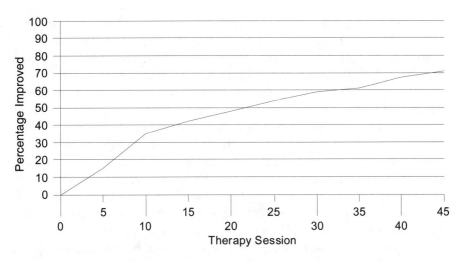

Figure 5.2. The relationship of number of sessions of psychotherapy with improvement in symptoms, interpersonal problems, and social role functioning. From "Patient-Focused Research: Using Patient Outcome Data to Enhance Treatment Effects," by M. J. Lambert, N. B. Hansen, and A. E. Finch, 2001, *Journal of Consulting and Clinical Psychology, 69,* p. 164. Copyright 2001 by the American Psychological Association.

It is unfortunate that their study was limited by reliance on pre–post estimates of patient improvement rather than session-by-session ratings of improvement. Reliance on pre–post ratings makes it difficult to identify the exact time to recovery for individual patients. More recently, Anderson and Lambert (2001) and Hansen and Lambert (2003) collected data from large samples of patients undergoing treatment in routine care who rated their symptoms, interpersonal relations, social role performance, and quality of life on a weekly basis before each treatment session. Thus, patient outcome was assessed from the beginning of treatment until it was completed or they withdrew. These authors studied clients' progress over time and used statistical methods to model the number of sessions needed for patients to return to a normal state of functioning (i.e., to have no more symptoms than people in the general population). Figure 5.2 presents the percentage of outpatients who recovered after each session of treatment. As can be seen, about one third of patients recovered by the 10th session, 50% by the 20th session, and 75% by the 55th session.

Current research in this area suggests that earlier reviews (e.g., Howard et al., 1986) overestimated the speed of recovery and the relationship between initial levels of distress and time to recovery, with more disturbed patients reaching criteria for recovery at a slower rate. Using a lesser standard of improvement (reliable change) and including patients who began treatment in the functional range, an estimated 50% of patients were expected to improve following 7 sessions of treatment, with 75% improving following 14 sessions of psychotherapy (Anderson & Lambert, 2001).

It also appears that rates of improvement vary as a function of the targets of treatment. For example, different sets of interpersonal problems (i.e., control, detachment, and self-effacing) were found to respond differently over the course of treatment (Maling, Gurtman, & Howard, 1995) "and in a manner inverse to their apparent salience in patients" (p. 71). Control problems responded rapidly to treatment, with nearly 50% of the clients improving in the first 10 sessions and a steady monotonic rate of change following a clear inflection point at Session 10. Problems of social detachment improved at a slower rate (30% improved in the first 17 sessions), with a clear inflection point at Session 17 and a steady rate of change thereafter increasing to approximately 55% after 38 sessions. Items tapping the self-effacing problems were unresponsive to therapy. By Session 4, about 25% of the patients had improved, but beyond that little improvement was observable.

In a similar way, some classes of symptoms have been found to respond more quickly than others in depressed clients involved in psychodynamic–interpersonal or CBT treatment, and "change occurred more rapidly when tighter time limits were imposed" (Barkham et al., 1996, p. 933). In addition, the relationship between rapid early response to treatment and maintenance of treatment gains at follow-up have been evaluated, with results suggesting that early (i.e., within the first three sessions) extreme positive response to psychotherapy predicted final treatment status as well as follow-up status (Haas, Hill, Lambert, & Morrell, 2002). About 80% of the patients who made clinically significant gains were rapid responders. Haas et al. suggested that this finding argued against the idea that early treatment response was merely a placebo effect. Many patients who respond to therapy make gains early on, and these gains precede rather than follow the specific techniques deemed to be essential by most theories of psychotherapeutic intervention. These findings also underscore the general findings on the dose–response relationship and phase model of psychotherapy—more improvement comes from earlier rather than later treatment sessions.

Research on the efficiency of psychotherapy can help therapists and patients make reasonable decisions for treatment planning. It can inform policy decisions about the amount of services that are necessary for sufficient medical coverage. It also allows for theory-driven exploration of variables that modify dosage models. Significant progress has been made in this area over the past decade and a half. Research suggests that a sizable portion of patients reliably improve after 10 sessions and that 75% of patients will meet more rigorous criteria for success after about 50 sessions of treatment. Limiting treatment sessions to fewer than 20 will mean that about 50% of patients will not achieve a substantial benefit from therapy (as measured by standard self-report scales). Aspects of patient functioning show differential responses to treatment, with more characterological and interpersonal aspects of functioning responding more slowly than psychological symptoms. Future research may illuminate which, if any, specific interventions are more efficient in producing patient change. At this point in time, it appears that most patients are being underserved by current session limits. Managed care, if it is interested in quality care, should do more to encourage greater, not less, utilization of psychotherapy services.

PSYCHOTHERAPY: FOR BETTER AND FOR WORSE

Despite the overall positive findings, a portion of patients who enter treatment are worse off when they leave treatment than when they entered. Estimates show that about 5% to 10% of patients deteriorate during treatment, and an additional 15% to 25% show no measured benefit (Lambert & Ogles, 2004; Mohr, 1995). This does not mean that all instances of worsening are the product of therapy. Some cases may be on a progressive decline that no therapist effort can stop. The extent or rate of negative change or of "spontaneous" deterioration in untreated groups has never been determined, so no baseline exists from which to judge deterioration rates observed in treated groups. The alternative is to observe negative change in experiments using treated versus control conditions and in studies of specific connections between therapy processes and patient responses.

It appears that negative outcomes can be observed across a variety of treatment modalities, including group and family therapies, as well as across theoretical orientations. Studies that use control groups usually show that deterioration is lower in control groups than in treated samples. For example, a reanalysis of the NIMH TDCRP data showed that 8% of the clients in the completer sample (the 162 clients who completed at least 12 sessions and 15 weeks of treatment) deteriorated as measured with the Hamilton Rating Scale for Depression (Ogles, Lambert, & Sawyer, 1995). None of the clients who deteriorated participated in the placebo plus clinical management control group. It is worth noting that clinical trials such as the NIMH study pay considerable attention to selecting, training, and monitoring therapists for both conformity and competence in treatment delivery. Even higher rates of negative outcome may be expected in routine care, where less outside attention is focused on therapist performance, dosages of treatment are substantially less, and clients who are being treated cannot be carefully selected and often have substantial comorbidity. As disheartening as it is to know that psychotherapy may be harmful for a small portion of patients and impotent for many others, it also points to the need for quality assurance mechanisms that reduce these occurrences to their lowest possible levels.

REDUCING NEGATIVE OUTCOMES

Among the most promising methods for reducing patient deterioration is one based on so-called patient-focused research. This research paradigm endeavors to improve psychotherapy outcomes by monitoring patient progress and providing this information to clinicians to guide ongoing treatment, especially for patients who are not having a favorable response to treatment. Patient-focused research is an extension of quality assurance and represents one effort to bridge the gap between research and practice and to enhance patient outcomes before treatment termination. It is also well suited to models of care in which clinicians attempt to step up or step down the intensity of treatments after assessing a patient's treatment response (Otto, Pollack, & Maki, 2000).

Four large-scale studies aimed at evaluating the effects of providing research-based feedback on patient progress have been conducted in the United States (Hawkins, Lambert, Vermeersch, Slade, & Tuttle, 2004; Lambert et al., 2001, 2002; Whipple et al., 2003). Each of the studies required about 1 year of data collection and evaluated the effects of providing therapists (and sometimes patients) with feedback about patients' improvement using progress graphs and warnings for patients who were not demonstrating expected treatment responses (called signal-alarm cases).

The primary question was, Does formal feedback to therapists (or patients) on patient progress improve psychotherapy outcomes? It was hypothesized that patients identified as signal-alarm cases (those predicted to have a poor final treatment response) whose therapists received feedback would show better outcomes than similar patients whose therapists did not receive feedback. The results from the four studies were combined to provide the best estimate of the consequences of providing signal-alarm feedback to psychotherapists and are presented graphically in Figure 5.3. The patients identified as signal-alarm cases had a different outcome course depending on assignment to the feedback or no feedback treatment conditions. Up to the point that these signal-alarm cases were first signaled (or in the case of the no feedback cases, treatment as usual condition could have been signaled), the graph illustrates an average worsening of around 10 points (about 0.5 standard deviation on the Outcome Questionnaire—45; Lambert et al., 2004). From the point of the signal alarm, all the experimental (feedback) groups improved, whereas the control (no feedback) cases improved to an average score near 80 but were, as a group, slightly worse off than when they entered treatment.

In the individual studies themselves, the effect sizes (standardized mean differences) for the difference between signal-alarm patients receiving feedback and treatment as usual control participants ranged from .34 to .92. Such effect sizes are surprisingly large when one considers that an average effect for empirically supported therapy and comparison treatments is usually somewhere between .00 and .20 (Lambert & Ogles, 2004; Wampold et al., 1997). Given the large sample sizes of the individual studies in this summary and the combined overall sample size of over 2,500, the findings seem compelling.

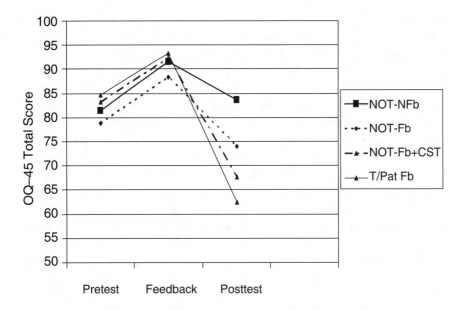

Figure 5.3. Comparison of change in Outcome Questionnaire—45 (OQ–45) scores over time in patients identified as signal-alarm cases whose therapist did not receive feedback (NOT-NFb), did receive feedback (NOT-Fb), or received feedback and used clinical support tools (NOT-Fb+CST) or for whom both therapist and patient received feedback (T/Pat Fb). Higher scores reflect more severe distress. Several acronyms are used to identify the treatment conditions. Patients not progressing as expected (signal-alarm cases) are termed *not on track* (NOT). Patients who progressed as expected during treatment are referred to as *on-track* (OT). If feedback was provided to therapists, *Fb* is used; *No-Fb* is used for patient groups when therapists did not receive feedback. NOT groups are further subdivided depending on whether therapists used clinical support tools (NOT-Fb+CST), and when therapists and patients received feedback (T/Pat Fb).

Early recognition of potential treatment failure (signal-alarm cases) may provide therapists with an indication that they need to re-examine the way they are proceeding. It seems likely that therapists become more attentive to such patients when they receive a signal that the patient is not progressing. Evidence across studies suggests that therapists tend to keep patients who are not on track in treatment for more sessions when they get feedback, further reinforcing the notion that feedback increases interest and investment in a patient.

CONCLUSION

The results of psychotherapy research with adults consistently show that psychotherapy, in its many variations, is highly effective and personally meaningful. About 75% of patients who undergo a course of treatment show some positive benefit, with 40% to 60% returning to a normal state of functioning. The benefits derived from psychotherapy depend largely on patient pretherapy characteristics such as degree of initial disturbance and diagnosis. These benefits also appear to be largely due to factors that are common across a variety of interventions.

Psychotherapy can be efficient, especially for patients who are not severely disturbed. Research on the amount of psychotherapy needed to return a patient to a state of normal functioning suggests that 50% of patients will improve to this degree after 20 sessions of treatment and that about 75% of patients will need at least 50 sessions. Rapid, dramatic treatment response foretells final positive outcomes, despite the fact that this response may occur before theoretically proposed mechanisms of change have been fully implemented. The effects of psychotherapy are often sustained for long periods of time following treatment.

Despite these positive evaluations, it is also true that therapists have a long way to go in assuring the value of treatment for all who participate. Not only is there no measured benefit from treatment in a sizable minority of patients but a negative outcome is found in some (around 8%). Research aimed at improving outcomes for these patients suggests that identifying negatively responding patients before they leave treatment can substantially increase the likelihood of success. It is unfortunate that monitoring patient treatment response in comparison with expected treatment response is seldom mentioned or applied for the purpose of enhancing treatment response and reducing treatment failure or nonresponse. Future research that examines the real-time treatment response of patients in routine care promises to make considerable contributions to the welfare of persons with psychological disorders.

Over the past 75 years, psychotherapy research has consistently supported the value of psychotherapy for reducing symptomatic disturbance and returning patients to states of healthy functioning. Psychotherapy research has helped to soften the claims of those who overstate its benefits and those who mislead the public with sham interventions. Such research has become more and more sophisticated in its methodology and analytic tools and more likely than ever to affect clinical practices.

REFERENCES

Abramowitz, J. S. (1996). Variants of exposure and response prevention in the treatment of obsessive–compulsive disorder: A meta-analysis. *Behavior Therapy, 27*, 583–600.

Anderson, E., & Lambert, M. (2001). A survival analysis of clinically significant change in outpatient psychotherapy. *Journal of Clinical Psychology, 57*, 875–888.

Andrews, G. (1983). A treatment outline for depressive disorders: The Quality Assurance Project. *Australian and New Zealand Journal of Psychiatry, 17*, 129–146.

Bakker, A., van Balkom, A. J. L. M., Spinhoven, P., Blaauw, B. M. J. W., & van Dyck, R. (1998). Follow up on the treatment of panic disorder with or without agoraphobia. *The Journal of Nervous and Mental Disease, 186*, 414–419.

Barkham, M., Rees, A., Stiles, W. B., Shapiro, D. A., Hardy, G. E., & Reynolds, S. (1996). Dose effect relations in time limited psychotherapy for depression. *Journal of Consulting and Clinical Psychology, 64*, 927–935.

Carlson, C. R., & Hoyle, R. H. (1993). Efficacy of abbreviated progressive muscle relaxation training: A quantitative review of behavioral medicine research. *Journal of Consulting and Clinical Psychology, 61*, 1059–1067.

Critelli, J. W., & Neumann, K. F. (1984). The placebo: Conceptual analysis of a construct in transition. *American Psychologist, 39*, 32–39.

Elkin, I. (1994). The NIMH treatment of depression collaborative research program: Where we began and where we are. In A. E. Bergin & S. L. Garfield (Eds.), *Handbook of psychotherapy and behavior change* (4th ed., pp. 114–142). New York: Wiley.

Emmelkamp, P. M. G. (2004). Behavior therapy with adults. In M. J. Lambert (Ed.), *Bergin and Garfield's handbook of psychotherapy and behavior change* (5th ed., pp. 393–446). New York: Wiley.

Feske, U., & Chambless, D. L. (1995). Cognitive–behavioral versus exposure only treatment for social phobia: A meta-analysis. *Behavior Therapy, 26*, 695–720.

Flor, H., Fydrich, T., & Turk, D. C. (1992). Efficacy of multidisciplinary pain treatment centers: A meta-analytic review. *Pain, 49*, 221–230.

Froyd, J. E., Lambert, M. J., & Froyd, J. D. (1996). A review of practices of psychotherapy outcome measurement. *Journal of Mental Health, 5*, 11–15.

Gloaguen, V., Cottraux, J., Cucherat, M., & Blackburn, I.-M. (1998). A meta-analysis of the effects of cognitive therapy in depressed patients. *Journal of Affective Disorders, 49*, 59–72.

Gould, R. A., Otto, M. W., Pollack, M. H., & Yap, L. (1997). Cognitive–behavioral and pharmacological treatment of generalized anxiety disorder: A preliminary meta-analysis. *Behavior Therapy, 28*, 285–305.

Haas, E., Hill, R., Lambert, M. J., & Morrell, B. (2002). Do early responders to psychotherapy maintain treatment gains? *Journal of Clinical Psychology, 58*, 1157–1172.

Hansen, N. B., & Lambert, M. J. (2003). An evaluation of the dose–response relationship in naturalistic treatment settings using survival analysis. *Mental Health Services Research, 5*, 1–12.

Hawkins, E. J., Lambert, M. J., Vermeersch, D., Slade, K., & Tuttle, K. (2004). The effects of providing patient progress information to therapists and patients. *Psychotherapy Research, 31*, 308–327.

Herbert, J. D., & Gaudiano, B. A. (2005). Introduction to the special issue on the placebo concept in psychotherapy. *Journal of Clinical Psychology, 61*, 787–790.

Howard, K. I., Kopta, S. M., Krause, M. S., & Orlinsky, D. E. (1986). The dose–effect relationship in psychotherapy. *American Psychologist, 41,* 159–164.

Jacobson, N. S., Roberts, L. J., Berns, S. B., & McGlinchey, J. B. (1999). Methods for defining and determining the clinical significance of treatment effects: Description, application, and alternatives. *Journal of Consulting and Clinical Psychology, 67,* 300–307.

Jacobson, N. S., & Truax, P. (1991). Clinical significance: A statistical approach to defining meaningful change in psychotherapy research. *Journal of Consulting and Clinical Psychology, 59,* 12–19.

Kendall, P. C., Marrs-Garcia, A., Nath, S. R., & Sheldrick, R. C. (1999). Normative comparisons for the evaluation of clinical significance. *Journal of Consulting and Clinical Psychology, 67,* 285–299.

Lambert, M. J. (2005). Early response in psychotherapy: Further evidence for the importance of common factors rather than "placebo effects." *Journal of Clinical Psychology, 61,* 855–869.

Lambert, M. J., Hansen, N. B., & Finch, A. E. (2001). Patient-focused research: Using patient outcome data to enhance treatment effects. *Journal of Consulting and Clinical Psychology, 69,* 159–172.

Lambert, M. J., Morton, J. J., Hatfield, D., Harmon, S. C., Hamilton, S., Reid, R. C., et al. (2004). *Administration and scoring manual for the Outcome Questionnaire—45.* Orem, UT: American Professional Credentialing Services.

Lambert, M. J., & Ogles, B. M. (2004). The efficacy and effectiveness of psychotherapy. In M. J. Lambert (Ed.), *Bergin and Garfield's handbook of psychotherapy and behavior change* (5th ed., pp. 139–193). New York: Wiley.

Lambert, M. J., Whipple, J. L., Smart, D. W., Vermeersch, D. A., Nielsen, S. L., & Hawkins, E. J. (2001). The effects of providing therapists with feedback on patient progress during psychotherapy: Are outcomes enhanced? *Psychotherapy Research, 11,* 49–68.

Lambert, M. J., Whipple, J. L., Vermeersch, D. A., Smart, D. W., Hawkins, E. J., Nielsen, S. L., & Goates, M. K. (2002). Enhancing psychotherapy outcomes via providing feedback on patient progress: A replication. *Clinical Psychology and Psychotherapy, 9,* 91–103.

Lipsey, M. W., & Wilson, D. B. (1993). The efficacy of psychological, educational, and behavioral treatment: Confirmation from meta-analysis. *American Psychologist, 48,* 1181–1209.

Maling, M. S., Gurtman, M. B., & Howard, K. I. (1995). The response of interpersonal problems to varying doses of psychotherapy. *Psychotherapy Research, 5,* 63–75.

McRoberts, C. H., Burlingame, G. M., & Hoag, M. J. (1998). Comparative efficacy of individual and group psychotherapy: A meta-analytic perspective. *Group Dynamics: Theory, Research, and Practice, 59,* 101–111.

Mohr, D. C. (1995). Negative outcome in psychotherapy: A critical review. *Clinical Psychology: Science and Practice, 2,* 1–27.

Munoz, R. F., Hollon, S. D., McGrath, E., Rehm, L. P., & VandenBos, G. R. (1994). On the AHCPR Depression in Primary Care guidelines: Further considerations for practitioners. *American Psychologist, 49*, 42–61.

Murtagh, D. R. R., & Greenwood, K. M. (1995). Identifying effective psychological treatments for insomnia: A meta-analysis. *Journal of Consulting and Clinical Psychology, 63*, 79–89.

Nicholson, R. A., & Berman, J. S. (1983). Is follow up necessary in evaluating psychotherapy? *Psychological Bulletin, 93*, 261–278.

Nietzel, M. T., Russell, R. L., Hemmings, K. A., & Gretter, M. L. (1987). Clinical significance of psychotherapy for unipolar depression: A meta-analytic approach to social comparison. *Journal of Consulting and Clinical Psychology, 55*, 156–161.

Norcross, J. C. (Ed.). (2002). *Psychotherapy relationships that work*. New York: Oxford University Press.

Oei, T. P. S., & Shuttlewood, G. J. (1996). Specific and nonspecific factors in psychotherapy: A case of cognitive therapy for depression. *Clinical Psychology Review, 16*, 83–103.

Ogles, B. M., Lambert, M. J., & Sawyer, J. D. (1995). Clinical significance of the National Institute of Mental Health Treatment of Depression Collaborative Research Program data. *Journal of Consulting and Clinical Psychology, 63*, 321–326.

Ogles, B. M., Lunnen, K. M., & Bonesteel, K. (2001). Clinical significance: History, definitions and applications. *Clinical Psychology Review, 21*, 421–446.

Otto, M. W., Pollack, M. H., & Maki, K. M. (2000). Empirically supported treatments for panic disorder: Costs, benefits, and stepped care. *Journal of Consulting and Clinical Psychology, 68*, 556–563.

Parloff, M. R. (1986). Placebo controls in psychotherapy research: A sine qua non or a placebo for research problems? *Journal of Consulting and Clinical Psychology, 54*, 79–87.

Robinson, L. A., Berman, J. S., & Neimeyer, R. A. (1990). Psychotherapy for the treatment of depression: A comprehensive review of controlled outcome research. *Psychological Bulletin, 108*, 30–49.

Rosenthal, D., & Frank, J. D. (1956). Psychotherapy and the placebo effect. *Psychological Bulletin, 53*, 294–302.

Shadish, W. R., Matt, G. E., Navarro, A. M., Siegle, G., Crits-Christoph, P., Hazelrigg, M. D., et al. (1997). Evidence that therapy works in clinically representative conditions. *Journal of Consulting and Clinical Psychology, 65*, 355–365.

Shadish, W. R., Montgomery, L. M., Wilson, P., Wilson, M. R., Bright, L., & Okwumabua, T. (1993). Effects of family and marital psychotherapies: A meta-analysis. *Journal of Consulting and Clinical Psychology, 61*, 992–1002.

Shadish, W. R., & Sweeney, R. B. (1991). Mediators and moderators in meta-analysis: There's a reason we don't let dodo birds tell us which psychotherapies should have prizes. *Journal of Consulting and Clinical Psychology, 59*, 883–893.

Shapiro, D. A., & Shapiro, D. (1982). Meta-analysis of comparative therapy outcome studies: A replication and refinement. *Psychological Bulletin, 92*, 581–604.

Sharpe, D. (1997). Of apples and oranges, file drawers and garbage: Why validity issues in meta-analysis will not go away. *Clinical Psychology Review, 17,* 881–901.

Sherman, J. J. (1998). Effects of psychotherapeutic treatments for PTSD: A meta-analysis of controlled clinical trials. *Journal of Traumatic Stress, 11,* 413–435.

Smith, M. L., Glass, G. V., & Miller, T. I. (1980). *The benefits of psychotherapy.* Baltimore: Johns Hopkins University Press.

Stanton, M. D., & Shadish, W. R. (1997). Outcome, attrition, and family–couples treatment for drug abuse: A meta-analysis and review of the controlled, comparative studies. *Psychological Bulletin, 122,* 170–191.

Steinbrueck, S. M., Maxwell, S. E., & Howard, G. S. (1983). A meta-analysis of psychotherapy and drug therapy in the treatment of unipolar depression with adults. *Journal of Consulting and Clinical Psychology, 51,* 856–863.

Taylor, S. (1996). Meta-analysis of cognitive–behavioral treatment for social phobia. *Journal of Behavior Therapy and Experimental Psychiatry, 27,* 1–9.

Thase, M. E., & Jindal, R. D. (2004). Combining psychotherapy and psychopharmacology for treatment of mental disorders. In M. J. Lambert (Ed.), *Bergin and Garfield's handbook of psychotherapy and behavior change* (5th ed., pp. 743–766). New York: Wiley.

Tillitski, C. J. (1990). A meta-analysis of estimated effect sizes for group versus individual versus control treatments. *International Journal of Group Psychotherapy, 40,* 215–224.

Trull, T. J., Nietzel, M. T., & Main, A. (1988). The use of meta-analysis to assess the clinical significance of behavior therapy for agoraphobia. *Behavior Therapy, 19,* 527–538.

Wampold, B. E., Mondin, G. W., Moody, M., Stich, F., Benson, K., & Ahn, H. (1997). A meta-analysis of outcome studies comparing bona fide psychotherapies: Empirically, "all must have prizes." *Psychological Bulletin, 122,* 203–215.

Watson, J. C., & Geller, S. M. (2005). The relation among the relationship conditions, working alliance, and outcome in both process–experiential and cognitive–behavioral psychotherapy. *Psychotherapy Research, 15,* 25–33.

Whipple, J. L., Lambert, M. J., Vermeersch, D. A., Smart, D. W., Nielsen, S. L., & Hawkins, E. J. (2003). Improving the effects of psychotherapy: The use of early identification of treatment failure and problem-solving strategies in routine practice. *Journal of Counseling Psychology, 58,* 59–68.

6

EVIDENCE-BASED PRACTICE AND PSYCHOLOGICAL TREATMENTS

JONATHAN D. HUPPERT, AMANDA FABBRO, AND DAVID H. BARLOW

A revolution in health care is occurring around the world. Health care strategies that have been the community standard for decades have been brought into question by research evidence, which has led to rapidly changing health care practices (see Barlow, 2004). Psychology has declared itself a health care profession (American Psychological Association [APA], 2001), and the diverse and heterogeneous practice of psychotherapy and related assessment procedures are being influenced by these changes. This chapter outlines historical developments leading to the emergence of the evidence-based practice (EBP) of psychology and summarizes related research and issues. We describe the psychological treatments, their efficacy and effectiveness. Then scientific evidence related to advances in clinical psychology that support the notion of EBP are discussed. These advances include the progress in psychological research informing treatment selection, the specificity of treatments for individual disorders or problems, recent findings suggesting that specific techniques interact with therapist factors, data suggesting that positive therapy characteristics should be complemented with effective techniques, and the development of treatment manuals to assist in the dissemination of psychological treatments and principles. Following the discussion of these advances, we make a number of suggestions to further improve psychological EBP, including incorporating more process research into clinical trials; ensuring that supervision accompanies the use of treatment manuals and that new treatment manuals include more flexibility and principle-based direction; establishing practice networks; improving the design and reporting of clinical trials; and using stronger, ecologically valid control or comparison groups in research designs. Finally, we describe a possible emerging consensus that EBP will be most effective when integrating therapist skills with specific techniques for specific disorders.

DEVELOPMENTS LEADING TO EVIDENCE-BASED PRACTICE

It is a fairly recent development in the history of clinical psychology and indeed in all of health care[1] that treatments are now described in the context of EBP. Why is there a growing emphasis on EBP? Or, stated another way, why is more attention now being given to practitioners' accountability for the effectiveness and efficiency of health care practices? Several trends have converged in recent years. First, there has been a rapid advancement in the understanding of the nature of various pathologies in recent years, which has in turn led to the development of new, more precisely targeted interventions. Second, clinical research methodologies have improved substantially and have produced new evidence for the effectiveness of interventions. Third, and most important, governments around the world and their health care systems, faced with spiraling costs and specific inadequacies in health care quality, have decided that the quality of health care must improve and that it should be evidence based (Barlow, 1996; Institute of Medicine, 2001).

The costs of health care have steadily increased throughout the past 50 years. In the 1980s, costs reached new heights and appeared to continue increasing at rapid rates, which led stakeholders to the realization that something had to be done. The delivery of health care (including behavioral health care) quickly developed from an industry dominated by independent practitioners and fee-for-service arrangements into a highly organized, commercial industry (Hayes, Barlow, & Nelson-Gray, 1999). Managed care was initially somewhat successful in curbing the rise of health care costs, though often through denial of services. By reducing costs, it has altered nearly every aspect of health care provision, including the services and providers available, the types and numbers of service settings accessible to patients, and the "doses" of treatments that are reimbursable (e.g., the number of sessions for outpa-

---

[1]Historically, the notion that psychotherapy needs to be evidence based can be traced to Eysenck's (1957) classic work on the effectiveness of psychotherapy, which was first received with great controversy. Since then, efforts have grown to demonstrate the efficacy of psychotherapy. In this section we specifically describe how those efforts have converged with health care policy and practice in general.

tient mental health). As is true for all business models, the viability of managed care depends on the maximization of profits. To increase profits while limiting costs and prices, in the early days managed care allowed compromises in or even abandonment of considerations of quality. As quality regulations have begun to be mandated through legislation and enforced through litigation, this issue is beginning to be addressed (National Committee for Quality Assurance, 2004). Many governments around the world have adopted far more active roles in the regulation of health care systems. In the United States, the hope is that the competitive nature of capitalistic enterprises will improve quality; as managed care organizations compete for larger market shares, those offering the best quality at the lowest price will win out. It is not yet clear that this strategy will work in the context of current systems of delivering health care.

The focus on quality of services has led to an increasing emphasis on evaluating the effectiveness of services (Hayes et al., 1999). Clinical practice guidelines for all areas of health care that have the government's stamp of approval are now easily accessible to professionals via the Internet (http://www.guideline.gov), and practitioners following these guidelines may in some instances reap various advantages such as increased referrals, differential reimbursements, or exemptions from malpractice liability in an increasing number of states (Barlow, Levitt, & Bufka, 1999). The President's New Freedom Commission on Mental Health (2003) recommended that the nation "advance evidence-based practices using dissemination and demonstration projects and create a public–private partnership to guide their implementation; [and] improve and expand the workforce providing evidence-based mental health services and supports" (p. 25).

Recent developments in psychological health care in the United Kingdom may provide a glimpse of future directions in the United States (keeping in mind, of course, the substantial differences in the organization of health care systems in these two countries). In 1988, the government outlined a policy for mental health services that reinforced the importance of ensuring high-quality evidence-based services for the population and followed it up with a National Service Framework that described how people should be able to gain access to primary care more quickly. In 1996 the National Health System (NHS) Executive Review described the variety of "psychological therapies" used to treat adults and children in the NHS and reviewed evidence for the effectiveness of these treatments. This group concluded that these approaches were effective on the basis of evidence available at that time and offered advice to commissioners, providers, employers, and trainers about how to promote the agenda to provide evidence-based psychological services. This review also acknowledged that access to psychological therapies was limited and uncoordinated and that this situation required increased attention.

In 2001 the NHS underwent a substantial reorganization based on perceptions that quality of care was diminishing, particularly in regard to other countries with national health services, and the National Institute for Clinical Excellence was established with a mandate to create guidelines for the United Kingdom (see http://www.nice.org.uk). The NHS plan that emerged took the process a step further and provided an extra annual investment of over £3,000,000 by 2003 or 2004 to push forward these ambitious goals. Because of the strong evidence for the effectiveness of psychological treatments, and partly because of diminished roles envisioned for psychiatrists in providing psychological treatments, the NHS projected a sizeable gap between supply and demand for psychologists in the near term. To address this problem, the British Psychological Society, in collaboration with the Department of Health and the Home Office, attempted to specify the extent of this projected gap (British Psychological Society, 2004). They concluded that the demand for psychological care had grown significantly and was likely to increase again substantially with the implementation of the National Service Framework. They recommended that the number of clinical psychologists be increased 15% each year over the near term. As a result of the enhanced visibility and demand for clinical psychologists in the NHS, a proposal is now on the table to increase their compensation to bring it on a par with that of physicians in many instances. If clinical psychology in the United States were to fully embrace EBP of psychological treatments, U.S. clinical psychologists may have greater success in receiving increased funding, recognition, and parity with psychiatry.

Definition of Evidence-Based Practice

EBP is the aspiration today for all health care professionals, third-party payers, and policymakers. Evidence-based practice should be differentiated from "empirically supported treatments," which are only one part of EBP. EBP was defined early on as the "conscientious, explicit and judicious use of current best evidence in making decisions about the care of individual patients" (Sackett, Rosenberg, Gray, Haynes, & Richardson, 1996, p. 71). More recently, this definition has been broadened to include the integration of clinical expertise and patient values with the best research evidence available (Institute of Medicine, 2001; Sackett, Straus, Richardson, Rosenberg, & Haynes, 2000). By *clinical expertise*, Sackett et al. (2000) referred to advanced clinical skills to assess, diagnose, and treat disorders; by *patient preferences and values*, they meant the full inclusion of the patient in an analysis of the likelihood of benefit and risk of failure in EBP using quantitative presentations where possible.

EBP in our view does not mean practice based on probabilistic evidence alone; rather, our current conceptualization of EBP recognizes that clinical skills and experience are necessary to apply the relevant research evidence to individual patients with unique preferences and needs. The expert ability of clinical psychologists to evaluate the strength of the available research evidence, and from this determine the course of treatment most likely to benefit their specific patients, sets them apart from other behavioral health care practitioners who may also have considerable clinical expertise and sensitivity to patients' individual values.

Clinical Practice Guidelines

EBP was quickly embraced by health care services and policymakers, and the methods for ascertaining empirically supported procedures that emerged, often with the involvement of government agencies, were called "best practice algorithms" or, more frequently, "clinical practice guidelines." The creation of new guidelines has flourished around the world, and they are becoming increasingly sophisticated. Nevertheless, it became apparent early on that it would be necessary to develop procedures to evaluate the adequacy of these guidelines, particularly early guidelines emanating from managed care companies that were little more than thinly disguised cost-cutting mechanisms. Anticipating these problems, the APA created a task force to develop criteria for evaluating guidelines pertaining to psychological interventions (APA, 1995) and updated this effort in 2002 (APA, 2002). The criteria created by the original task force and organized by the dimensions of treatment efficacy and clinical utility are presented in Exhibit 6.1.

PSYCHOLOGICAL TREATMENTS

Psychology is a health care profession, and the evidence base that has developed on the efficacy of psychological treatments points to psychologists as the principal purveyors of these procedures. Elsewhere (Barlow, 2004) it has been suggested that psychologists delineate the heterogeneous nature of psychotherapy to better distinguish the subgroup of procedures that are particularly applicable, on the basis of the best available evidence, to individuals with pathology (either physical or psychological) severe enough to gain entry into the health care system. The proposal is to term these techniques "psychological treatments" (Barlow, 2004) to distinguish them from more generic psychotherapy with a different target such as promoting growth, the ability to love and be loved, and the ability to pursue an integrated and happy life. This endeavor is a very noble undertaking with a history going back thousands of years to Socrates, who stated that "an unexamined life is not worth living," as recorded by Plato (trans. 1996) in his Apology (4th century BC, section 38a). However, despite the best efforts of the psychology profession, it is likely that without directly targeting the remediation or prevention of psychopathology or pathophysiology, procedures for addressing this target will not be included in most health care systems. The potential market for life-enhancing psychotherapy certainly exceeds that for psychological treat-

EXHIBIT 6.1
Criteria for Evaluating Treatment Guidelines

TREATMENT EFFICACY CRITERIA

1. Guidelines should be based on broad and careful consideration of the relevant empirical literature.
2. Recommendations on specific interventions should take into consideration the level of methodological rigor and clinical sophistication of the research supporting the intervention.
3. Recommendations on specific interventions should take into consideration the treatment conditions to which the intervention has been compared.
4. Guidelines should consider available evidence regarding patient–treatment matching.
5. Guidelines should specify the outcomes the intervention is intended to produce, and evidence should be provided for each outcome.

CLINICAL UTILITY CRITERIA

6. Guidelines should reflect the breadth of patient variables that may influence the clinical utility of the intervention.
7. Guidelines should take into account data on how differences between individual health care professionals may affect the efficacy of the treatment.
8. Guidelines should take into account information pertaining to the setting in which the treatment is offered.
9. Guidelines should take into account data on treatment robustness.
10. Guidelines should take into account the intervention's level of acceptability to the patients who are to receive the service.

Note. From "Criteria for Evaluating Treatment Guidelines," by the American Psychological Association, 2002, American Psychologist, 57, pp. 1054–1057. Copyright 2002 by the American Psychological Association.

ments in emerging health care systems but will likely need alternative models for remuneration.

Efficacy of Psychological Treatments

In accord with the APA Task Force on evaluating guidelines, we now turn to a discussion of the evidence for first the efficacy and then the effectiveness, or clinical utility, of psychological treatments. In the case of psychological interventions, there is now enough evidence on efficacy to influence policy. More and more studies using sophisticated methodological designs and statistical analyses and broad inclusion criteria to maximize generalizability have shown robust effects of psychological treatments for specific psychopathology. The Task Force on Promotion and Dissemination of Psychological Procedures of APA's Division 12 (Society of Clinical Psychology) made an early effort to outline the criteria necessary to determine the extent of empirical support for a particular psychological treatment (APA, 1995). Using these criteria, treatments were classified as "well-established treatments," "probably efficacious treatments," or "experimental treatments."

This effort has been updated several times (Chambless et al., 1996, 1998). Well-established treatments now exist for a wide range of disorders and problems, including anxiety disorders, depression, behavioral problems of childhood, marital discord, sexual dysfunction, chemical abuse and dependence, eating disorders, schizophrenia (in combination with medication), smoking cessation, various physical disorders, and borderline personality disorder, to name a few (Barlow et al., 1999; for descriptions and analyses of specific psychological treatments, see extensive reviews by Barrett & Ollendick, 2003; Kazdin & Weisz, 2003; Nathan & Gorman, 2002; Roth & Fonagy, 2004).

Some of this research on the efficacy of specific psychological treatments in comparison to medication or alternative treatments has been published in the most rigorously reviewed medical journals, from which health care policy often emanates (see Barlow, 2004). When one also considers the vast amount of accumulating evidence in the top journals in psychology and psychiatry, it is clear that the state of the science is impressive and continually improving. Furthermore, as governments and health care systems increasingly support EBP efforts with extensive funding, the infrastructure for extending research into practice is slowly but surely developing.

Treatments that have proven to be efficacious vary in many ways, but they share at least two characteristics. First, these treatments are specific: They are targeted to the particular manifestations of psychopathology or psychological aspects of physical pathology that are distressing the patient and impairing his or her functioning. Second, the techniques are grounded in knowledge gleaned from basic psychological science laboratories and thus incorporate approaches from across schools of psychotherapy on the basis of their evidentiary support. As more psychological treatments are developed and tested in such ways, the lines distinguishing "pure" theoretical camps are blurring. Psychologists now have the tools and research available to select treatments on the basis of what works, rather than what they believe is consistent with their own theories. Unfortunately, policy and practices are only slowly catching up with the research evidence (e.g., see Olfson et al., 2002).

Clinical Effectiveness of Psychological Treatments

In addition to treatment efficacy, which focuses on internal validity, or whether a treatment works in a controlled research setting, it is important in any discussion of practice to consider clinical utility, or effectiveness, which refers to the generalizability, feasibility, and usefulness of interventions in the local settings where they are offered to the public (APA, 2002). Although at this point more evidence is available for efficacy than for effectiveness, the existing effectiveness evidence is promising. For example, in trials of treatments for social phobia and obsessive–compulsive disorder, patients excluded from randomized controlled trials evidenced improvements comparable to patients included when they received the identical intervention (Franklin, Abramowitz, Kozak, Levitt, & Foa, 2000; Juster, Heimberg, & Engelberg, 1995). Other studies have examined exporting treatments to frontline clinical practice with great success in both acute and long-term outcomes. For example, patients treated with cognitive–behavioral therapy (CBT) for panic disorder in a community mental health center by current staff had remarkably similar outcomes to those reported in research studies, despite the absence of exclusionary criteria (Stuart, Treat, & Wade, 2000; Wade, Treat, & Stuart, 1998). Similar studies for a variety of disorders are either now published or in progress (e.g., Merrill, Tolbert, & Wade, 2003), and the results appear quite consistent: Treatments established in the laboratory also apply to the real world. Continued research in this area is essential.

Funding for collaborative efficacy and effectiveness research also illustrates the increasing recognition of the need to advance knowledge about the generalizability of efficacious interventions and of the importance of continual communication between research and service settings. For example, the Substance Abuse and Mental Health Services Administration (2003) has established the National Child Traumatic Stress Network specifically to develop and disseminate empirically supported interventions to ameliorate trauma-related distress and impairment in children and their families. This initiative is unique in its balance of attention to efficacy and effectiveness research. It funds two types of centers, some for treatment development and evaluation and some for treatment delivery, feedback, and adaptation. Part of the centers' funding is specifically allocated to collaboration with other centers. This collaboration ensures that all treatment development centers are in continual communication with clinical service centers and that all clinical service centers have access to research expertise and the ability to provide feedback to influence treatment adaptations and refinements. The innovative structure of this initiative should enable it to serve eventually as an invaluable example of the most useful ways to link research and practice and to disseminate empirically supported treatments directly to the front lines of patient care. Other large-scale efforts to study and implement EBP have been funded by the National Institute of Drug Abuse in its clinical trials network initiative and by various state governments (e.g., Chorpita et al., 2002).

THE SCIENTIFIC BASE FOR EVIDENCE-BASED PRACTICE IN PSYCHOLOGY

Having considered evidence for efficacy and effectiveness of psychological treatments, we turn now to specifics about these interventions that will help integrate psychology into EBP more broadly construed. EBP should not widen the divide between practice and research, nor should it seed discord among therapists of different orientations; rather, it should protect and advance psychology by putting the profession's best evidence forward and cementing the role of psychologists in emerging health care systems around the world. A number of individuals have written cogent articles in support of EBP in psychology (e.g., Beutler, 2004; Chambless & Ollendick, 2000; Weissman & Sanderson, 2002). We do not repeat these points, except when pertinent to our discussion. Our purpose is to delineate a number of important points derived from research that should facilitate the integration of psychology with EBP.

Psychological Model of Treatment Outcome

A psychological model of treatment constitutes best practice within psychology. We advocate for a psychological model of psychotherapy, which is a middle ground between the contextual and medical models (c.f. Wampold, 2001). This model not only allows for the existence of therapist effects, allegiance effects, and common factors but also underscores specific treatment effects, the importance of flexible adherence, and differential efficacy. At the same time, it advocates and allows for an interface between psychologists and their medical colleagues and health service policymakers and increases the probability that psychological treatments will be seen as relevant to health care.

One method of facilitating relationships with other health care professionals is to present evidence for the effectiveness of psychological treatments, particularly in comparison to medications. Through such evidence, psychologists can persuade their colleagues in psychiatry and psychopharmacology to support psychotherapy, making a significant impact on behavioral health care policy. Many collaborative studies including psychological and drug treatments (e.g., Davidson et al., 2004; Foa et al., 2005) have demonstrated the efficacy of psychological treatments and may lead health care delivery systems to increase training in and dissemination of these treatments. Furthermore, the collaboration of psychologists with medicine extends far beyond psychiatry: Many treatments developed in the field of health psychology have been collaborative efforts with physicians and other health care practitioners to deal with many aspects of physical illness. These studies have yielded promising results (see Smith, Kendall, & Keefe, 2002, for a review) and are likely to be integrated into the health care system.

Specific Treatments for Specific Disorders

Some specific treatments have particular efficacy for specific disorders. When well-designed psychological treatments are matched to specific forms of psychological pathology, robust effects are apparent. Although some have suggested that all treatments are equally effective (Wampold, 2001), more fine-grained analyses suggest otherwise (e.g., Beutler, 2002; Crits-Christoph, 1997). Even those who suggest that treatments may be equally effective still support the superiority of specific treatments for anxiety disorders, health-related behavioral pathology, or other problems (e.g., Lambert & Ogles, 2004). Providing further support for the notion that specific techniques matter, Howard (1999) reported findings from a managed health care system indicating that clinicians who reported having received specialty training in cognitive–behavioral treatments had better outcomes with patients with an anxiety disorder than clinicians who reported having no such training. It is clear that more research is required to better understand such findings. Fortunately, a number of newer studies are aimed at clarifying such questions within well-controlled studies (e.g., Addis et al., 2004; Merrill et al., 2003).

From the standpoint of EBP, it is more helpful and credible to specify treatments for specific disorders than to contend that a whole range of treatments under a single rubric (e.g., "psychotherapy works") are effective for any complaint. Such a notion leaves one without guidelines regarding what strategies to use and leads to the uncomfortable and unlikely conclusion that past life regression therapy, thought field therapy, or similar approaches without evidence are as effective as interpersonal psychotherapy for depression due to common factors operative in each. In medicine, a belief that "surgery works" would not guide the surgeon to know which procedure to select for any given condition or even whether to operate. Thus, analyses need to be conducted carefully with an understanding of the underlying complexities of the disorders and the treatments. Grouped analyses across treatments and conditions that ignore these interactions are at risk of obfuscating benefits.

The Importance of Therapist Techniques

The outcomes of psychological treatments are determined by the manner in which therapists execute specific techniques. Several researchers have suggested that only 10% of treatment effects are accounted for by techniques, and that more than 50% can be accounted for by the therapist (Lambert & Barley, 2002; but see Beutler, 2004, for a lower estimate). However, the definition of *therapist effects* is complex and may include aspects of technique not well captured in many discussions of the notion of therapist effects. We maintain that the interaction of a skilled therapist with effective techniques is crucial. Depending on the disorder, some treatments may show differential benefits of techniques and therapists immediately during treatment, whereas others are more likely to show such effects in the longer term. For example, in a recent study on the relative efficacy of CBT and medications for obsessive–compulsive disorder (OCD; Foa et al., 2005), therapist effects in CBT accounted for approximately 12% of the outcomes, whereas treatment effects (compared with placebo) accounted for 60% of the outcomes (Huppert, Franklin, Foa, Simpson, & Liebowitz, 2003). For this chapter, we examined therapist and treatment effects at posttreatment and 1 year after acute treatment for panic disorder from a large clinical trial (Barlow, Gorman, Shear, & Woods, 2000). Therapist effects remained at approximately 10% between posttreatment and follow-up, but the treatment effects rose from 10% to approximately 40% (Huppert, 2004; Huppert et al., 2001). More data are needed to identify and understand the factors that contributed to outcomes. These data certainly suggest that researchers should not be quick to dismiss the importance of techniques simply because therapist effects may be found. We use an analogy from surgery: There is documented evidence of differential surgeon effects (New York State Department of Health, 2001) and hospital effects (e.g., Birkmeyer et al., 2002). Surgeons and hospitals with higher volumes of specific types of surgery tend to have better outcomes. Of course, the right techniques need to be in the right hands before this analysis can be done. Until researchers understand the specifics of what variables (i.e., what specific therapist actions) account for therapist effects, one cannot be sure that competency using a technique or the methods used to motivate a patient to comply with treatment are not what accounts for such effects when they are found (c.f. Huppert, Barlow, Gorman, Shear, & Woods, in press).

Therapeutic Relationship: Necessary but Not Sufficient

The therapeutic alliance, empathy, expectancy, and motivation are necessary, but they are not sufficient factors in producing positive therapeutic outcomes. The data support the notion that the alliance or other common factors are related to outcomes for many disorders or treatments, but most analyses ignore the important interactions with techniques that are possible reasons for such findings. In one study (Lindsay, Crino, & Andrews, 1997), patients with OCD who received exposure and response prevention benefited significantly more from treatment than patients who received stress management training, even though the two treatments were seen by the patients as highly credible and alliance was high in both conditions. In a study of treatments for cocaine abuse, Carroll, Nich, and Rounsaville (1997) found that alliance was not correlated with outcome within structured treatments, although it was strongly related to outcome in supportive psychotherapy. Others have found that some treatment factors, such as level of emotional arousal, are most effective in facilitating change in the context of a positive alliance (Beutler, Clarkin, & Bongar, 2000). Still others have found that both techniques and alliance are related to outcome (Klein et al., 2003; Pos, Greenberg, Goldman, & Korman, 2003). In a study of CBT for generalized anxiety disorder, alliance was related to immediate outcomes, but it was unrelated to long-term outcomes, suggesting that it is important to examine the long-term impact of alliance on outcomes (Durham et al., 2005).

More important, the mechanisms producing a good alliance are not clear, despite attempts to clarify this issue (e.g., Horvath & Bedi, 2002; Lambert & Ogles, 2004). Some studies have suggested that a positive alliance leads to better treatment compliance (Blackwell, 1997), which suggests that the more powerful the treatment strategies, the greater the benefit from a strong alliance. However, the reverse is also possible: The more effective the strategy, the better developed the alliance may become. For example, providing psychoeducation about the nature of panic attacks and realistic treatment expectations based on outcome data may greatly improve the therapeutic alliance because the patient now feels understood and understands some of his or her experiences better and because psychoeducation provides an excellent framework for a realistic, hopeful relationship in which the patient expects to improve. Thus, empirically supported techniques (Castonguay & Beutler, 2005) that comprise the foundation of the empirically supported treatments used in EBP (Chambless et al., 1998) are likely to positively affect empirically supported relationships (Norcross, 2002). This is the essence of evidence-based practice.

Value of Treatment Manuals

Treatment manuals can help ensure that therapists are using appropriate techniques for a given disorder. Manuals and manualized treatment are tools and guidelines for practitioners, not fixed, unalterable software programs (c.f. Sackett et al., 1996). A treatment manual (e.g., Craske, Barlow, & Meadows, 2000) is meant to serve as a tool that provides clinicians with both the basic psychological principles that will help most patients with a specific problem and a combination of techniques that are proved to accomplish these principles. There are, of course, times that these techniques do not work and that the treatment plans need to be adjusted (e.g., Huppert & Baker-Morissette, 2003). In this regard, manualized psychological treatments can be viewed as similar to surgery (i.e., therapist as surgeon and treatment as tools for surgery). It is understood that no one can simply read a manual in any of these areas and apply the treatment proficiently or with expertise; furthermore, clinicians must be able to deal expertly with complications that may arise. Training, supervision, and practice are all necessary. There are a growing number of published efforts encouraging therapists to learn how to use manuals appropriately, with flexibility and sensitivity, while still adhering to the general psychological principles appropriate for the condition under treatment (see Huppert & Abramowitz, 2003).

IMPROVING RESEARCH IN PSYCHOLOGY TO ADVANCE EVIDENCE-BASED PSYCHOTHERAPY

To inform the continuing discussion regarding the best way to conceptualize and improve EBP, we have identified five issues that may allow for better integration of psychological research into EBP and that should thereby improve quality of care. The paragraphs that follow outline these issues.

First, process research should be incorporated into clinical trials. In pursuit of the best evidence for the efficacy of psychological treatments and to retain the credibility of the psychology profession in developing health care policy, well-controlled randomized controlled trials (RCTs) are necessary, but they may not be sufficient to elucidate mechanisms of action. A significant amount of process research has been conducted from the National Institute of Mental Health Treatment for Depression Collaborative Research Project (TDCRP; a PsycLIT search of articles from 1987–2004 yielded 73 articles and dissertations involving the study), and other studies are beginning to report important process results (e.g., Arnow et al., 2003; Klein et al., 2003; Nemeroff et al., 2003). However, clinical trials should include measures of both common factors and specific techniques so that researchers can examine not only which treatment works but also why and for whom.

Second, treatment manuals should include a caveat about the need for expert supervision to maximize the benefits of their use. All manualized treatments from a variety of theoretical persuasions were developed by expert clinicians who put great effort into documenting what they believed were the core principles and efficacious techniques of their treatments (e.g., Clarkin, Yeomans, & Kernberg, 1999; Linehan, 1993). However, these treatments still require supervision. Under expert supervision, therapists learn to incorporate aspects of the treatment that are not articulated in the manual (e.g., Huppert & Abramowitz, 2003). This transmission of unwritten knowledge is similar to what happens in the training of physician specialists through their residencies or beginning psychology students in their clinical practica. Fortunately, a number of manuals already published or currently in progress attempt to clarify this unwritten knowledge (e.g., Segal, Williams, & Teasdale, 2002).

Third, practice research networks should be established to further evaluate techniques and disseminate them in clinical practice while informing future research directions (Borkovec, 2004; Borkovec, Echemendia, Ragusea, & Ruiz, 2001). Some have suggested that rather than developing a new generation of treatments and manuals from the laboratory, researchers should shift their focus to discerning what works in real-world practice (Westen, Novotny, & Thompson-Brenner, 2004). It would definitely be interesting to see the fruits of such an endeavor. At the same time, significant progress has been made using the incremental scientific paradigm, in which treatments evaluated in well-controlled RCTs to establish efficacy are then tested in real-world clinical settings and appropriate modifications made. Of course, many interventions ultimately tested in RCTs originated in practice settings, so it is something of a two-way street already (c.f. Clark, 2004). Nevertheless, several notable recent studies have suggested that usual and typical treatments in the real world (treatment as usual) are not as effective as those conducted in research settings (Bickman, Noser, & Summerfelt, 1999; Hansen, Lambert, & Forman, 2002; Weisz, 2004).

Psychological treatments will best be advanced by a combination of information integration from psychological science (c.f. Bouton, Mineka, & Barlow, 2001; Foa & Kozak, 1997) and systematic study of techniques based on theory and science (Clark, 2004). Of course, knowledge gained from clinical practice should be fully integrated into treatment development at every stage, with practitioners as full partners in the process (Hollon et al., 2002), and studying outcomes in the real world after training can provide important results. It is fortunate that organized systems are arising to facilitate communication and interconnection between research facilities and clinical service settings. Practice research networks such as the Pennsylvania Practice Research Network are developing in an effort to create organized infrastructures for effectiveness research collaboration between researchers and practitioners (Borkovec et al., 2001), and government research initiatives are also promoting such efforts.

Fourth, improvements are needed in the design and reporting of clinical trials. Westen et al. (2004) suggested that improving the reporting of clinical trials in psychology is necessary to determine whether findings are generalizable to clinical practice. One would be hard-pressed to find a dissenter to that opinion. A recent study showed that most patients in community health centers would in fact meet criteria for at least one clinical trial (Stirman, DeRubeis, Crits-Cristoph, & Brody, 2003). Many patients are reasonably excluded because their disorders are not the primary focus of the study or sufficiently severe. Although there have been recent calls to include more suicidal patients in protocols (Hollon et al., 2002; Westen et al., 2004), such steps should be taken with extreme care so as not to increase the risk of harm for a patient in a trial.

In the meantime, promising results have been reported from case series and other studies on the generalizability of empirically supported treatments to excluded populations, such as those with comorbid alcohol abuse and panic disorders (Lehman, Brown, & Barlow, 1998) or schizophrenia and social anxiety (Halperin, Nathan, Drummond, & Castle, 2000). Furthermore, there are large bodies of research on a number of treatments that have been applied to multiple real-world settings (e.g., Program of Assertive Community Treatment [PACT]; Stein & Santos, 1998) for individuals with severe mental illness (Bond, Drake, Mueser, & Latimer, 2001; Gold et al., 2003). Overall, most data support the generalizability of these treatments into clinical practice (see Shadish, Matt, Navarro, & Phillips, 2000; see http://www.psych.upenn.edu/~dchamb/ESTs/effect2.html).

It is important to report clinical trials according to Consolidated Standards of Reporting Trials (CONSORT) guidelines (Moher, Schultz, & Altman, 2001), which stipulate the kinds of data from randomized clinical trials that should be reported. Westen et al. (2004) recently called for a similar guideline, perhaps with additional information such as completer response and dropout analyses, to account for all patients from study inception through follow-up. In addition to learning about patient selection for the studies, one may also learn important additional information about the treatment-seeking samples (e.g., Huppert, Franklin, Foa, & Davidson, 2003). However, it is an overstatement to suggest that because studies have not had 5-year follow-ups and reported on every patient excluded from the study, their results cannot guide practice (Westen et al., 2004), because results thus far suggest otherwise (see the section on Clinical Effectiveness of Psychology, this chapter).

Finally, attention must be paid to the use of proper control groups. Researchers should compare study treatments with those in widespread use in practice (Wampold, 2001; Westen et al., 2004). We wholeheartedly agree that ideal studies should include expert therapists performing both the treatment under evaluation and the "control treatment," which should be treatment as usual in the community. It is essential that collaborative efforts such as those with psychiatry be undertaken with practitioners of psychodynamic, experiential, and eclectic treatments in the community to avoid any confounding allegiance effects accounting for differences that may occur (c.f. Luborsky et al., 1999), which has begun to happen (see Clarkin, Levy, Lenzenweger, & Kernberg, 2004; Crits-Christoph et al., 1999; Weersing & Weisz, 2002). Unfortunately, the dearth of non-CBT researchers and the difficulty in obtaining funding for such studies make this endeavor more difficult.

CONCLUSION

Governments and health care policymakers around the world have evaluated the evidence for the psychological treatment of various physical and psychological pathologies and have accepted this evidence as sufficient to include these procedures in a variety of officially authorized clinical treatment guidelines. Although the data have at times been misused by managed care organizations to limit reimbursement for continued treatment and also can lead to a clinician applying treatment manuals without considering the individual needs of the specific patient, such issues are against the principles of EBP in psychology as we see them. We have suggested in this chapter that emerging psychological treatments with proved efficacy are made up of an integral relationship between therapist skill and technique in the context of treating a specific disorder (or vulnerabilities for a disorder) and that these two factors cannot be usefully separated. Although much additional evidence needs to be developed, particularly focusing on the clinical utility or generalizability of these procedures to frontline clinical settings, many government agencies are invested in promoting this research. Fortunately, the results thus far are very encouraging, although researchers have a very long way to go to fully understand this process. It is also clear that a full elucidation of clinical utility or effectiveness will depend on a close working relationship between clinical scientists developing these techniques and practitioners using them in the community. An iterative process is required whereby newly developed techniques are beta tested in the community with a resulting process of feedback and refinement that will lead to either the establishment of the procedures as useful in frontline practice settings or the abandonment of the procedures as not feasible. In this way, practitioners will become full partners in the research process (Barlow, Hayes, & Nelson, 1984; Hayes et al., 1999). The beginnings of this type of effort are found in practice research networks such as that established by the Pennsylvania Psychological Association (Borkovec et al., 2001). Indeed, perhaps it is time for the APA to establish its own nationwide practice research network.

Although health care systems in the United States are more disorganized than in a number of other nations, it seems clear to many observers (e.g., Richmond & Fien, 2003) that this country will ultimately move toward a more unified and perhaps even a single-payer system of health care. With the further development of evidence-based psychological treatments, the psychology profession will be poised to take advantage of these advances and to play a major role in the nation's health and well-being.

REFERENCES

Addis, M. E., Hatgis, C., Krasnow, A. D., Jacob, K., Bourne, L., & Mansfield, A. (2004). Effectiveness of cognitive–behavioral treatment for panic disorder versus treatment as usual in a managed care setting. *Journal of Consulting and Clinical Psychology, 72*, 625–635.

American Psychological Association. (1995). *Template for developing guidelines: Interventions for mental disorders and psychosocial aspects of physical disorders.* Washington, DC: Author.

American Psychological Association. (2001). Amendment to bylaws accepted. *Monitor on Psychology, 32.* Retrieved October 31, 2005, from http://www.apa.org/monitor/julaug01/amendaccept.html

American Psychological Association. (2002). Criteria for evaluating treatment guidelines. *American Psychologist, 57*, 1052–1059.

Arnow, B. A., Manber, R., Blasey, C., Klein, D. N., Blalock, J. A., Markowitz, J. C., et al. (2003). Therapeutic reactance as a predictor of outcome in the treatment of chronic depression. *Journal of Consulting and Clinical Psychology, 71*, 1025–1035.

Barlow, D. H. (1996). Health care policy, psychotherapy research, and the future of psychotherapy. *American Psychologist, 51*, 1050–1058.

Barlow, D. H. (2004). Psychological treatments. *American Psychologist, 59*, 869–878.

Barlow, D. H., Gorman, J. M., Shear, M. K., & Woods, S. W. (2000, May 17). Cognitive–behavioral therapy, imipramine, or their combination for panic disorder: A randomized controlled trial. *Journal of the American Medical Association, 283,* 2529–2536.

Barlow, D. H., Hayes, S., & Nelson, R. (1984). *The scientist–practitioner.* Elmsford, NY: Pergamon Press.

Barlow, D. H., Levitt, J. T., & Bufka, L. F. (1999). The dissemination of empirically supported treatments: A view to the future. *Behaviour Research and Therapy, 37,* S147–S162.

Barrett, P. M., & Ollendick, T. H. (Eds.). (2003). *Handbook of interventions that work with children and adolescents.* West Sussex, England: Wiley.

Beutler, L. E. (2002). The dodo bird is extinct. *Clinical Psychology: Science and Practice, 9,* 30–34.

Beutler, L. E. (2004). The empirically supported treatments movement: A scientist–practitioner's response. *Clinical Psychology: Science and Practice, 11,* 225–229.

Beutler, L. E., Clarkin, J. F., & Bongar, B. (2000). *Guidelines for the systematic treatment of the depressed patient.* New York: Oxford University Press.

Bickman, L., Noser, K., & Summerfelt, W. T. (1999). Long-term effects of a system of care on children and adolescents. *Journal of Behavioral Health Services and Research, 26,* 185–202.

Birkmeyer, J. D., Siewers, A. E., Finlayson, E. V. A., Stukel, T. A., Lucas, F. L., Batista, I., et al. (2002). Hospital volume and surgical mortality in the United States. *New England Journal of Medicine, 346,* 1128–1137.

Blackwell, B. (Ed.). (1997). *Treatment compliance and the therapeutic alliance.* Amsterdam: Harwood Academic.

Bond, G. R., Drake, R. E., Mueser, K. T., & Latimer, E. (2001). Assertive community treatment for people with severe mental illness: Critical ingredients and impact on patients. *Disease Management and Health Outcomes, 9,* 141–159.

Borkovec, T. D. (2004). Research in training clinics and practice research networks: A route to the integration of science and practice. *Clinical Psychology: Science and Practice, 11,* 211–215.

Borkovec, T. D., Echemendia, R. J., Ragusea, S. A., & Ruiz, M. (2001). The Pennsylvania Practice Research Network and future possibilities for clinically meaningful and scientifically rigorous psychotherapy effectiveness research. *Clinical Psychology: Science and Practice, 8,* 155–167.

Bouton, M. E., Mineka, S., & Barlow, D. H. (2001). A modern learning-theory perspective on the etiology of panic disorder. *Psychological Review, 108,* 4–32.

British Psychological Society. (2004). *English survey of applied psychologists in health & social care and in the probation & prison service.* Leicester, England: Author.

Carroll, K. M., Nich, C., & Rounsaville, B. J. (1997). Contribution of the therapeutic alliance to outcome in active versus control psychotherapies. *Journal of Consulting and Clinical Psychology, 65,* 510–514.

Castonguay, L. G., & Beutler, L. E. (2005). Empirically supported principles of therapy change. New York: Oxford University Press.

Chambless, D. L., Baker, M. J., Baucom, D. H., Beutler, L. E., Calhoun, K. S., Crits-Christoph, P., et al. (1998). Update on empirically validated therapies: II. *The Clinical Psychologist, 51*, 3–16.

Chambless, D. L., & Ollendick, T. H. (2000). Empirically supported psychological interventions: Controversies and evidence. *Annual Review of Psychology, 52*, 685–716.

Chambless, D. L., Sanderson, W. C., Shoham, V., Bennett Johnson, S., Pope, K. S., Crits-Christoph, P., et al. (1996). An update on empirically validated therapies. *The Clinical Psychologist, 49*, 5–18.

Chorpita, B. F., Yim, L. M., Donkervoet, J. C., Arensdorf, A., Amundsen, M. J., McGee, C., et al. (2002). Toward large-scale implementation of empirically supported treatments for children: A review and observations by the Hawaii Empirical Basis to Services Task Force. *Clinical Psychology: Science and Practice, 9*, 165–190.

Clark, D. M. (2004). Developing new treatments: On the interplay between theories, experimental science and clinical innovation. *Behaviour Research and Therapy, 42*, 1089–1104.

Clarkin, J. F., Levy, K. N., Lenzenweger, M. F., & Kernberg, O. F. (2004). The Personality Disorders Institute/Borderline Personality Disorder Research Foundation randomized control trial for borderline personality disorder: Rationale and methods. *Journal of Personality Disorders, 18*, 52–72.

Clarkin, J. F., Yeomans, F., & Kernberg, O. F. (1999). *Psychotherapy of borderline personality*. New York: Wiley.

Craske, M. G., Barlow, D. H., & Meadows, E. (2000). *Mastery of your anxiety and panic: Therapist guide for anxiety, panic, and agoraphobia (MAP–3)*. Boulder, CO: Graywind Publications.

Crits-Christoph, P. (1997). Limitations of the dodo bird verdict and the role of clinical trials in psychotherapy research: Comment on Wampold et al. (1997). *Psychological Bulletin, 122*, 216–220.

Crits-Christoph, P., Siqueland, L., Blaine, J., Frank, A., Luborsky, L., Onken, L. S., et al. (1999). Psychosocial treatments for cocaine dependence: National Institute on Drug Abuse Collaborative Cocaine Treatment Study. *Archives of General Psychiatry, 56*, 493–502.

Davidson, J. R. T., Foa, E. B., Huppert, J. D., Keefe, F. J., Franklin, M. E., Compton, J. S., et al. (2004). Fluoxetine comprehensive cognitive–behavioral therapy (CCBT) and placebo in generalized social phobia. *Archives of General Psychiatry, 61*, 1005–1013.

Durham, R. C., Chambers, J. A., Dow, M. G. T., Gumley, A. I., Macdonald, R. R., Major, K. A., et al. (2005). Long-term outcome of cognitive behaviour therapy clinical trials in central Scotland. *Health Technology Assessment, 9*(42), 1–174.

Eysenck, H. J. (1957). The effects of psychotherapy: An evaluation. *Journal of Consulting Psychology, 16*, 319–324.

Foa, E. B., & Kozak, M. J. (1997). Beyond the efficacy ceiling? Cognitive behavior therapy in search of theory. *Behavior Therapy, 28*, 601–611.

Foa, E. B., Liebowitz, M. L., Kozak, M. J., Davies, S., Campeas, R., Franklin, M. E., et al. (2005). Clomipramine, exposure and response prevention, and their combination for OCD. *American Journal of Psychiatry, 162,* 151–161.

Franklin, M. E., Abramowitz, J. S., Kozak, M. J., Levitt, J. T., & Foa, E. B. (2000). Effectiveness of exposure and ritual prevention for obsessive–compulsive disorder: Randomized compared with nonrandomized samples. *Journal of Consulting and Clinical Psychology, 68,* 594–602.

Gold, P. B., Meisler, N., Santos, A. B., Keleher, J., Becker, D. R., Knoedler, W. H., et al. (2003). The Program of Assertive Community Treatment: Implementation and dissemination of an evidence-based model of community-based care for persons with severe and persistent mental illness. *Cognitive and Behavioral Practice, 10,* 290–303.

Halperin, S., Nathan, P., Drummond, P., & Castle, D. (2000). A cognitive–behavioural, group-based intervention for social anxiety in schizophrenia. *Australian and New Zealand Journal of Psychiatry, 34,* 809–813.

Hansen, N. B., Lambert, M. J., & Forman, E. M. (2002). The psychotherapy dose–response effect and its implications for treatment delivery services. *Clinical Psychology: Science and Practice, 9,* 329–343.

Hayes, S. C., Barlow, D. H., & Nelson-Gray, R. O. (1999). *The scientist practitioner: Research and accountability in the age of managed care* (2nd ed.). Boston: Allyn & Bacon.

Hollon, S. D., Munoz, R. F., Barlow, D. H., Beardslee, W. R., Bell, C. C., & Bernal, G. (2002). Psychosocial intervention development for the prevention and treatment of depression: Promoting innovation and increasing access. *Biological Psychiatry, 52,* 610–630.

Horvath, A. O., & Bedi, R. P. (2002). The alliance. In J. C. Norcross (Ed.), *Psychotherapy relationships that work: Therapist contributions and responsiveness to patients* (pp. 37–69). London: Oxford University Press.

Howard, R. C. (1999). Treatment of anxiety disorders: Does specialty training help? *Professional Psychology: Research and Practice, 30,* 470–473.

Huppert, J. D. (2004). [Treatment and therapist effects after follow-up in the Multi-Center Collaborative Treatment Study for Panic Disorder]. Unpublished raw data.

Huppert, J. D., & Abramowitz, J. A. (2003). Introduction to special section: Going beyond the manual. *Cognitive and Behavioral Practice, 10,* 1–2.

Huppert, J. D., & Baker-Morissette, S. L. (2003). Going beyond the manual: An insider's guide to Panic Control Treatment. *Cognitive and Behavioral Practice, 10,* 2–12.

Huppert, J. D., Barlow, D. H., Gorman, J. M., Shear, M. K., & Woods, S. W. (in press). The interaction of motivation and therapist adherence predict outcome in cognitive behavioral therapy for panic disorder: Preliminary findings. *Cognitive and Behavioral Practice.*

Huppert, J. D., Bufka, L. F., Barlow, D. H., Gorman, J. M., Shear, M. K., & Woods, S. W. (2001). Therapists, therapist variables, and cognitive–behavioral therapy outcome in a multicenter trial for panic disorder. *Journal of Consulting and Clinical Psychology, 69,* 747–755.

Huppert, J. D., Franklin, M. E., Foa, E. B., & Davidson, J. R. T. (2003). Study refusal and exclusion from a randomized treatment study of generalized social phobia. *Journal of Anxiety Disorders, 17,* 683–693.

Huppert, J. D., Franklin, M. E., Foa, E. B., Simspon, H. B., & Liebowitz, M. R. (2003). *Therapist effects in the treatment of OCD: Results from a randomized trial.* Paper presented at the annual conference of the Association for the Advancement of Behavior Therapy, Boston.

Institute of Medicine. (2001). *Crossing the quality chasm: A new health system for the 21st century.* Washington, DC: National Academy Press.

Juster, H. R., Heimberg, R. G., & Engelberg, B. (1995). Self-selection and sample selection in a treatment study of social phobia. *Behaviour Research and Therapy, 33,* 321–324.

Kazdin, A. E., & Weisz, J. R. (2003). *Evidence-based psychotherapies for children and adolescents.* New York: Guilford Press.

Klein, D. N., Schwartz, J. E., Santiago, N. J., Vivian, D., Vocisano, C., Castonguay, L. C., et al. (2003). Therapeutic alliance in depression treatment: Controlling for prior change and patient characteristics. *Journal of Consulting and Clinical Psychology, 71,* 997–1006.

Lambert, M. J., & Barley, D. E. (2002). Research summary on the therapeutic relationship and psychotherapy outcome. In J. Norcross (Ed.), *Psychotherapy relationships that work: Therapist contributions and responsiveness to patient needs* (pp. 17–36). New York: Oxford University Press.

Lambert, M. J., & Ogles, B. M. (2004). The efficacy and effectiveness of psychotherapy. In M. J. Lambert (Ed.), *Bergin and Garfield's handbook of psychotherapy and behavior change* (5th ed., pp. 139–193). New York: Wiley.

Lehman, C. L., Brown, T. A., & Barlow, D. H. (1998). Effects of cognitive–behavioral treatment for panic disorder with agoraphobia on concurrent alcohol abuse. *Behavior Therapy, 29,* 423–433.

Lindsay, M., Crino, R., & Andrews, G. (1997). Controlled trial of exposure and response prevention in obsessive–compulsive disorder. *British Journal of Psychiatry, 171,* 135–139.

Linehan, M. M. (1993). *Cognitive–behavioral treatment of borderline personality disorder.* New York: Guilford Press.

Luborsky, L., Diguer, L., Seligman, D. A., Rosenthal, R., Johnson, S., & Halperin, G., et al. (1999). The researcher's own therapeutic allegiance: A "wild card" in comparisons of treatment efficacy. *Clinical Psychology: Science and Practice, 6,* 95–132.

Merrill, K. A., Tolbert, V. E., & Wade, W. A. (2003). Effectiveness of cognitive therapy for depression in a community mental health center: A benchmarking study. *Journal of Consulting and Clinical Psychology, 71,* 404–409.

Moher, D., Schultz, K. F., Altman, D., for the CONSORT Group. (2001, April 18). The CONSORT statement: Revised recommendations for improving the quality of reports of parallel-group randomized trials. *Journal of the American Medical Association, 285,* 1987–1991.

Nathan, P. E., & Gorman, J. M. (2002). Efficacy, effectiveness, and the clinical utility of psychotherapy research. In P. E. Nathan & J. M. Gorman (Eds.), *A guide to treatments that work* (2nd ed., pp. 643–654). New York: Oxford University Press.

National Committee for Quality Assurance. (2004). *NCQA's mission, vision, and values.* Retrieved August 14, 2004, from http://www.ncqa.org/about/about.htm

Nemeroff, C. B., Heim, C. M., Thase, M. E., Klein, D. N., Rush, A. J., Schatzberg, A. F., et al. (2003). Differential responses to psychotherapy versus pharmacotherapy in patients with chronic forms of major depression and childhood trauma. *Proceedings of the National Academy of Sciences of the United States of America, 100,* 14293–14296.

New York State Department of Health. (2001). *Coronary artery bypass surgery in New York State 1996–1998.* Albany, NY: Author.

Norcross, J. C. (Ed.). (2002). *Psychotherapy relationships that work: Therapist contributions and responsiveness to patient needs.* New York: Oxford University Press.

Olfson, M., Marcus, S. C., Druss, B., Elinson, L., Tanielian, T., & Pincus, H. A. (2002, January 9). National trends in the outpatient treatment of depression. *Journal of the American Medical Association, 287,* 203–209.

Plato. (1996). *Apology* (H. N. Fowler, Trans.). Cambridge, MA: Harvard University Press.

Pos, A. E., Greenberg, L. S., Goldman, R. N., & Korman, L. M. (2003). Emotional processing during experiential treatment of depression. *Journal of Consulting and Clinical Psychology, 71,* 1007–1016.

President's New Freedom Commission on Mental Health. (2003). *Achieving the promise: Transforming mental health care in America. Final report* (DHHS Publication No. SMA 03-3832). Rockville, MD: U.S. Department of Health and Human Services.

Richmond, J. B., & Fien, R. (2003, September 26). Health insurance in the USA. *Science, 301,* 1813.

Roth, A., & Fonagy, P. (2004). *What works for whom? A critical review of psychotherapy research* (2nd ed.). New York: Guilford Press.

Sackett, D. L., Rosenberg, W. M., Gray, J. A., Haynes, R. B., & Richardson, W. S. (1996). Evidence-based medicine: What it is and what it isn't. *British Medical Journal, 312,* 71–72.

Sackett, D. L., Straus, S. E., Richardson, W. S., Rosenberg, W., & Haynes, R. B. (2000). *Evidence-based medicine: How to practice and teach EBM.* New York: Churchill Livingstone.

Segal, Z., Williams, M., & Teasdale, J. (2002). *Mindfulness-based cognitive therapy for depression: A new approach to preventing relapse.* New York: Guilford Press.

Shadish, W. R., Matt, G. E., Navarro, A. M., & Phillips, G. (2000). The effects of psychological therapies under clinically representative conditions: A meta-analysis. *Psychological Bulletin, 126,* 512–529.

Smith, T. W., Kendall, P. C., & Keefe, F. J. (2002). Behavioral medicine and clinical health psychology [Special issue]. *Journal of Abnormal Psychology, 70*(3).

Stein, L. I., & Santos, A. B. (1998). *Assertive community treatment of persons with severe mental illness.* New York: Norton.

Stirman, S. W., DeRubeis, R. J., Crits-Cristoph, P., & Brody, P. E. (2003). Are samples in randomized controlled trials of psychotherapy representative of community outpatients? A new methodology and initial findings. *Journal of Consulting and Clinical Psychology, 71,* 963–972.

Stuart, G. L., Treat, T. A., & Wade, W. A. (2000). Effectiveness of an empirically based treatment for panic disorder delivered in a service clinic setting: 1-year follow-up. *Journal of Consulting and Clinical Psychology, 68,* 506–512.

Substance Abuse and Mental Health Services Administration. (2003). *SAMHSA agency overview.* Retrieved October 31, 2005, from http://www.samhsa.gov/news/newsreleases/031009nr_childtrauma.htm

Wade, W. A., Treat, T. A., & Stuart, G. L. (1998). Transporting an empirically supported treatment for panic disorder to a service clinic setting: A benchmarking strategy. *Journal of Consulting and Clinical Psychology, 66,* 231–239.

Wampold, B. E. (2001). *The great psychotherapy debate: Models, methods, and findings.* Hillsdale, NJ: Erlbaum.

Weersing, V. R., & Weisz, J. R. (2002). Community clinic treatment of depressed youth: Benchmarking usual care against CBT clinical trials. *Journal of Consulting and Clinical Psychology, 70,* 299–310.

Weissman, M. M., & Sanderson, W. C. (2002). Problems and promises in modern psychotherapy: The need for increased training in evidence-based treatments. In B. Hamburg (Ed.), *Modern psychiatry: Challenges in educating health professionals to meet new needs* (pp. 1–40). New York: Josiah Macy Foundation.

Weisz, J. R. (2004). *Psychotherapy for children and adolescents: Evidence-based treatments and case examples.* Cambridge, England: Cambridge University Press.

Westen, D., Novotny, C. M., & Thompson-Brenner, H. (2004). Empirical status of empirically supported psychotherapies: Assumptions, findings, and reporting in controlled clinical trials. *Psychological Bulletin, 130,* 631–663.

7

ASSESSMENT AND EVALUATION IN CLINICAL PRACTICE

ALAN E. KAZDIN

There is a long-standing hiatus between research and clinical practice. Among the many issues in the context of psychotherapy is that treatment research is conducted in well-controlled laboratory settings and conditions that depart from many conditions in clinical practice (e.g., Borkovec & Rachman, 1979; Heller, 1971; Kazdin, 1978). Efficacy and effectiveness research have been distinguished to reflect these differences (Hoagwood, Hibbs, Brent, & Jensen, 1995). Efficacy studies are conducted in controlled settings and under conditions that depart from clinical practice. Effectiveness studies are conducted in clinical settings with a diverse set of patient, therapist, and treatment administration characteristics. Evidence-based treatments (EBTs) are based almost exclusively on studies in highly controlled settings, and this fact has been repeatedly discussed as a concern about the generalizability of the findings to clinical practice (e.g., Persons & Silberschatz, 1998; Westen, Novotny, & Thompson-Brenner, 2004).

Whether the substantive findings from research ought to serve as a basis for clinical practice has been argued repeatedly. There is, in my view, a

This work was supported, in part, by a grant from the National Institute of Mental Health (MH59029).

much greater problem in relation to the gap between treatment research and clinical practice: The problem pertains to the sharply different ways of evaluating information in research and clinical settings and the use of the information to draw conclusions. Mental health researchers and clinicians are well familiar with the methods of treatment research, with emphasis on evaluating treatment effects on the basis of mean differences among various treatment and control conditions. The way in which treatment is evaluated in the tradition of quantitative research and hypothesis testing has no useful parallel in evaluating whether a particular patient seen in treatment gets better or has improved. Also, multiple patients in a group study are evaluated with standardized measures, none of which may capture their particular problems very well. Standardization in this way is very useful for research but not so clearly relevant for therapy in practice.

Clinical practice focuses on the individual rather than on groups. The case study has dominated clinical work; the therapist describes in a narrative way possible causes of the problem, how he or she formulated or conceived the case, the patient's clinical course, and the treatment provided. Typically, therapists in clinical practice do not evaluate cases in a systematic way. They may complete evaluations in relation to reimbursement or required clinical and hospital documentation. However, the information clinicians usually use to evaluate patient progress over the course of treatment is based on their views, experiences, and impressions. When these impressions are not systematically codified, they constitute the familiar anecdotal case study, in which the therapist constructs narrative information to draw inferences and to make connections in relation to possible etiologies, treatment course, and intervention effects.

In this chapter, I discuss the importance of systematic evaluation in clinical practice, illustrate steps that therapists can use, and highlights critical clinical and research issues that need to be addressed to provide the necessary underpinnings of evaluation. Although I focus on concrete steps to conduct evaluation, I also raise broader issues that pertain to features of clinical training that may unwittingly undermine evaluation. The focus of the chapter is on *systematic evaluation*, by which I mean evaluation by methods or instruments that begin with a construct and seek to operationalize that construct in ways that can be scrutinized, validated, and replicated by others in similar circumstances.

THE NEED FOR SYSTEMATIC EVALUATION IN CLINICAL WORK

Systematic evaluation is critically important in clinical practice. First, the therapist cannot assume that any given treatment will be effective in any given case. It is important to monitor treatment effects in an ongoing way to make decisions about continuing or terminating treatment and altering treatment on the basis of how the patient is responding. Some patients make rapid changes quite early in treatment, so-called sudden therapeutic gains (Tang & DeRubeis, 1999); others do not make expected changes and do not respond to treatment, so-called signal-alarm cases (Lambert et al., 2003). Of course, change can occur in some areas but not in others, and change may occur at different rates in the different areas. Systematic evaluation permits finer delineation of therapeutic changes than would be possible with more global clinical judgments and unsystematic assessment.

Second, systematic evaluation is intended to add to clinical evaluation or judgment. There is no need to abandon clinical judgment. However, the need for systematic evaluation stems in part from the limitations of judgment. A discussion of clinical judgment begins with the selectivity of perception, cognitive heuristics, and the utility of clinical predictions. These are weighty concepts, but they point to therapist limitations in perception and cognition in gathering information and drawing conclusions. Systematic measures have their own artifacts and biases, but these can be evaluated and even corrected or taken into account in systematic ways.

Third, clinicians are wont to note the complexity of clinical cases. Clients bring multiple problems to treatment, the problems change as treatment begins, and new problems emerge. Complexity is an argument for systematic evaluation as well. Are the goals of treatment being achieved? Which goals, and to what degree? Are there new goals? Is the patient actually functioning better in everyday life? Systematic evaluation can improve decision making in light of the complexity of the case.

Fourth, systematic information obtained with individuals in clinical practice can greatly contribute to the knowledge base. Systematic assessment and the accumulation of cases can yield new insights even when experimental designs cannot be invoked. Over time, as cases accumulate, analyses can identify client characteristics that may influence outcomes and the course of change in treatment among individuals with different types of problems. Examples of contributions to the knowledge base from accumulated clinical information are evident in private practice (e.g., Clement, 1999), clinics (e.g., Fonagy & Target, 1994), and research settings (e.g., Lambert, Hansen, & Finch, 2001; Lambert et al., 2003). Patient information gathered systematically over the course of treatment can be useful for both generating and testing hypotheses.

STEPS FOR ASSESSMENT AND EVALUATION IN CLINICAL WORK

Suggestions that therapists engage in the systematic evaluation of the individual case are not new and include recommended ways of assessing and reporting cases to improve clinical care and contribute to the knowledge base (e.g., Cone, 2000; Fishman, 2001; Hayes, Barlow, & Nelson, 1999; Kazdin, 1993, 1996; Meier, 2003). These recommendations focus on bridging the methodological gap between clinical work and research. Evaluation can include multiple components including assessment, research design, and data analyses and interpretation. All are relevant to clinical work. However, assessment, as a component of evaluation, includes the most pivotal step for improving clinical work. For present purposes *systematic assessment* refers to the use of measures that provide replicable information and that have evidence in their behalf in relation to various types of reliability and validity as pertinent to their use (e.g., test–retest reliability if used repeatedly, concurrent validity in relation to symptoms or functioning beyond the measurement device).

Systematic assessment and evaluation of the effects of treatment in clinical practice have as their main goal to foster high-quality patient care. Introducing systematic assessment to clinical practice is not merely the addition of a few measures to supplement clinical judgment. Several steps are essential, as summarized in Table 7.1 and elaborated in the sections that follow.

Specifying and Assessing Treatment Goals

Identifying treatment goals is a prerequisite for the selection of measures for assessment and evaluation. Therapy can have many different goals (e.g., reduction of symptoms, improved functioning at home and at work), and these are tailored to individual clients. Prioritizing the goals is important to permit initial assessment and to make treatment decisions. Treatment goals may vary over time on the basis of changing priorities and progress in treatment. For example, excessive dieting and maladaptive food consumption may serve as the initial treatment focus for a young adult referred for an eating disorder. The focus may later shift toward less immediate but no less important domains such as body image, management of stress, and relations with peers.

The notion of goals may unwittingly suggest that treatment always is aiming toward something concrete or a specific end. Therapy may have as a goal helping individuals cope, vent, or tell their stories. Making the goals of treatment explicit is important whether or not the goals are concrete. Explicitness is a condition for assessment of progress over the course of treatment.

Specifying and Assessing Procedures and Processes

Ideally, clinical evaluation specifies the means of achieving the goals. *The means* may refer to the procedures used in treatment—that is, what the therapist does and what he or she asks the client to do in or outside of the sessions. Alternatively, the means may reflect emergent processes or rela-

TABLE 7.1

Five Key Steps for Systematic Evaluation in Clinical Practice

Step	Description
1. Specify and assess treatment goals	Explicitly identify the initial focus of treatment and the goals or changes that are desired. Select or develop a measure that reflects the current status of the individual on these characteristics (e.g., symptoms, functioning).
2. Specify and assess procedures and processes	Explicitly identify the means or processes (procedures, tasks, activities, and experiences) that are expected to lead to therapeutic change. Measure the extent to which these means or their performance, execution, or implementation are achieved during treatment.
3. Select measures	Identify or develop the instruments, scales, or measures that will be used to assess progress over the course of treatment. Identifying the measure of process or procedures depends heavily on whether the procedures are straightforward (e.g., execution of tasks in the session) or emergent processes (e.g., alliance, bonding) that require separate measures.
4. Assess on multiple occasions	Measure performance on the measure of functioning toward which treatment is directed before treatment begins and then on a regular, ongoing basis over the course of treatment. Ongoing assessment may be every session, every other session, or some other regimen that allows the therapist to see any patterns or trends over time.
5. Evaluate the data	Display the information obtained from the assessment to examine changes, patterns, or other features of progress that can directly inform treatment decisions (e.g., changing or ending treatment, shifting the focus of treatment). Graphic displays are especially useful.

tionship issues (e.g., experiencing emotions, developing a therapeutic alliance). Specifying procedures or processes is not an end in itself. The primary goal is to use the information to benefit the client on the basis of how well treatment was implemented and the ends that were achieved.

Ongoing assessment of client progress may reveal that there is no therapeutic change. Assessment of procedures or processes that the therapist believes are important may provide useful information regarding how to proceed. The information may reveal that treatment procedures (e.g., addressing certain topics, engaging in role-play during the sessions) were not implemented very well or that processes within sessions (e.g., developing an alliance, dealing with a particular conflict) did not succeed. Hence, it is reasonable to try different strategies to alter these processes.

Assessment may reveal that the processes have been evoked fairly well but that no therapeutic changes are evident. Of course, patients do not change at the same rate. When enough time has elapsed to question whether change is still likely to occur is not known. (Indeed, data to guide clinical work on this question could readily emerge from systematic data accumulated from clinical practice.) In any case, when the patient has not changed or change is not progressing well, it might be reasonable to try a different treatment. In advance, the therapist needs assurances that he or she tried the procedures or that the processes he or she identified were successful.

Selecting Measures

The next step is to operationalize the constructs by noting the specific measure or measures the therapist will use. Selecting measures requires decisions about the source of information (e.g., self- or clinician report) and assessment method (e.g., objective measures of personality or psychopathology, client diaries, card sorts, interviews, direct observation, biological markers or indexes). In principle, available measures include the full range of psychological instruments.

A few measures are now available that have been well tested in clinical work. For example, the Outcome Questionnaire—45 (OQ–45; Lambert et al., 1996) is a self-report measure designed to measure client progress (e.g., weekly) over the course of treatment and at termination. The measure requires approximately 5 minutes to complete and provides information on four domains of functioning: symptoms of psychological disturbance (primarily depression and anxiety), interpersonal problems, social role functioning (e.g., problems at work), and quality of life (e.g., facets of life satisfaction). Total scores across the 45 items present a global assessment of functioning; the subscales target more specific areas. Research has evaluated different types of reliability and validity, with more than 10,000 patients included in the various reports (see Lambert et al., 2001, 2003).

Another example is the COMPASS Outpatient Treatment Assessment System (Howard, Brill, Lueger, & O'Mahoney, 1992; Lueger et al., 2001), a measure that includes 68 items in three broad scales: Current Well-Being (e.g., health, adjustment, stress, life satisfaction), Current Symptoms (e.g., various symptoms for psychiatric diagnoses), and Current Life Functioning (e.g., work, leisure, family, self-management). Careful psychometric evaluation in the context of clinical application supports the use of the measure in outpatient treatment with adults.

The OQ–45 and the COMPASS System provide a fixed set of items that are quite broad and cover domains likely to be relevant for most adults who come to treatment. Goal Attainment Scaling, alternatively, is an assessment strategy that individualizes treatment goals. The measure is based on collaboration between the patient and therapist at the outset of treatment about the goals and expectations of treatment (Kiresuk & Garwick, 1979; Kiresuk, Smith, & Cardillo, 1994). This measure has been widely used, applied, and validated and is illustrated in a case example later in this chapter.

These three measures are major options that have been carefully studied and have wide applicability to patients seen in outpatient or inpatient treatment. Other measures useful in clinical work that draw on a variety of different assessment methods have been identified elsewhere (e.g., Alter & Evens, 1990; Faulkner & Gray Health Care Information Center, 1997; Meier, 2003). Rating scales are a particularly useful format that allow an endless array of options to be developed and evaluated (see Aiken, 1996). Diverse measures have been developed and formatted to facilitate their use in clinical settings (Clement, 1999; Wiger, 1999).

In addition to measurement of client functioning, measurement of treatment means or processes is important as well. The specific types of treatment and putative processes or features leading to change dictate the assessment focus. The therapist proposes (hypothesizes) that specific means are central to therapeutic change. If these means (e.g., quality of the relationship with the client, completion of specific homework assignments) can vary with treatment administration, their assessment is likely to be useful. The assessment priority is evaluating clinical outcomes and systematically collecting information on whether the client is changing over the course of treatment.

Assessing on Multiple Occasions

The major change that is needed in clinical practice is ongoing, continuous assessment during the course of treatment. Ongoing assessment can be used to chart where the client is at the beginning of treatment and to see whether changes are made over time. Several data points are needed not only to assess the mean level of functioning over time but also to give an idea of variability and trends on the measure. There are many opportunities for flexible application of continuous assessment. Ideally, but perhaps unrealistically, pretreatment assessment would include two or three assessment occasions to provide a baseline to help evaluate subsequent progress. Also, at initial assessment the client's level of performance on the measure may be at an extreme because of stress or crisis, and marked changes from the first to second assessment occasion can be expected because of statistical regression, passing of the crisis, and repeat testing (see Kazdin, 2003). Assessment before beginning the intervention may even show improvement in the client's status and hence has implications for reevaluating the goals of treatment, the means to obtain them, and the measures to evaluate progress.

The initial assessment provides descriptive information (baseline) about the client's level of performance and its variation. Perhaps only one assessment occasion is feasible, or indeed no assessment may be feasible because of the urgent nature of the treatment. For most psychotherapy clients, it is not clear that intervention is absolutely essential at the first contact. Usually, assessment can begin while efforts to manage the situation are under way. When treatment begins immediately, it may be possible to obtain a retrospective baseline in which the client and others in his or her life provide an estimate of the client's recent functioning. Apart from baseline assessment, evaluation during the treatment phase is pivotal to gauge whether any changes are being made and whether the magnitude and rate of these changes are important clinically.

Evaluating the Data

Data evaluation refers to the use and interpretation of the assessment information. Two issues emerge in clinical care. First, one must decide whether change has occurred, is reliable, and departs from the fluctuations one would expect without the intervention. Second, are the changes important, and do they make a difference in the patient's life?

Ongoing assessment provides data before and during the course of treatment that serve as the basis for evaluating whether the changes are reliable and beyond routine fluctuations. Several methods are available to evaluate the reliability of the information (Kazdin, 2003). Of all methods, graphic display (e.g., a simple line graph) is particularly useful for seeing the pattern in the data obtained over time. Nonstatistical data evaluation methods (changes in means, levels, slope, latency of change over time) are used extensively in single-case research (applied behavior analysis) focused on interventions for diverse client and community populations and can be used for clinical evaluation (see Kazdin, 1982; Parsonson & Baer, 1978). Nonstatistical data evaluation does not require complex computations but follows directly from graphic presentation of the data. Other methods of graphing than a simple line graph (e.g., stem-and-leaf plots, box plots), usually used for multiple subjects from group research, might also be used to plot multiple data points from individual clients (see Meier, 2003; Rosenthal & Rosnow, 1991). If a patient's data are entered regularly on a database or office management system, then graphical presentation and simple slope or trend lines (e.g., regression lines) can be plotted automatically, as illustrated later.[1]

In addition, there is interest in evaluating whether the changes made in treatment are clinically significant—that is, whether they make a difference to the client. Several measures of clinical significance have been used in treatment research, including whether level of functioning at the end of treatment falls within the normative range of individuals functioning adequately to well in everyday life, whether the individual makes a change that is large (e.g., in standard deviation units) on the measure, and whether the individual no longer meets criteria for a diagnosis that were met at intake (see Kazdin, 1999; Kendall, 1999). These measures all have interpretative

---

[1]Statistical tests are available as well to consider changes over time and whether these changes are reliable according to the usual standards of research (Kazdin, 1982). I mention these only to note their availability. The value of identifying whether a particular change is or is not statistically significant is questionable in research (see Kazdin, 2003). Few would lobby for the use of statistical significance in clinical applications with individual patients. Yet some means of identifying whether the change is reliable is needed.

problems insofar as there are little or no data showing that someone who has made a change labeled as clinically significant is in fact functioning palpably better in the world (Kazdin, 2001). That said, these measures, especially the one in which a large change in the measure is required, have been applied in clinical work (Lambert et al., 2003; Lueger et al., 2001).

Some effort is needed to evaluate whether the treatment goals are approached or attained and whether the changes make a difference. With some clinical problems (e.g., panic attacks, tics), elimination of the problem can be taken as a clinically important change. With other problems (e.g., obesity), clinically important change may involve reduction of the problem to levels that improve health consequences (risk). These types of clinical problems are exceptions in the course of psychotherapy, however. Whether impairment declines, symptoms improve, marriages are better, and the experience of loss is alleviated are matters of degree, and whether the amount of change is helpful or enough is difficult to discern. Indeed, the same amount of change on a measure (e.g., of marital satisfaction) or set of measures may be experienced quite differently among patients and may have a varied impact on everyday life (e.g., whether they remain or do not remain married).

CASE ILLUSTRATION

The following case study highlights the steps outlined in previous sections and illustrates how they can be applied. The description emphasizes assessment and evaluation, rather than the details of the intervention itself.

Brief Background

Gloria was a European American, 39-year-old woman who referred herself for outpatient treatment. She was married and had two children (ages 16 and 17). She and her husband were both college educated; on the basis of her education and income and her husband's occupation, they were middle class. Gloria was not employed outside of the home; her husband was a manager of a computer software firm. She and her husband had been married for 18 years.

Gloria scheduled an appointment because she said she was depressed and needed to talk to someone. During the initial interview at the clinic, Gloria saw a male therapist, who asked, with open-ended questioning, about the reasons she sought treatment, sources of satisfaction and dissatisfaction in her life, relationships with significant others, symptoms, and related matters. Toward the end of this discussion, the therapist queried Gloria about what she expected and wished to obtain from treatment.

During the interview, Gloria indicated that she had been treated for depression on two separate occasions in her life, once during college and once after the birth of her first child. On each occasion she was placed on medication. She reported some relief but also complained about side effects and did not feel really helped overall with her problems. Currently, she said, she was depressed again. She reported feeling "empty and lost" about her life and marriage. She said that she lacked meaning and direction in her life. She felt alienated from her husband and her children. In the case of her husband, she felt great emotional distance because of years of reduced intimacy, joint activity, and time together. Her children were very important to her, but she felt they did not need her very much now that they were teenagers. Gloria identified as her own goals for treatment simply feeling better about her life, not being depressed, having some direction, and improving relations with her spouse and others.

Assessment

In the initial interview, the therapist introduced systematic assessment after the open-ended discussion provided an initial formulation of the focus. He explained that the assessment procedures would help make the goals and directions of treatment more explicit and quantify the domains that were to be the foci. The therapist used three measures. The first measure was adapted from Goal Attainment Scaling (Kiresuk et al., 1994), which was developed decades ago as a general method to evaluate outcomes of mental health treatment, has been widely applied and tested, and has extensive information on psychometric properties, training, and use. The scale identifies individualized goals of treatment to reflect the domains pertinent to the patient. The therapist adapted the method to focus on the domains Gloria identified as important. Toward the end of the interview, the therapist identified four major concerns, themes, or areas as a beginning for them to work on (a) depressive thoughts and feelings, (b) little involvement in meaningful and fulfilling activities, (c) disengagement from her family, and (d) lack of supportive contacts outside of the home. The therapist and Gloria discussed these to see if they captured Gloria's experience, because they did not follow exactly from her original formulation of the problems.

For each theme, the therapist asked Gloria to help construct statements that they then graded to indicate different levels of functioning. The goal was to compose a 4-point scale for each theme in which 1 = *worsening of the problem*, 2 = *no change in current functioning or feelings*, 3 = *some improvement*, and 4 = *attainment of goal of functioning and feeling on this domain*. The therapist referred to this as the Gloria Scale (G Scale for short) and explained that it would help guide them during treatment. The therapist conveyed the concept of the 4-point scale, but Gloria provided the content of each of the statements. The therapist asked her to describe a way to characterize her current functioning or where she was now, what it would be like if she became worse, what some improvement might look like, and how things would

TABLE 7.2
TABLE 7.2
Four Themes and Items for the Gloria Scale

Theme	Items
Depressive thoughts and feelings	1. I feel more depressed and dejected than I did before I started treatment. 2. I feel about the same level of depression and dejection as I did when I started. 3. I feel a little better about my mood, and things are not as bad as before. 4. I feel a lot better, I do not think about my feelings as negative, and I have more energy to get out and do things.
Involvement in meaningful and fulfilling activities	1. I really feel paralyzed about doing anything any more. 2. I am not doing anything differently now or anything special I like compared with when I started treatment. 3. I feel better that I have some direction and focus in what to do. 4. I am totally involved in some things, such as a career, that give me good feelings about life.
Disengagement from family	1. I do less with my husband and children than before and don't seem to care about doing things with them. 2. Things really have not changed about my feelings. Everyone at home does his or her own thing, and my husband and I mostly just eat meals together. 3. My husband and I are a little better. We go out once in a while and are a couple again. 4. My husband and I are really "together." We are intimate in many ways, and I can feel that he cares for me.
Supportive contacts outside the home	1. I am isolated from people in general, including my relatives who live in town. 2. Once in a while I see someone when I shop or at a school event with my children. We chat a bit, but nothing beyond the superficial. 3. I meet someone to have coffee with or to go to an event or shopping with during the day. 4. I meet a few people by myself or some couples that my husband and I can get together with, and we do this on a regular basis.

Note. The theme areas were derived from an open-ended interview with Gloria. The specific statements were generated by her to reflect what it would be like to become worse, to remain the same, to improve a little, and to achieve her goal for that theme. These alternative outcomes reflect Items 1 through 4 respectively under each theme. Each time she completed this measure, Gloria selected the statement under each theme that was closest to how she had felt during the previous week. From *Research Design in Clinical Psychology* (4th ed., p. 320), by A. E. Kazdin, 2003, Boston: Allyn & Bacon. Copyright 2003 by Allyn & Bacon. Reprinted with permission.

be if she really made the kind of change she wanted. Table 7.2 presents the four themes and the graded statements Gloria and the therapist constructed. For the assessment on the G Scale, she was instructed to select the statement under each theme that characterized how she had felt during the previous week. After they had developed the scale in the initial session, the therapist asked Gloria specifically if the second statement of each theme area really captured her current feelings; she reported that it did.

The therapist described two other measures and gave them to Gloria to complete. The Beck Depression Inventory (BDI; Beck, Steer, & Garbin, 1988) addressed the severity of her depressive symptoms. This measure includes 21 items; for each item, the client selects 1 of 5 statements reflecting differing severity of depressive symptoms (each item is scored 1–3). Gloria also completed the Quality of Life Inventory (QOLI; Frisch, 1998), a self-report scale that assesses overall quality of and satisfaction with life in 17 domains (e.g., love relationship, home, learning, recreation, friendships, philosophy of life, work, health, neighborhood). The weighted score is used for each domain on the basis of the client's rating of the importance of that domain in his or her life (0 = *not at all important*, 2 = *very important*) then multiplied by the satisfaction derived from that domain (–3 = *very dissatisfied* to +3 = *very satisfied*). The BDI and QOLI took approximately 20 minutes total to complete.

The initial contact with Gloria lasted about 2 hours. The interview and development of the G Scale took about 1.5 hours, and completion of the BDI and QOLI took the rest of the time. Gloria was scheduled to return the following week and was asked to come 20 minutes before the session. Before the second session began, she completed the BDI and QOLI and brought them to the therapist.

The therapist began the session by asking Gloria to select one statement from each of the four theme areas that they had discussed. The material had now been typed in a format similar to that of Table 7.2. They briefly discussed whether the areas were still important to her and whether she felt that their last interview had missed critical material. The therapist conveyed that the initial goals were a place to begin and that the information within the sessions and from the assessments would be important to make any midcourse corrections as needed.

At this point, the therapist described the treatment and said that it would take place on a weekly basis. The therapist selected treatment that combined cognitive therapy with interpersonal psychotherapy. Cognitive therapy focused on Gloria's maladaptive cognitions about herself related to her depressive affect, poor self-esteem, feelings that life was not worthwhile, and internal attributions regarding her views of herself (see Beck, Rush, Shaw, & Emery, 1979). Interpersonal psychotherapy focused on her interpersonal relations, her roles and the sources of satisfaction and emotion associated with each, and her feelings about herself as a spouse and parent (see Klerman, Weissman, Rounsaville, & Chevron, 1984). The therapy integrated these treatments and included assignments (e.g., shared activities with her husband) carried out between the sessions.

Each week, Gloria came about 20 minutes before the session to complete the G Scale, BDI, and QOLI. At the first and second sessions, the full scales were administered. However, there were symptoms and domains within the two standardized scales that were not problematic or not seemingly relevant to Gloria. The therapist constructed abbreviated versions of the BDI (15 items) and the QOLI (13 domains) by eliminating selected items, and they used these versions throughout treatment. From each scale, the therapist quantified Gloria's performance with a summary total score for each measure to examine whether any systematic pattern or change was evident as treatment progressed. The assessment information is graphed in Figure 7.1. The two assessment occasions before treatment were delineated as baseline (Weeks B1 and B2 in the figure). The therapist added a linear regression line to each graph to characterize the slope that best fit the data. Overall, the individual data points and regression line suggest that Gloria showed improvement over time.

Although the overall scores are useful in summary form, the mean for all of the items of a given measure (e.g., BDI) with an individual case can suffer the same liability as means in group research—namely, they can obscure critical information. In Gloria's case, the G scale and the QOLI indicated that she had made little progress in her relationship with her husband. The relationship issues emerged more fully in the treatment session of Week 14. At the beginning of the session, the therapist indicated that he thought this would be a good time to discuss at length the original goals of treatment and how she had been doing on the basis of the assessment information and Gloria's appraisal of treatment.

Gloria indicated that she had felt much better about herself and her life. Her thoughts about her life, what she saw as important, and her direction were much better. Over the course of treatment, she had initiated a number of activities. She had begun a class at a local university and now planned to obtain a degree in nursing. She had developed greater interaction with a neighbor, a woman similar to her in age, whom she met almost daily to engage in routine activities (e.g., exercise, shopping). Also, from her class she met a few people whom she enjoyed. Finally, time with her children was more enjoyable. In general, she felt much better about her overall well-being. At the same time, she felt that her relationship with her husband had not been helped at all by treatment. Although she and her husband had gone out on a couple of dates, she felt that this was merely time together with no connection or closeness. She said she loved her husband and could not imagine being without him but that there seemed to be none of the closeness or contact they had experienced in the past. The therapist suggested that they focus more on this issue for a few sessions but that the immediate goal would be for her and her husband to consider joint steps toward improving their marriage. They then used the same method as that for developing the G Scale to identify theme areas within her marriage that were significant and to set anchor points and added this measure to Gloria's routine assessments.

Treatment continued for 5 more weeks. Gloria no longer completed the BDI and QOLI weekly, instead completing them every other week. Weekly

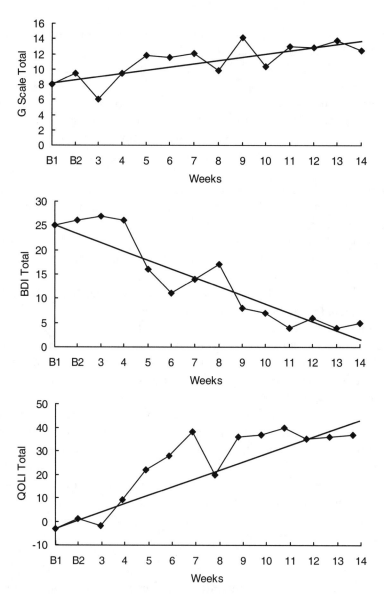

Figure 7.1. Session-by-session scores for Gloria on three measures including the Gloria Scale (G Scale, upper panel), the modified Beck Depression Inventory (BDI, middle panel), and the modified Quality of Life Inventory (QOLI, lower panel). The scores for each measure (BDI and QOLI) include items that were selected as relevant to the client and do not reflect the complete scales. Data are presented for 14 sessions (weeks). The first week was devoted entirely to interview and assessment. The second week began with completion of assessments followed by the initiation of treatment. The first two weeks (B1, B2) refer to baseline or pretreatment assessment. Given the direction of scoring of the measures, improvement would be reflected in increases for the G Scale and QOLI and a decrease in the BDI. Fitted to each graph is a linear regression line over the course of all data points. From *Research Design in Clinical Psychology* (4th ed., p. 322), by A. E. Kazdin, 2003, Boston: Allyn & Bacon. Copyright 2003 by Allyn & Bacon. Reprinted with permission.

assessment continued for the original G Scale and for the scale related specifically to her marital relationship. After 5 weeks, Gloria and her husband agreed to begin marital counseling, and Gloria ceased individual treatment.

Discussion

There are useful features of this case that illustrate evaluation in clinical practice. First, the therapist made efforts to make the initial goals of treatment explicit and to quantify them. Second, the therapist used systematic, clinically relevant, and user-friendly assessments. The assessment procedures included a highly individualized scale, the Gloria Scale. The therapist altered the two standardized measures (BDI, QOLI) to address the specific domains that seemed relevant to the client. Finally, he charted the information to evaluate Gloria's progress and used this information both to alter treatment and to suggest the need for further assessment and treatment.

Many limitations are apparent as well. First, the three measures overlapped in method (all self-report), and all were conducted in the treatment setting. Other methods (e.g., spouse ratings, daily log of activities during the week) may have been useful as well. Second, the therapist might have identified the issue of marital dissatisfaction earlier and given it a more central role early in treatment. Perhaps the marital issues became more salient as treatment progressed precisely because the client felt progress in other domains. Third, the regression lines must be interpreted cautiously. The lines suggest an overall improvement and hence are very useful in conveying a pattern, but the changes over time cannot be interpreted as being the result of treatment. Finally, the case description does not give an idea of how well Gloria adhered to the tasks in the session or performed the homework assignments. Whether she adhered to assignments and whether the therapist felt that cognitive issues and interpersonal functioning were suitably addressed within each session are important considerations.

Overall, the case illustration highlights the use of systematic assessment and evaluation. The assessment was individualized but also included standardized measures pertinent to the treatment focus. The measures required 20 minutes to complete before each session. Other measures are available that encompass multiple areas of functioning but require much less time for administration (e.g., 5 minutes for the OQ–45). Also, the data obtained during treatment were useful not only in evaluating progress but also in making decisions about the focus of treatment over time.

ISSUES AND LIMITATIONS IN
SYSTEMATIC ASSESSMENT AND EVALUATION

Systematic assessment and evaluation can be readily implemented in clinical work to improve the therapist's inferences about whether change occurs, the importance or extent of the change, and even the likelihood that treatment is responsible for the change. Yet there remain some obstacles to implementation.

Methodological Issues

Few measures are available that are clinically feasible and validated for clinical work. *Feasible* means user friendly and brief; *validated* refers to all of the usual concepts of validity but also to validity over time with multiple and repeated assessments. Progress has been made in identifying measures that can be used in individual therapy, that can be applied widely across clinical settings and clients, and that can provide information that contributes to the knowledge base more generally (e.g., Barkham et al., 2001; Kordy, Hannöver, & Richard, 2001).

Another issue pertains to evaluation of what factors might contribute to change. Valuable additions to evaluation efforts include assessment of the therapeutic process (e.g., relationship and alliance), of the various activities or exercises that treatment may depend on, and of other aspects of treatment. Clearly, the initial priority is to identify whether a given patient does improve and improves adequately. As this aspect of evaluation becomes more routine, the therapist might make more effort to evaluate possible mediators of change.

Finally, how to evaluate the data obtained from the measures raises several issues. Descriptive statistics (e.g., changes in means, slope) can be used for inferential purposes. Various data management programs can be used to enter data, to provide graphic displays, and to document progress in user-friendly ways (e.g., OPTAIO, 1997). Yet what decisions ought to be made from the data, and on the basis of what criteria? The patient may have made a clinically significant and important change, but with only rare exceptions researchers do not yet know how changes on measures used to evaluate treatment translate to actual changes in everyday life (Kazdin, 2001). Research is needed to understand the amount and type of change in treatment that constitute effects that genuinely benefit individual patients.

Clinical Issues and Concerns

Several concerns and objections may emerge in clinical practice about the utility of systematic assessment and evaluation. First, therapists are often concerned that assessment may interfere with the therapeutic relationship. The therapist is responsible for treatment; adding to that the role of the assessor or evaluator may, on conceptual grounds, mix roles and be viewed as antitherapeutic. Yet the presumption that evaluation harms is arguable; indeed, alternative assumptions are plausible as well (e.g., that not evaluating the patient can permit harm to occur, that evaluation may have no impact, that evaluation may help). How clients perceive systematic evaluation probably depends on the therapist's views of evaluation and presentation of the evaluation objectives and methods. If evaluation is presented as a matter of course, as central to treatment, and as purposeful, then the client's views are likely to be positive.

Second, measures of a clinical problem may oversimplify the problem. Yet for a measure to be useful, it need not capture all there is about the construct. A measure provides a key sign, correlate, or sample of the problem—that is, an operational definition. Therapists usually are not interested in measures, but rather in constructs, or the characteristics the measures were designed to assess. They use measures even though they do not cover the entire scope of the problem.

A third and related concern is that assessment seemingly ignores the individuality or uniqueness of the client. Yet systematic assessment can be quite individualized, as exemplified in the case example. The clinician can decide with the patient which domains of functioning are most relevant and can build the assessment devices to reflect those domains. Clinical practice, unlike the usual research context, permits individualization of both assessment and treatment. Standardized assessment may still play a critically important role in therapy and can complement individualized assessment in critical ways. A client's profile on a standardized measure and his or her standing relative to a normative group of peers of the same age, sex, and ethnicity, for example, can provide meaningful data that may also guide treatment. The standardized nature of a measure is not a threat to patient individuality, but rather an opportunity to examine that individuality against a broader backdrop.

Fourth, an objection to evaluation in clinical work is based on the dynamic nature of treatment. In much of psychotherapy, there is not a single, simple patient problem that remains constant. Indeed, over half of clients seen in therapy add new target complaints over the course of treatment (Sorenson, Gorsuch, & Mintz, 1985). The changing focus of treatment and the multifaceted nature of the foci are not arguments against assessment. Rather, they make systematic assessment all the more important. It is critical to identify changes in problem domains and priorities from the standpoint of the patient and therapist. Therapists and clients can set new goals and present or withdraw assessments to reflect these changes.

If the goal of clinical work is to help patients and to address the concerns of a specific individual, here and now, then the case for systematic evaluation is easily made. In fact, the case does not need to be made for systematic assessment and evaluation. Just the opposite—in clinical work, where the individual patient is so important and direct benefits are the goal, unsystematic evaluation is difficult to justify. There are clearly urgent circumstances in which intervention must proceed immediately (e.g., disasters, suicide attempts in progress). The important exceptions certainly preclude collecting baseline data, but they do not preclude evaluating the impact after the crises have abated.

IMPEDIMENTS TO CLINICAL EVALUATION

Introducing systematic evaluation into clinical practice can be readily accomplished. The steps are not too complex or onerous, assessment tools are available, and the yield from these tools has been shown to be useful in large-scale evaluations with many individual cases. Systematic evaluation is not in the mindset of most clinicians, clinic directors, residency and internship training directors, and clinical supervisors who oversee treatment. Clinicians are often faulted for their disinterest in evaluation in clinical work. Yet clinical training, whether in psychology, psychiatry, social work, or counseling, does not equip individuals to evaluate their cases in user-friendly and methodologically sound ways.

Psychotherapy Outcome Research

Psychotherapy outcome research is dominated by randomized controlled clinical trials (RCTs). Such trials are recognized to have special status with regard to testing interventions effects. My comments are not intended to impugn such trials. However, pivotal features of these trials make them not very relevant for clinical practice. Endless discussions have been provided about the conditions of testing treatment (e.g., efficacy studies) and how the results may not be generalizable to clinical practice. I wish to convey a point different from this now well-worn path: The methods, as well as the results, of RCTs are not generalizable to clinical practice. Methodological features of RCTs make them largely of little relevance to clinical work and unwittingly may impede evaluation in clinical practice.

RCTs of psychotherapy are characterized by pre- and posttreatment assessment and comparison of means between conditions (e.g., treatment and control groups) using statistical analyses of the data. These methodological features have no useful counterpart for treatment evaluation in clinical practice. In clinical work, therapists do not wish to give a fixed regimen of treatment and see how the patient has done after treatment has ended. To be sure, they do want to know how the patient is doing at the end of treatment, but they care just as much about assessment during treatment so they can make changes if and as needed or indeed stop the treatment because of early gains. RCTs do not provide methods that can be extended to address the priorities of clinical care. Therapists in any of the clinical disciplines who have been trained in research methods can extend few or none of the methods they have learned to clinical work.

A relatively recent development in treatment outcome studies is referred to as *patient-oriented research* (Howard, Moras, Brill, Martinovich, &

Lutz, 1996; Lambert et al., 2003). The key to patient-oriented research is ongoing assessment and monitoring of individual patients from the beginning to the end of treatment and use of the information to chart progress and make decisions about treatment. Unlike RCTs, patient-oriented research does not involve an extensive battery of pre- and posttreatment assessments. Rather, therapists conduct assessment at each session with a brief measure that captures functioning in diverse domains. The OQ–45 (Lambert et al., 1996) is one such brief measure. The measure requires only minutes to complete and provides information about multiple domains. The therapist evaluates the treatment by discerning the extent to which the client makes a change or fails to make a change. During treatment, different criteria can be used to guide treatment decisions (see Lambert et al., 2001, 2003). Patient-oriented research greatly reduces the gap between research and practice. The methods used in clinical research and practice become one and the same. Patient-oriented research provides a methodology that could be added to training to help would-be therapists become more interested in systematic evaluation of the treatment they provide.

Training in Alternative Methodologies

My comments on RCTs focused narrowly on the common model for psychotherapy outcome research. The comments apply more broadly to quantitative research methods involving group designs, null hypothesis testing, and statistical evaluation. But there are other research methods routinely omitted from training that offer great promise for and applicability to clinical work. The following paragraphs highlight three alternatives.

First, qualitative research methods are extremely relevant to clinical work. Qualitative research has its own methodology, including strategies for assessment, design, and data evaluation.[2] Qualitative research seeks knowledge in ways that are systematic, replicable, and cumulative. The methods look at phenomena in ways that are intended to reveal many of those facets of human experience that the quantitative tradition has been designed to circumvent—the human experience, subjective views, and how people represent (perceive, feel) and react to their situations in context. For example, quantitative research has elaborated many of the factors that contribute to or are associated with homelessness. Predictors of homelessness, the relative weight of these predictors, and the short- and long-term effects of homelessness (e.g., medical, psychiatric) on adults, children, and families have been elaborated in quantitative research. A qualitative study is likely to focus on the

---

[2]In clinical work, *qualitative* is sometimes used to refer to descriptive, anecdotal, and case study material. That is, the term has been inappropriately adopted to refer to any nonquantitative evaluation. This is a misuse—*qualitative* is not a synonym for loose or unsystematic data or "my opinions." Indeed, it is an antonym for these characteristics. Qualitative research is rigorous, scientific, disciplined, and replicable and can both test and generate theory.

experience of being homeless, the details of the frustrations, and the conflicts and demands the experience raises in ways that are not captured by quantitative studies (e.g., Lindsey, 1998). Clinical psychology and related disciplines that have clinical practice as a career path rarely train students in qualitative research methods. This is unfortunate, because the methodology and its many rich variations provide options that would be well suited to promote understanding of the individual experience of patients, to systematically codify treatment changes, and to do so in replicable ways.

Second, single-case experimental designs have features that are readily adaptable to clinical work. Single-case experiment designs emerged from laboratory research with humans and other animals to study such basic processes as learning and performance. They have been used quite extensively in an area referred to as *applied behavior analysis* in which interventions are used to address goals of clinical dysfunction, education, rehabilitation, health, and scores of domains of functioning in everyday life (e.g., the home, business, and industry; see Kazdin, 2001). The designs are rigorous and can yield causal inferences, as that term is used in science. Among their key features, single-case experiments consist of multiple observations with one or a few cases, in sharp contrast to typical group experiments in which few observations (e.g., pretreatment, posttreatment) are made with multiple subjects. User-friendly variations of the designs provide tools that can be used to evaluate and to improve patient care in clinical work (e.g., Hayes et al., 1999; Kazdin, 1981, 2003). As with qualitative research, these designs are rarely included in clinical training in the mental health professions.

Finally, the case study, with all of its problems, can provide useful information and even permit strong inferences (see Sechrest, Stewart, Stickle, & Sidani, 1996). Among the issues with this methodology is understanding what sorts of influences compete with drawing inferences about events that happen with the case, how these influences might be combated or made implausible, and when and how can inferences be drawn as a result. The anecdotal case study as traditionally conceived and implemented is not the only alternative. There is much a clinician can do to bolster the quality of the inferences he or she draws about patient change and the reasons for change, but these techniques are rarely taught (Kazdin, 1981). Learning about the strengths of the case study and the underlying thought processes that can increase its yield would be enormously helpful in clinical training and ultimately in patient care.

I mention three methodologies here in addition to the quantitative tradition. These other three methodologies are much more readily adaptable to the questions and conditions of clinical practice than the methods in which mental health professionals are routinely trained. It is quite easy to point to a seeming antidata and antievaluation mindset among those in clinical practice. But probing a little deeper conveys that the training necessary for therapists to do evaluation in clinical work has not been and is not being provided.

General Comments

Training in psychology and science more generally is designed to teach substance (content areas of interest), methods (assessment, design), and a broader approach to science. This broader approach is a way of thinking about phenomena and systematizing the information one obtains to draw inferences. The thought processes reflect concerns about ways of operationalizing critical constructs, posing hypotheses about interventions and processes leading to change, and testing assumptions about interventions and their impact. Assessment, research design, and evaluation are not alien to clinical practice. Invariably, practitioners are drawing inferences, actively or passively making decisions regarding what they perceive, and so on. Introducing systematic assessment into clinical work brings these practices in harmony with tenets of science (e.g., testing hypotheses, operationalizing critical concepts, fostering replication). The special feature is to use evaluation concepts and practices to advance the therapeutic progress of individual clients.

The priority of the client and concerns for client well-being have been used as arguments for not evaluating treatment progress systematically. I would argue a fortiori that when the goal is to help someone and to address the needs, concerns, or desperation often evident in clinical work, assessment, evaluation, and drawing informed inferences are more important than ever. Much of the thinking underlying training appears to foster dichotomies in which research tenets and priorities (e.g., careful and systematic observation, collection of replicable data, focus on group designs) are contrasted with the priorities of clinical practice (e.g., concern for individuals and their unique circumstances, narrative and in-depth evaluation that is more qualitative). There is no need for these dichotomies, and patient care is the victim when they are fostered.

CONCLUSION

This chapter has advocated and illustrated systematic evaluation in clinical practice as a means to improve the quality of clinical care. Several steps for systematic evaluation were discussed, including specifying and assessing treatment goals, specifying and assessing procedures and processes, selecting measures, assessing on multiple occasions, and evaluating the data. A clinical case illustrated the use of these steps to convey the use of systematic evaluation in clinical work. Methodology and evaluation are not just for empirical research; they are for instances in which the clinician wants to know whether there is a change, difference, or effect and to isolate possible reasons.

An important point of departure for evaluation in clinical practice is the goal of the benefit of the individual patient. Assessment methods must be able to accommodate a wide range of clinical problems and situations. There are two major challenges. First, psychologists must develop practices and procedures that can easily be integrated into clinical practice. Much progress has been made on this front; a few well-validated measures are available for clinical use. Technological innovations using various everyday gadgets (e.g., scheduling devices, cell phones with cameras) are likely to increase assessment options. The challenge of implementing evaluation in clinical work is not related to the paucity of tools, even though more and better tools will always be welcome.

Currently, the training of clinicians is a huge impediment to integrating evaluation into practice. Clinical evaluation needs to be conveyed as pivotal to patient care. Patient care and high-quality clinical work demand that clinicians use the best treatments and evaluation tools to evaluate their impact. The personal judgment and experience of a therapist, although clearly valuable, are not a substitute for the collection of systematic information and the use of that information in making critical decisions.

There is a seeming resistance among clinicians to conduct systematic evaluation or to use their scientific thinking for clinical work. In this regard, I very much favor the so-called medical models. In the context of medical problems, it would be poor practice, if not unethical, to conduct an evaluation without using medical tests and a thorough workup to provide solid information about the problem, where possible. A physician who has experience with many patients with similar symptoms is of great benefit. It would be of even more benefit if that physician drew on the amazing array of systematic assessments (e.g., blood work, scans of various sorts) that can rule in or rule out problems and that can be used to monitor whether the intervention, once initiated, is having any effect. One would not think of administering chemotherapy or surgery without evaluating over time the impact and durability of their effects. Unsystematic and loose assessment has its place too; "How are you feeling? Can you get around very much? How was your week?" are all part of bedside manner and could be recorded systematically, but usually are not. In the clinical practice of psychotherapy, there is little evaluation that is systematic. The stereotype of clinicians is that they enter clinical work in part because they care for people and are less interested in data and research. Let us hope this stereotype is a straw person. Clinicians want evaluation in clinical practice precisely because they care about the individual patient.

REFERENCES

Aiken, L. R. (1996). *Rating scales and checklists: Evaluating behavior, personality, and attitude.* New York: Wiley.

Alter, C., & Evens, W. (1990). *Evaluating your practice: A guide to self-assessment.* New York: Springer.

Barkham, M., Margison, F., Leach, C., Lucock, M., Mellor-Clark, J., Evans, C., et al. (2001). Service profiling and outcomes benchmarking using the CORE–OM: Toward practice-based evidence in the psychological therapies. *Journal of Consulting and Clinical Psychology, 69,* 184–196.

Beck, A. T., Rush, A. J., Shaw, B. F., & Emery, G. (1979). *Cognitive therapy of depression.* New York: Guilford Press.

Beck, A. T., Steer, R. A., & Garbin, M. G. (1988). Psychometric properties of the Beck Depression Inventory: Twenty-five years of evaluation. *Clinical Psychology Review, 8,* 77–100.

Borkovec, T., & Rachman, S. (1979). The utility of analogue research. *Behaviour Research and Therapy, 17,* 253–261.

Clement, P. W. (1999). *Outcomes and incomes: How to evaluate, improve, and market your practice by measuring outcomes in psychotherapy.* New York: Guilford Press.

Cone, J. D. (2000). *Evaluating outcomes: Empirical tools for effective practice.* Washington, DC: American Psychological Association.

Faulkner & Gray Health Care Information Center. (1997). *The 1997 behavioral outcomes and guidelines sourcebook.* New York: Author.

Fishman, D. B. (2001). From single case to database: A new method for enhancing psychotherapy, forensic, and other psychological practice. *Applied & Preventive Psychology, 10,* 275–304.

Fonagy, P., & Target, M. (1994). The efficacy of psychoanalysis for children with disruptive disorders. *Journal of the American Academy of Child and Adolescent Psychiatry, 33,* 45–55.

Frisch, M. B. (1998). Quality of life therapy and assessment in health care. *Clinical Psychology: Science and Practice, 5,* 19–40.

Hayes, S. C., Barlow, D. H., & Nelson, R. O. (1999). *The scientist–practitioner: Research and accountability in clinical and educational settings* (2nd ed.). New York: Pergamon Press.

Heller, K. (1971). Laboratory interview research as an analogue to treatment. In A. E. Bergin & S. L. Garfield (Eds.), *Handbook of psychotherapy and behavior change: An empirical analysis* (pp. 126–153). New York: Wiley.

Hoagwood, K., Hibbs, E., Brent, D., & Jensen, P. J. (1995). Efficacy and effectiveness in studies of child and adolescent psychotherapy. *Journal of Consulting and Clinical Psychology, 63,* 683–687.

Howard, K. I., Brill, P. L., Lueger, R. J., & O'Mahoney, M. T. (1992). *Integra Outpatient Tracking Assessment.* Radnor, PA: Integra.

Howard, K. I., Moras, K., Brill, P. L., Martinovich, Z., & Lutz, W. (1996). Efficacy, effectiveness, and patient progress. *American Psychologist, 51,* 1059–1064.

Kazdin, A. E. (1978). Evaluating the generality of findings in analogue therapy research. *Journal of Consulting and Clinical Psychology, 46,* 673–686.

Kazdin, A. E. (1981). Drawing valid inferences from case studies. *Journal of Consulting and Clinical Psychology, 49,* 183–192.

Kazdin, A. E. (1982). *Single-case research designs: Methods for clinical and applied settings.* New York: Oxford University Press.

Kazdin, A. E. (1993). Evaluation in clinical practice: Clinically sensitive and systematic methods of treatment delivery. *Behavior Therapy, 24,* 11–45.

Kazdin, A. E. (Ed.). (1996). Special section: Evaluation in clinical practice. *Clinical Psychology: Science and Practice, 3,* 144–181.

Kazdin, A. E. (1999). The meanings and measurement of clinical significance. *Journal of Consulting and Clinical Psychology, 67,* 332–339.

Kazdin, A. E. (2001). Almost clinically significant ($p < .10$): Current measures may only approach clinical significance. *Clinical Psychology: Science and Practice, 8,* 455–462.

Kazdin, A. E. (2003). *Research design in clinical psychology* (4th ed.). Needham Heights, MA: Allyn & Bacon.

Kendall, P. C. (Ed.). (1999). Special section: Clinical significance. *Journal of Consulting and Clinical Psychology, 67,* 283–339.

Kiresuk, T. J., & Garwick, G. (1979). Basic Goal Attainment Scaling procedures. In B. R. Compton & B. Gallaway (Eds.), *Social work processes* (Rev. ed., pp. 412–420). Homewood, IL: Dorsey.

Kiresuk, T. J., Smith, A., & Cardillo, J. E. (1994). *Goal Attainment Scaling: Applications, theory, and measurement.* Hillsdale, NJ: Erlbaum.

Klerman, G. L., Weissman, M. M., Rounsaville, B. J., & Chevron, E. (1984). *Interpersonal psychotherapy of depression.* New York: Basic Books.

Kordy, H., Hannöver, W., & Richard, M. (2001). Computer-assisted feedback-driven quality management for psychotherapy: The Stuttgart-Heidelberg Model. *Journal of Consulting and Clinical Psychology, 69,* 173–183.

Lambert, M. J., Hansen, N. B., & Finch, A. E. (2001). Client-focused research: Using client outcome data to enhance treatment effects. *Journal of Consulting and Clinical Psychology, 69,* 159–172.

Lambert, M. J., Hansen, N. B., Umphress, V., Lunnen, K., Okiishi, J., Burlingame, G., et al. (1996). *Administration and scoring manual for the Outcome Questionnaire (OQ 45.2).* Wilmington, DE: American Professional Credentialing Services.

Lambert, M. J., Whipple, J. L., Hawkins, E. J., Vermeersch, D. A., Nielsen, S. L., & Smart, D. W. (2003). Is it time for clinicians to routinely track patient outcome? A meta-analysis. *Clinical Psychology: Science and Practice, 10,* 288–301.

Lindsey, E. W. (1998). The impact of homelessness and shelter life on family relationships. *Family Relations, 47,* 243–252.

Lueger, R. J., Howard, K. I., Martinovich, Z., Lutz, W., Anderson, E. E., & Grissom, G. (2001). Assessing treatment progress of individual patients using expected treatment response models. *Journal of Consulting and Clinical Psychology, 69,* 150–158.

Meier, S. T. (2003). *Bridging case conceptualization, assessment, and intervention.* Thousand Oaks, CA: Sage.

OPTAIO. (1997). *Provider's desktop*. San Antonio, TX: Psychological Corporation.

Parsonson, B. S., & Baer, D. M. (1978). The analysis and presentation of graphic data. In T. R. Kratochwill (Ed.), *Single-subject research: Strategies for evaluating change* (pp. 101–165). New York: Academic Press.

Persons, J. B., & Silberschatz, G. (1998). Are results of randomized controlled clinical trials useful to psychotherapists? *Journal of Consulting and Clinical Psychology, 66*, 126–135.

Rosenthal, R., & Rosnow, R. L. (1991). *Essentials of behavioral research: Methods and data analysis* (2nd ed.). New York: McGraw-Hill.

Sechrest, L., Stewart, M., Stickle, T. R., & Sidani, S. (1996). *Effective and persuasive case studies*. Cambridge, MA: Human Services Research Institute.

Sorenson, R. L., Gorsuch, R. L., & Mintz, J. (1985). Moving targets: Patients' changing complaints during psychotherapy. *Journal of Consulting and Clinical Psychology, 53*, 49–54.

Tang, T. Z., & DeRubeis, R. J. (1999). Sudden gains and critical sessions in cognitive–behavioral therapy for depression. *Journal of Consulting and Clinical Psychology, 67*, 894–904.

Westen, W., Novotny, C. M., & Thompson-Brenner, H. (2004). The empirical status of empirically supported psychotherapies: Assumptions, findings, and reporting in controlled clinical trials. *Psychological Bulletin, 130*, 631–663.

Wiger, D. E. (1999). *The psychotherapy documentation primer*. New York: Wiley.

8

THE RESEARCH–PRACTICE TANGO AND OTHER CHOREOGRAPHIC CHALLENGES: USING AND TESTING EVIDENCE-BASED PSYCHOTHERAPIES IN CLINICAL CARE SETTINGS

JOHN R. WEISZ AND MICHAEL E. ADDIS

Professionals in clinical practice and those in clinical research have important goals in common. Both groups seek to identify, understand, and ameliorate dysfunction and distress, and both are continually working to improve what they do. On this broad foundation, there is room for a great deal of shared understanding and complementary activity. One such activity, the focus of this chapter, is extending treatments that have been tested in research settings into clinical practice settings for testing under clinically representative conditions and for everyday clinical use, if they prove to be effective in clinical application. This has been a focus of our research in practice with youths (Weisz) and adults (Addis). In this chapter, we describe

The research described in this chapter was supported by the John D. and Catherine T. MacArthur Foundation (Research Network on Youth Mental Health [Weisz]) and by grants from the National Institute of Mental Health (R29 MH57778 [Addis]; R01 MH57347 [Weisz]; R01 MH 49522 [Weisz]; R01 68806 [Weisz]), all of which we gratefully acknowledge.

179

this work, some of what we have learned from it, and what it suggests about broader efforts to bring evidence-based treatments (EBTs) into clinical practice. Because our research has focused on clinics that use multiple practitioners, our comments may fit such settings better than other service contexts, but we suspect that a number of our comments are applicable to a range of clinical care settings.

TWO WORLDS:
CLINICAL PRACTICE AND CLINICAL RESEARCH

Clinical practice and research do have much in common, but our collaborative work with colleagues in practice settings has taught us that there are also profound differences between the practice and research worlds. Indeed, some of the differences between the two contexts are almost as profound as differences between national cultures. The relevant dimensions include goals and objectives, incentive systems, constraints, pressures, work products, and the nature of daily life.

Goals and Objectives

Goals and objectives in clinical practice settings tend to be focused on services to clients and their families. The services provided often include assessment, diagnosis, and intervention, delivered in ways that must be consistent with clinic, agency, or provider mandates or contractual obligations. Particular significance attaches to client and payer satisfaction with services; dissatisfied clients may be no-shows or terminate care prematurely, and the contracts that form a financial base for some clinics may emphasize meeting consumer needs. In research as in practice, the services provided to individuals may include assessment, diagnosis, and intervention; but the primary goal of the investigator is typically to expand understanding of a clinical phenomenon or test the effects of new procedures. The arbiters of how effectively this goal has been met are usually scientific authorities, frequently represented by peer reviewers and journal editors; thus, much of what clinical researchers do is done in ways designed to ensure the scientific integrity needed to pass the eventual scrutiny of peer reviewers and editors.

Incentive Systems, Constraints, and Work Pressures

Markedly different incentive systems, constraints, and work pressures impinge on clinical practitioners and clinical researchers. The way most mental health service incentive systems are structured tends to emphasize quantity of care, but in rather different ways depending on payment systems. When services are provided through fixed-price contracts that dictate a particular quantity of care, a principal way in which contracts may be lost (or adjusted downward in cost) is that the quantity of care provided in a particular year is below the goal set in that year's contract; this produces pressure to maintain a particular annual number of clients served or hours of care provided. In traditional indemnity plans, the provider agency or clinician receives income based on number of hours of care provided, so the incentive system argues for more care; however, for the payer in such plans, the incentives are reversed in that less care equals higher profit. These and other incentive systems prevail across most provider clinics and agencies around the country, currently, and the financial fragility of many of these institutions means that funding is a highly potent incentive. Most of the practitioners we know are committed to providing quality care that will improve the mental health of those they treat, but the incentive systems within which the practitioners work may emphasize quality and outcomes less than quantity and reimbursability. In contrast, the incentive system that prevails for researchers is one in which findings and results are critical to success. Thus, in clinical trials, a premium is placed on findings showing that a particular treatment both is delivered exactly as designed and produces better outcomes than those found in control or comparison groups. A trial that does not result in such findings may be considered a failure. These pressures have a financial dimension, as well. Research and research careers often depend on grant funding, which depends, in turn, on the scientific quality of investigators' proposed studies and on their record of completed research. Promotion and tenure decisions may depend on both research quality and success in generating grant support. Such pressures may lead to clinical trial procedures that emphasize experimental control and the likelihood of good results, sometimes at the expense of clinical representativeness and relevance to everyday clinical care (see Weisz, 2004). It is clear that the incentive systems, constraints, and pressures that drive so much of the daily behavior of practitioners and researchers show little overlap across the two professional groups.

Work Products and Nature of Daily Life

Given all these differences, it is not surprising that work products and the nature of daily life are remarkably different for practitioners and researchers. Among the diverse work products of practitioners, a central element is total hours of clinical care provided, and increasingly the emphasis is on billable hours. For administrators, development of new service programs (e.g., for substance abuse) or new ways of delivering care (e.g., home- or school-based treatment) may be an important work product. For researchers, scientifically sound studies, grant support to fund those studies, and publications in peer-reviewed journals are important products. The daily work of those in clinical practice emphasizes providing direct care and developing and refining the forms of care and means of delivery. The daily work of those in research settings heavily emphasizes writing proposals, obtaining funding for studies, overseeing the conduct of studies to ensure their scientific integrity, analyzing study findings, and writing for a scientific audience. Thus, as with the other domains previously discussed, work products and daily activities in clinical practice and clinical research are quite different.

PRACTITIONERS' AND RESEARCHERS' VIEWS ON THE RELATION BETWEEN PRACTICE AND RESEARCH

Given the numerous differences between the worlds of clinical practitioners and researchers, questions arise as to what the two groups know about each other and think about each other's work. The venerable Boulder model of clinical training and practice has always envisioned a mutually beneficial relationship in which many of the same individuals do both kinds of work and in which research and clinical practice inform and support each others' pursuits (Shakow, 1976; Stricker & Trierweiler, 1995). In contrast, what has evolved over the last several decades has been a significant divide between the activities of clinical researchers and practitioners (see Westen, Novotny, & Thompson-Brenner, 2004). Some have gone so far as to argue that the values and goals of practitioners and researchers are orthogonal (Fensterheim & Raw, 1996; Silverman, 1996). Reflecting on the emotional intensity of debates over EBTs, Addis (2002) suggested that a particularly toxic stereotype has emerged in which practitioners are characterized by some researchers as mindless true believers incapable of critical thinking and researchers are characterized by some practitioners as ivory tower rat runners out of touch with the realities of clinical practice.

In contrast to the abundance of opinions and rhetoric, there is surprisingly little empirical data on how researchers and clinical practitioners view each other's work. However, some empirical attention has focused recently on practitioners' perceptions of psychotherapy research products, particularly the treatment manuals associated with EBTs. Addis and Krasnow (2000) conducted a survey of over 800 practicing doctoral-level psychotherapists and found widely varying attitudes toward treatment manuals. Respondents rather strongly endorsed the views that manuals can help keep therapists on track during therapy and if used appropriately, will enhance the average outcomes of clients, but many also endorsed the views that manuals force individual clients into arbitrary categories and ignore the contributions of individual therapists. Attitudes were partly associated with therapists' theoretical orientation. For example, psychodynamically oriented clinicians reported significantly more negative attitudes toward treatment manuals than did clinicians who used cognitive–behavioral therapy (CBT). In a multisite cocaine treatment trial, Najavits and colleagues (2004) similarly found that psychodynamic (supportive–expressive) therapists reported less satisfaction with using a treatment manual than the other therapists in the study (i.e., those using CBT, individual drug counseling, and group drug counseling). Others who have examined therapist use of manuals in clinical practice have also found generally positive reactions among CBT therapists (e.g., Morgenstern, Morgan, McCrady, Keller, & Carroll, 2001; Najavits, Weiss, Shaw, & Dierberger, 2000). This pattern may reflect, in part, the fact that cognitive–behavioral approaches are well-represented among the manuals, whereas psychodynamic approaches are not.

The studies cited in this section are only the tip of the iceberg compared with the useful information that could be gathered in the future. For example, Addis (2002) suggested that research–practice relationships could fruitfully be studied from a social psychology perspective focusing on the effects of attitudes, beliefs, and stereotypes on the different ways research–practice relationships operate. One useful starting point would be to assess the extent to which both researchers and practitioners actually hold common stereotypes about the other group. It is possible that positive perceptions of researchers by practitioners (and vice versa) are more common than one would suspect from the largely impressionistic literature. The recent emergence of larger-scale research–practice networks suggests that this might be the case (e.g., Borkovec, 2004). In addition, although some have suggested that some clinical researchers have colluded with third-party payers to constrain practice (Wampold & Bhati, 2004), it should be stressed that research can assist practitioners in coping with health care reimbursement challenges by providing scientific documentation that psychotherapy can be effective and by disseminating tested treatments. Indeed, one of us recently helped a practitioner become a preferred provider for a panel by documenting the clinician's participation in research that included training in empirically supported treatment for anxiety disorders.

EXTENT OF SPREAD OF RESEARCH-TESTED TREATMENTS INTO CLINICAL TRAINING AND PRACTICE

Most of what we know about current patterns in clinical training and clinical practice suggests that the impact of EBTs on clinical training and practice has been modest. In the training domain, relevant evidence comes from a survey carried out by Woody, Weisz, and McLean (in press) as a part of the work of the American Psychological Association (APA) Division 12 (Society of Clinical Psychology) Committee on Science and Practice (CSP). This survey was a 10-year follow-up to a nearly identical survey conducted in 1993. In both surveys, directors of doctoral graduate programs in clinical psychology and directors of clinical psychology predoctoral internship programs were given a list of EBTs and asked to report the extent to which each treatment was taught in coursework and covered in supervised training. For the 22 EBTs that were included in both surveys, both graduate programs and internship programs reported more inclusion in their course content in 2003 than in 1993, although a great deal of the coverage was described as "brief." However, in terms of actual supervised training, the picture had changed in a negative direction over the decade. For both graduate and internship programs, supervised training had actually declined over the decade for more EBTs than it had increased. If we assume that skill in actual clinical use of these treatments is more closely related to supervised training than to coursework, the Woody et al. findings suggest the possibility that expertise in the use of scientifically tested treatments may have declined over time. Of course, the survey applies only to the discipline of clinical psychology, not to other fields (e.g., social work, marriage and family therapy). But given that clinical psychology is the discipline most responsible for the development of EBTs, it seems unlikely that these treatments are more thoroughly trained and disseminated within other disciplines.

Our own contact with clinical practice settings and the limited research evidence of which we are aware also suggest that EBTs are not very evident in everyday clinical practice. This is the impression conveyed by therapists' reports of their treatment methods with children and adolescents (Weersing, Weisz, & Donenberg, 2002) and by observer coding of treatment as usual or usual care therapy sessions with children and adolescents (McLeod & Weisz, 2005). It is also the impression conveyed by evidence from adult patient self-reports (Goisman, Warshaw, & Keller, 1999) and from content analyses of usual care psychotherapy sessions with adults (Addis et al., 2004). These findings are not consistent with the apparently increasing popularity of the term *cognitive–behavioral* in therapists' self-described theoretical orientation. CBT treatments for youths and adults constitute a very large portion of the manualized EBTs. It is possible that such treatments (e.g., CBT for anxiety and depression in youths and adults) or elements of the treatments (e.g., identifying and altering unrealistic negative cognitions) are more widely used than the available data would suggest. It is also possible that certain terms, such as *cognitive–behavioral,* are used rather liberally in everyday practice— for example, to refer to any intervention in which cognitions are discussed and not just to interventions that have all the features and procedures of standard CBT protocols. A useful question for discussion is just what level of adherence—ranging from exclusive manual use to a mixture of manual elements with nonprotocol procedures—is required for an EBT to have been appropriately implemented in a practice setting. The question will be difficult to answer fairly until researchers are able to identify the active ingredients in particular EBTs (see, e.g., Kazdin, 2000; Weersing & Weisz, 2002) and thus to determine what is needed to effect genuine change.

Although findings show a limited impact of EBTs on clinical training and clinical practice to date, numerous efforts are now afoot in the public and private sectors to support the use of tested interventions. Federal funding has been made available to providers to build practice-based research infrastructures and train community therapists in evidence-based interventions (e.g., U.S. Department of Health and Human Services, 2004a, 2004b). Policymakers at the national level have endorsed the importance of evidence-based quality mental health care (National Institute of Mental Health [NIMH], 2001; Office of the Surgeon General, 1999; President's New Freedom Commission on Mental Health, 2003). Family advocacy groups and patient organizations have become increasingly vocal in advocating for access not only to mental health care but also to interventions with demonstrated effectiveness and high patient satisfaction (Allness & Knoedler, 2003; Flynn, 2005; Hoagwood, 2005; National Alliance for the Mentally Ill, 2003), and states have developed initiatives to support the use of effective mental health services (National Association of State Mental Health Program Directors, 2004).

In summary, it appears that research-tested treatments have shown rather limited spread into clinical training and practice to date but that there is considerable interest within the public and private sectors in promoting such spread. What may be needed at this point is a genre of research testing various approaches to bridging the research–practice gap that spans the two cultures in ways designed to bring tested interventions into clinical care contexts. We have tried to help shape and promote this genre of research, in part by conducting effectiveness trials within practicing clinics. In the next sections of this chapter, we will summarize these trials and discuss what we have learned by conducting them. An important theme in this discussion will be the two-way nature of the process. In our view, efforts to bring research-based treatments into practice can succeed only if they draw on the experience, expertise, and wisdom of practitioners, as well as their insights into what is possible in their work settings.

EFFORTS TO TEST EMPIRICALLY SUPPORTED TREATMENTS IN PRACTICE SETTINGS: EFFECTIVENESS TRIALS

Our efforts to bring empirically supported treatments into real-world practice contexts are part of a broader effort encompassing other investigators. Although others have not used the same approach we have followed, their work is valuable and an important context for ours. Examples include the Community Reinforcement Approach (Budney & Higgins, 1998) for treatment of adult drug abuse; the Program of Assertive Community Treatment (Stein & Santos, 1998) for adults with severe and persistent mental illness; and Multisystemic Therapy (Henggeler, Schoenwald, Borduin, Rowland, & Cunningham, 1998), Functional Family Therapy (Sexton & Alexander, 2004), and Multidimensional Treatment Foster Care (Chamberlain, 1998), all treatments for aggressive and antisocial behavior in youths.

Other efforts have focused on treatment of internalizing conditions, including depression (Mufson et al., 2004), panic disorder (Stuart, Treat, & Wade, 2000; Wade, Treat, & Stuart, 1998), and bulimia nervosa (Tuschen-Caffier, Pook, & Frank, 2001).

Our own work builds on the tradition established by these and other investigators. However, as best we can determine, what we have done differs from prior research in some significant ways. In our work with youths and adults, we have identified treatments that showed beneficial effects in prior randomized efficacy trials, helped randomly selected clinicians who are employed in clinical practice settings to learn and use those treatments in their settings, randomly selected other clinicians from the same settings to continue practicing usual care, and compared outcomes for clients of the different clinician groups to assess whether evidence-based care delivered by practitioners within everyday clinical practice settings leads to better outcomes than usual clinical care.

Our comparison of target treatments to usual clinical care warrants discussion. A limitation of this approach is that usual care tends to be a mixture of varied methods, to be different for each individual therapist, and not to be documented in ways that would make it possible to replicate the interventions (see Kazdin & Weisz, 1998; Weisz, 2004). It is possible, however, to train coders to reliably characterize usual care along particular dimensions of interest (see, e.g., Addis et al., 2004; McLeod & Weisz, 2005), so that the nature of the treatment processes need not be a complete mystery. An important advantage of the usual care comparison is that it is highly relevant to the concerns and goals of our clinical practice partners and to the clients and client families they serve. A critical question for those parties to the research–practice collaboration is how to achieve the best outcome possible. Thus, a key question for any new intervention is whether it can outperform the clinical care that is currently available in practice. In our experience, treatment approaches for which that question has not been addressed are of limited interest to those in the practice community. It is important to note that this question has not yet been addressed for most of the treatments that are currently considered to be evidence based.

The approach taken in our effectiveness trials, with efficacy-tested treatment compared with usual care, and with the other elements noted in this chapter is a particularly conservative way to test the effects of any treatment that is new to the clinical practice setting for at least five reasons. First, in tests pitting manualized treatments against control groups, by far the most common control group has been the wait-list or no-treatment group (see, e.g., review by Weisz, Doss, & Hawley, 2005); comparison of a manualized treatment to standard practice in which clinicians are working hard to benefit their clients almost certainly reduces the prospects for strong outcomes in favor of the manualized treatment, because treatment versus treatment comparisons generate smaller effect sizes than treatment versus control comparisons (see, e.g., Kazdin, Bass, Ayers, & Rodgers, 1990). Second, clinicians in the usual care condition are using the treatment procedures they know best and often have developed over many years of practice, whereas clinicians in the manualized treatment condition are being asked to learn and use unfamiliar procedures that in many cases conflict with their usual, preferred approaches.

Third, doing highly structured and prescriptive treatment is incompatible with the way many clinicians picture their role and with the expectations many had when they chose a clinical career; thus, asking clinicians to learn a detailed treatment manual and plan their sessions according to a structured flow chart is asking a lot. Fourth, the reality constraints we described earlier (e.g., time pressures and productivity requirements) limit the time and energy available to clinicians to learn and master entirely new treatment procedures, giving an additional advantage to therapists who need only use their familiar usual care approaches. Fifth, many characteristics of everyday clinical practice with referred clients and under managed care present a challenge to the use of structured, manual-guided treatments. For example, most such treatments are designed for individuals with a single diagnosis, but comorbidity is the rule in clinical practice. As another example, most manuals require a fixed minimum number of sessions, often 15 or more, but the average number of sessions attended in many practice settings is well below that number, and client no-show and unannounced dropout are common phenomena in everyday practice. Moreover, increasingly strict session limits are imposed by many managed care companies, and these limits often fall well below the number of sessions required for completion of most manualized treatments.

Notwithstanding these and other challenges, bringing structured, manualized protocols into everyday clinical practice presents a remarkable opportunity to learn. For anyone who believes that scientifically tested treatments can improve outcomes in clinical practice, the opportunity to test that proposition and to learn what is needed to put such treatments into practice is invaluable. Because we have each had that opportunity, we want to share a bit of what we have done, and what we have learned in the process.

Effectiveness Research With Youths in a Practice Context

This section describes Weisz's experience in a youth practice context. In the latter half of the 1990s, his research team at the University of California, Los Angeles, had just carried out a longitudinal study that tracked children and teens through their episodes of care in community mental health clinics. In the process, they met some very impressive clinic administrators and practitioners who were clearly devoted to the goal of quality mental health care. Because this was also a time of growing interest in EBTs, they looked for such treatments in the community care they were studying; they found little evidence that research-tested treatments had made their way into community practice. They became increasingly convinced that the worlds of research and practice had been so separate for so long that the field lacked good mechanisms for linking the two. Given the apparent potential of research-tested treatments to improve outcomes, they thought it would be useful to bring such treatments into the California clinics they knew well and test the impact on client outcomes. They conducted parallel studies of CBT for youth anxiety disorders (Kendall's 1994 Coping Cat program for separation anxiety disorder, generalized anxiety disorder, and social phobia) and CBT for youth depression (the PASCET program, developed by Weisz, Thurber, Sweeney, Proffitt, & LeGagnoux, 1997). Volunteer clinicians employed in each of the participating clinics were randomly assigned to either learn and receive weekly supervision in the manual-guided procedures (either Coping Cat or PASCET, depending on diagnosis) or continue doing treatment as they had done it prior to the study—that is, provide usual care. Children who were referred to the clinics through normal channels and who met diagnostic criteria (in standardized diagnostic interviews) for the appropriate anxiety or depressive disorders were randomized to the manual-guided treatment condition (Coping Cat for anxiety, PASCET for depression) or to the usual care condition. Outcomes were assessed at posttreatment and at a later follow-up.

Because usual care had no defined end point, and because some youths with certain public entitlements remained in treatment for extended periods, the research team has only recently completed final data collection; thus, there are no findings to report yet. However, they have learned a great deal already, and some of this is described elsewhere by research team members (Connor-Smith & Weisz, 2003; Southam-Gerow, Weisz, & Kendall, 2003; Weisz, Southam-Gerow, Gordis, & Connor-Smith, 2003). However, brief comments are warranted on lessons learned in relation to the clients, practitioners, clinic administrators, and research team. An overarching theme that emerged quite clearly is that the interplay of these four perspectives has a profound impact on the course of effectiveness research.

Clients

Understanding client perspectives is important regardless of client age, but the challenge is compounded in youth treatment because multiple clients are involved in each case. Parents or guardians typically initiate the referral, and other family members may also be involved. The consent from adults and assent from minors that are required for internal review board (IRB) approval of research pose special challenges in effectiveness research. The screening process and the multipage, legalistic language the university required was off-putting to parents, appearing to suggest many risks and conveying the idea that something very complex and perhaps quite sinister was being proposed. Parents had contacted the clinics seeking the best care for their children, and some declined to consent because the IRB document implied a risk of something other than the best care. The youths, in general, had not sought care on their own; most had only a vague idea of what clinic care would involve, and some declined assent for the project because the IRB procedures made the process even more confusing.

For those youths and parents who did agree to participate, an assessment challenge arose: Parent and child responses to questionnaires and diagnostic interviews showed poor agreement. Faced with substantial parent–child differences in what measures showed, the team opted to admit youths into the project when *either* parent report *or* youth report placed the youth above threshold for study entry. At study entry, the team thought it important to understand the concerns that had led to clinic referral, and here they faced another challenge: Referred youths and their parents tend to have quite different views on what the problems are that need attention and thus on what the goals of therapy should be (Hawley & Weisz, 2003; Yeh & Weisz, 2001). So team members collected lists of referral concerns from both youths and parents and tried to incorporate some of the concerns from both lists within the treatment plan for each youth. This, they believed, was important in engaging families. In general, the team found that the formal diagnoses on which both researchers and clinicians depend were of much less interest to youths and parents than the specific problems that interfere with effective daily living (e.g., school refusal, depressed mood that interferes with concentration on schoolwork, fear of leaving home for a sleepover with friends).

Practitioners

Practitioner responses to the project were rather different from what the published debates between proponents and opponents of EBTs might suggest. Open animosity and opposition to the use of empirically tested, manual-guided treatments were not a significant issue for most clinicians. Many found the project interesting in concept. Significant concerns did arise, however, regarding the scrutiny implied by videotaping sessions and the time commitment that would be involved in the project (e.g., learning the manual, preparing for sessions, taping sessions), whether participation would cut into the productivity the clinic required (in each clinic, a certain percentage ranging from 50%–75% of all clinician time was required to be billable), whether use of the manuals would rule out the use of therapists' clinical judgment, and whether the manualized treatments could actually be effective with the severe, complex, comorbid cases most often seen in the clinic.

For practitioners who decided to participate, the research team found it important to stay in regular contact, build interpersonal connections, respond quickly to any requests for information or assistance, and protect therapists' time so as to make participation feasible. The team took on all the paperwork and other research tasks they could handle themselves to avoid unduly cutting into client care or consultation time; for example, in each weekly consultation visit with each EBT therapist, the project supervisors asked a few questions that allowed them, rather than the therapists, to fill in session tracking forms. For therapists in the EBT condition, team members also tried to maximize opportunities to use and build on the therapists' current clinical skills (e.g., in engaging youth interest and parent participation), to show team members' respect, and to convey that joining the project represented continued professional development, not abandonment of all prior learning.

Clinic Administrators and Staff

For the administrative leaders and staff of the partner clinics, research participation required a delicate balancing act. Supporting the project, and thus the professional development of their clinical staff, needed to be balanced against maintaining clinic operations in ways that met contractual obligations and maintained solvency. It was impossible for research team members to avoid cutting into personnel time in the clinics, but team members tried to strictly limit activities that might take time away from efficient management of clinic operations; project personnel handled paperwork or logistics for the project whenever possible. Team members also tried to design project procedures to fit smoothly and unobtrusively into clinic operations; they delighted in one clinic CEO's comment that he had hardly noticed they were there. Team members also felt a special obligation to provide quality training and clinical consultation to ensure that they were adding genuine value to each clinic's operations.

On the administrative front, a critical role was played by the clinic staff who linked clients to clinicians. Included in this group were the phone screeners who received the initial calls from parents seeking services, the staff who scheduled assessment and intake appointments, and those who navigated the process of therapist assignment. These individuals were among the busiest in all of the clinics, and this research project clearly added to their list of duties. The fact that the roles they played were critical to identification of study participants made these individuals major partners in the project. From the outset, team members sought procedural guidance from these partners regarding the best ways to blend the study procedures with their procedures and the best ways to minimize extra work for them. Wherever possible, team members sought ways to support and show their appreciation to those who played these administrative roles.

The Research Team

As was true in the adult research described in the next section, the research team began the project focused intently on the scientific integrity of the study. However, as the project evolved, it became quite clear that the research would not succeed without an equally intense focus on the clinical practice setting and process within which the study operated. Increasingly, team members became immersed with their clinic partners in the details of the initial phone contact with potential clients, the clinic intake and assessment procedures, case assignment, supervision procedures, and the procedures each clinic used in responding to youth and family crises and handling concerns about risk (e.g., maltreatment, suicide). In each of these respects, research procedures and clinical care procedures intersected and interacted.

Because the project participants were, first and foremost, clinic clients, project procedures had to be shaped to fit clinic mandates and requirements. As an example, the project's therapist supervision procedures had to be complemented, in each clinic, by some process through which clinic-designated supervisors—who had to sign, and thus endorse, treatment plans and case notes—could monitor the treatment procedures used and the responses of clients. In one case, for example, a clinic supervisor attended the team's supervision sessions; in another, the project supervisor met with the clinic supervisor biweekly and reviewed case notes separately. Overall, team members found that clinic operations and research operations converged increasingly, creating an interactive process—a kind of research–practice tango—in which clinic staff and research staff learned to operate in ever closer synchrony with one another. In the process, team members and clinic staff learned more and more about each other's beliefs, perspectives, settings, and workplace.

Effectiveness Research With Adults in a Practice Context

This section describes the experience of the second author in an adult practice context. In 1995, he was a first-year assistant professor at Clark University, which was in the process of developing a psychotherapy research program. It had only been 2 years since the publication of APA's Division 12 Task Force on empirically validated treatments, and psychotherapy researchers were hopeful that the positive effects of EBTs demonstrated in controlled clinical trials would generalize to clinical practice. However, at that time there appeared to be no controlled studies testing the effectiveness of EBTs in "real-world" practice settings. Addis conducted what amounted to a randomized controlled effectiveness study of cognitive–behavioral treatment for panic disorder (Craske, Meadows, & Barlow, 1994) in a managed care setting. The design of the study provided for a very conservative test of effectiveness; therapists were masters-level practitioners with no prior experience in manual-based CBT treatments, medication use was left free to vary in both conditions, and treatment length was also left free to vary. Nonetheless, under conditions that should have watered down treatment effects, clients receiving the EBT showed modestly superior outcomes to clients receiving usual care and comparable outcomes to those clients treated in controlled efficacy studies (Addis et al., 2004). The outcome differences were even more pronounced for clients who attended at least six sessions; across outcome measures, an average of 43% of clients receiving the EBT achieved clinically significant change compared with 19% receiving treatment as usual.

It is fair to say that the research team learned as much from the process of conducting an effectiveness study as they did from the outcomes. The details of the team's experiences are summarized in an article coauthored by members of the research team, practitioners, and clinical administrators involved in the study (Hatgis et al., 2001). This section describes some of the more salient issues that arose when viewing the study from the perspectives of the clients, the practitioners, the clinic administrators, and the research team. The perspectives of these different players in the research process involved goals, values, costs and obstacles, and valued outcomes (Hatgis et al., 2001). If there is one overall lesson that the team gleaned from this experience, it is that conducting a successful effectiveness study requires regular and thoughtful consideration of the way these various perspectives converge and diverge as the research evolves.

Clients

It should go without saying that clients' primary goals are relief from distress, regardless of whether they are receiving treatment in the context of research or routine clinical practice. Nonetheless, team members found that it was easy to lose sight of this fact when the majority of their energy was devoted to maintaining the integrity of the research process. In effectiveness research, in which treatment is received in real-world practice settings, many clients lose sight of the fact, or even forget, that they are involved in research. Clients may therefore be more sensitive to costs and obstacles to participating, such as audiotaping sessions, participating in follow-up assessments, or completing self-report measures during treatment. At the same time, we found that many clients held values, such as helping others with similar problems, that coincided well with the perspective of the research team.

Practitioners

The research team's experiences working with frontline practitioners in a capitated managed care setting taught them a great deal about the contingencies affecting ability and willingness to participate in research. In capitated managed care, a clinical service organization contracts with a third-party payer to provide all mental health care services for a population of people covered by the payer. The service organization and the third-party payer must then "manage" care such that all individuals covered have access to care but the costs of care are contained in a way that both is profitable for the third-party payer (or allows them to break even in the case of a nonprofit entity) and allows the service organization to meet its contractual obligations in terms of access to and quantity of care provided. These systems of service delivery and compensation create contingencies that directly affect the ability and willingness of practitioners to participate in clinical treatment research.

Right from the start, several practitioners declined to participate in the research process. Some did not provide a reason, but others made it clear that they did not feel they had adequate time or that they were concerned about having their treatment monitored through audiotaping (despite the research team's reassurances that therapist-level data would never be shared with clinic administrators). It is important to note that not one of the roughly 30 practitioners the team approached expressed any negative attitudes toward research in general or toward the value of research for psychotherapy practice. Rather, it seemed clear that the demands of conducting clinical work within a capitated managed care system made it extremely difficult to collaborate with researchers; practitioners scheduled an average of 30 client contact hours per week, of which several were required to be new intakes. It seems that many contemporary clinical practice settings end up creating cultures of productivity rather than cultures of learning for frontline practitioners.

Fortunately for the research team, they were able to form relationships with several practitioners who were both interested in the research process and willing to participate. As a group, these practitioners had values and professional development goals that included career advancement, education, and work satisfaction. Nonetheless, they faced costs and obstacles, including lost wages for uncompensated research time, scheduling difficulties with study clients, and evaluation apprehension. In the end, these obstacles were offset by their clients' improvement and the new knowledge base and clinical skill sets they acquired. Developing a strong working alliance with these practitioners was critical to the success of the study; this was equally true for therapists conducting the EBT and those conducting treatment as usual. Team members sought feedback from therapists on a weekly basis to find out what the team members could do to make their participation easier and more rewarding. This became a delicate balance of team members making themselves available for consultation, or even a friendly chat over a cup of coffee, without being intrusive or creating yet more demands on the clinicians' time.

Clinic Administrators and Staff

The research team could not have conducted the study without the support of the clinic administrators. The team had no idea at the start that the key players would shift several times throughout the course of the research. First, mental health services had initially been provided by an "in-house" clinic run by the parent HMO. Team members had spent the year prior to the start of the grant developing collaborative relationships with practitioners and administrators in this clinic. Then, just before the project was to begin, mental health services were carved out by the HMO and subcontracted to a separate clinic. This made all the initial point people essentially irrelevant to the day-to-day conduct of the study. Such shifting structures, which are not at all uncommon in managed care settings, create significant challenges for researchers. An additional challenge was that the clinic was bought and sold three times during the study. Each time, the need for the study had to be rejustified and the relevant administrators assured that the research process would in no way interfere with practitioner or clinic productivity.

Clinical administrators within a managed care context typically seek to protect and expand the business side of things while assuring the best possible clinical care given the constraints inherent in a capitated system. In the research team's experience, the clinic administrators' values converged with the research process when it came to enhancing the quality of clinical services by providing the best EBT available. At the same time, the additional concrete burdens on staff, such as telephone time, paperwork tracking, and space allotment, created conflict. As with the therapists, the team found it essential to stay in continual contact with the administrators both to take their temperature regarding the study and to find ways to streamline the research process to create as few costs and obstacles as possible.

Research Team

Research team members did not begin the study conceptualizing themselves as an interested party to the process with particular goals and values. They simply saw themselves as researchers needing to conduct a study in a somewhat different setting than they were used to. Like most clinical researchers, this team was interested in conducting a good study, advancing clinical practice through science, advancing a particular program of research, and gaining some knowledge about the workings of particular practice settings. The practice setting was certainly important to this work, but team members perceived it as relatively external, an asset or an obstacle to be dealt with according to the research needs at any point in time.

This is probably where the most fundamental change occurred in the team's approach to effectiveness research. Rather than viewing the practice setting as an obstacle to be overcome or as an interesting object of study, team members came to view it as an essential component of the entire enterprise. In other words, it was simply impossible to do feasible and meaningful dissemination or effectiveness research without considering the vagaries of the practice setting at every choice point. Team members frequently found it necessary to relax some of the traditional methodological requirements for internally valid experiments in exchange for enhancing the generalizability of the findings. For example, it would have helped manipulation of the primary independent variable (the EBT) if the team had required practitioners to attend weekly supervision meetings. However, weekly attendance at group supervision was not typically required for these practitioners, and requiring it would not only have introduced limits on generalizability but also may have weakened team members' rapport with the practitioners and administrators. The team also chose to significantly reduce the assessment burden for clients. Although one of the research goals was rigorous measurement of the key outcome variables, it became apparent that clients were typically not willing to complete extensive measures that they did not perceive as central to their treatment. The bottom line was that the clinical practice setting switched from an obstacle to be conquered to an equal partner and shaper of the research process.

COMMON THREADS: SIMILAR THEMES IN YOUTH AND ADULT EFFECTIVENESS RESEARCH

From our descriptions of our youth and adult effectiveness research, a sampling of common themes can be identified as follows:

- Clients and client families contact clinics and practitioners to seek clinical care, not to participate in research. They are likely to participate in effectiveness research only to the extent that it emphasizes clinical care, not research procedures.
- Most practitioners chose clinical careers to do clinical practice, not to conduct research, and they often work under time and financial pressure. Effectiveness research is most likely to engage practitioners to the extent that it emphasizes respect for their skills, provides opportunities for professional development and support, and does not add unduly to time and financial pressures.
- Clinic administrators and staff must oversee the day-to-day operation of the clinic, ensure compliance with contracts and mandates, and maintain fiscal viability. Their support, essential to successful effectiveness research, may depend on the extent to which the research fits smoothly into ongoing clinic operations, does not conflict with existing contracts and mandates, and does not increase costs or limit clinic income.
- Research team members may well begin effectiveness research as clinic outsiders focused mainly on the scientific integrity of their project. However, the success of the research project is likely to require close interaction between research and clinic personnel and collaborative problem solving, with each party developing an understanding of the other's perspective and work demands.

LOOKING AHEAD: ADDRESSING CHALLENGES TO EFFECTIVENESS RESEARCH AND RESEARCH–PRACTICE COLLABORATION

Our experience in effectiveness research has helped us appreciate the challenges that will be faced by those who attempt such research in the future, as well as the challenges posed by broader efforts at research–practice collaboration. In this section we note a few of those challenges, together with our thoughts on how the challenges may be addressed. Table 8.1 summarizes these points.

Psychologists and Other Mental Health Professions

Psychologists are not alone; in fact, they are a distinct minority among mental health providers. Clinical psychology is an influential part of the mental health provider system and thus is one appropriate target for efforts to link science and practice. However, the psychology discipline provides only a small portion of the mental health care in the United States. Psychology's role is dwarfed by that of the social work profession, which has 2.5 times the number of active mental health providers, and by added numbers from the professions of psychiatry, marriage and family therapy, counseling, psychiatric nursing, school psychology, and psychosocial rehabilitation (National Mental Health Information Center, 2003). Nonpsychologists were certainly a majority among the staffs in our effectiveness trials. In addition, primary care physicians, family practitioners, and pediatricians operate as a kind of front line for many initial encounters between caring professionals and troubled and troubling individuals and their families, making the role of these medical specialists critical.

The various professions differ markedly in the degree to which their traditions favor reliance on scientific evidence as a basis for selecting interventions. Indeed, clinical psychology is unusual in the extent to which such thinking is embedded in graduate professional education in relation to psychotherapy. Thus, for the majority of providers, the gap between previous psychotherapy training and the elements of most EBTs is quite wide. To bridge this gap may require active consensus building across the mental health disciplines, as well as thoughtful attention to the rationale for evidence-based care and strategies for training and supervision that are sensitive to wide variations in therapist values, background, and previous graduate training.

Which Treatments Are Evidence Based?

Consensus is elusive as to what the "true EBTs" are. The diversity of the various mental health professions may also make it difficult to reach consensus on a central question critical to research–practice collaboration around

TABLE 8.1
Linking Clinical Science and Clinical Practice: Challenges for the Future

Challenge	Our thoughts
We (psychologists) are not alone.	Psychologists are a small minority among mental health disciplines and providers; movement toward evidence-based practice may require cross-disciplinary consensus building and variations in skill-building methods to address variations in professional backgrounds.
What are the "real" EBTs?	Various disciplines, and subdisciplines within psychology, differ in their views as to how evidence should be reviewed, what criteria should be applied, and what form practice recommendations should take; more consensus building is needed.
EBTs require EBAs.	Most EBTs are designed for specific disorders or conditions; current conditions in clinical practice make EBA and identification of disorders and conditions difficult, undermining efforts to create evidence-based practice.
Who will pay the bills?	Dissemination of empirically sound assessment and diagnosis and of empirically supported treatments is expensive; current fiscal conditions in the public and private sectors make it unclear where the resources will be found to meet the costs.
The assess–treat–reassess–refine dialectic is essential.	True evidence-based practice requires an ongoing assess–treat–reassess–refine treatment dialectic that goes well beyond the capacity of the current evidence base.
Can EBTs outperform usual care?	A fully developed case for the clinical use of EBTs requires evidence that EBTs outperform usual clinical care; researchers have provided little such evidence to date.
Science → practice must be complemented with practice → science.	The ideal collaboration between science and practice is a two-way street along which wisdom and learning travel in both directions.

Note. EBT = evidence-based treatment; EBA = evidence-based assessment.

EBTs: What *are* the evidence-based treatments? The professions that have used the evidence base to make recommendations for practice (e.g., clinical psychology, psychiatry, pediatrics) have developed different approaches and products, ranging from lists of empirically supported or evidence-based treatment to practice parameters to treatment guidelines, and the specific interventions identified within those products differ across the disciplines. Even within psychology, the various divisions and specialties produce different lists of best practices. A practitioner or potential client seeking the best treatment for a particular condition may experience frustration in deciding which professional discipline, criteria, or guidelines, parameters, or lists of treatments to turn to. To address this problem, researchers may well need to work toward a broad consensus across disciplines, and even within psychology, regarding (a) what procedures and criteria should be used to identify beneficial treatments, (b) what treatments are identified by those procedures and criteria, and (c) what form recommendations to practitioners and consumers should take.

Need for Evidence-Based Assessments

Evidence-based treatments require evidence-based assessments. Even if a broad consensus existed within psychology and across disciplines regarding which treatments are evidence based, the treatments could be expected to help only if paired with the conditions for which they were developed and tested. This may be a major challenge, particularly when it comes to the most universal basis for treatment decisions in North America: the *Diagnostic and Statistical Manual of Mental Disorders* (4th ed., DSM–IV; American Psychiatric Association, 1994). It certainly is true that the *DSM* taxonomy is widely used—this is guaranteed by a mental health delivery system in which a *DSM* diagnosis is required for reimbursement. However, dissemination of the diagnostic labels may not mean accurate use. A number of studies (e.g., Garb, 1998; Jensen & Weisz, 2002) have found very low levels of agreement between *DSM* diagnoses generated in everyday clinical practice and those obtained through standardized diagnostic interviews of the same individuals. A concern raised by such findings is that even if evidence-based treatments were available in most practice settings, clinicians might have real difficulty matching them to the individuals for whom they are best suited.

For evidence-based practice to be a reality, EBTs need to be paired with EBA and diagnosis. Implementing them will not be easy, given the time constraints placed on clinical practice. The standardized diagnostic interviews for which psychometric evidence is most encouraging require so much time to administer that they are probably not feasible in most clinical practice settings under current reimbursement schedules. More practice-friendly instruments are certainly available—the Child Behavior Checklist and its companion instruments (Achenbach & Rescorla, 2001), for example—but their use is eclipsed by both service system requirements and pressure from the agencies that fund clinical trials (e.g., NIMH) to link intervention choice to formal *DSM* diagnosis, thus perpetuating the conundrum. The fact that most EBTs are "evidence based" only for specific disorders and conditions means that true evidence-based treatment can be realized only if researchers find valid ways to identify those disorders and conditions in everyday clinical care.

Cost Factors

Effective implementation of empirically based assessment and treatment can initially be costly. Empirically sound assessment can be expensive, particularly diagnostic assessment that uses structured, standardized interviews. Training in EBTs is also expensive. Moreover, our experience suggests that training programs may not be very effective unless they are complemented by ongoing clinical consultation from individuals who are skilled in the treatment programs involved. We have covered these expenses through the grants that fund our research, but grants are not widely available to providers whose focus is on clinical service rather than research. Further complicating the picture for providers is the fact that the cost of training and ongoing consultation must be multiplied by the number of different disorders that are evident in their practice settings—because each disorder has its own protocols—and in turn by the number of staff who would need to receive the training and consultation.

Doing the math on these costs makes it clear that clinics, programs, agencies, and individual providers seeking to incorporate significant levels of EBA and EBT could run up massive bills. It is not at all clear who would pay these bills, given that so much of the mental health delivery system now operates on a break-even basis at best. Eventually, some relief may be found in more efficient forms of standardized diagnostic assessment (e.g., Lucas et al., 2001), in more streamlined or modular forms of treatment protocol design that build on common elements of separate treatments for different disorders (e.g., Chorpita, Delaiden, & Weisz, in press, 2005), and in the longer term from research identifying core mechanisms of action underlying treatment benefit (see Kazdin, 2000; Weersing & Weisz, 2002). But empirically sound assessment and intervention—whatever form they take—will always require training and monitoring, so that transporting them from research settings to practice settings will always carry costs. Inevitably, dissemination and effective use will depend on identifying the financial resources needed to absorb those costs on an ongoing basis.

Use of Evidence as a Guide Throughout the Treatment Process

Transcending routine application of EBTs will require an assessment–treatment–reassessment–adaptation dialectic. Although our own research has focused on implementation of specific EBTs in practice settings, we believe that empirically sound practice needs to entail much more than simply obtaining a valid diagnosis and choosing a matching treatment from a list of EBTs. Indeed, sound practice in our view is not a specific treatment or even a set of treatments but rather an orientation or value system, one that relies on evidence to guide the entire treatment process.

Assuming that the initial treatment target has been correctly identified, consulting a list of EBTs may be a useful first step in treatment. However, because clinical trials involve a focus on group differences, and other forms of outcome research (e.g., multiple baseline, single subject) tend to involve small numbers, each treatment on such lists is likely to be effective for some, but not all, clients with the target condition. Thus, a critical element of evidence-based care will need to be periodic assessment to gauge whether the treatment selected initially is in fact proving helpful. If it is not, adjustments in procedures will be needed, perhaps several times over the course of treatment. An episode of empirically sensitive care, then, would consist of a series of sessions interspersed with periodic assessments, followed by adjustments in treatment strategy when the evidence suggests such a need.

Specific EBTs could certainly provide an excellent reservoir from which to select treatment strategies over the course of such an episode. But the dialectic of assess–treat–reassess–refine is not yet a routine part of the treatment repertoire in the field. Indeed, the dialectic needs to be considered in the light of treatment manuals that require numerous sessions to be delivered in a fixed order before the intervention is complete. The strategy proposed here is more consistent with models of treatment design (e.g., Chorpita et al., in press, 2005) than with standard, fixed-order manuals. How the process is conceived and implemented will likely need to vary with treatment target, time required for various treatments to show an effect, reliability of the available assessments, and a variety of other factors. Still, it is worth noting that identifying lists of EBTs may be but the beginning of an extended process in the development of fully evidence-based care.

Testing Whether Evidence-Based Therapies Outperform Usual Care

Rather than simply assuming that EBTs will improve outcomes, researchers need to test the proposition fairly. An assumption guiding much of the movement for evidence-based mental health care is that bringing EBTs into clinical practice will improve client outcomes. A truly evidence-based perspective would regard this notion not as a given, but rather as a proposition in need of testing. As discussed elsewhere in detail (see Addis & Waltz, 2002; Weisz, 2004), there are reasons to suspect that moving treatments from efficacy trials into practice may often, but not always, improve outcomes beyond those found in usual clinical care. This evidence underscores the need to directly test the impact of efficacy-tested treatments in the practice contexts to which they are relocated and in direct comparison to the usual care procedures provided in the practice setting. After all, the bottom-line question is whether bringing EBTs into practice can in fact improve outcomes relative to those of current practice. If not, then why change current practice?

Attention to Practice Contributions to Science

The science → practice model needs to be complemented by a practice → science model. Most of this chapter has focused on moving the products of scientific research into clinical practice. In our view, this process is but one segment of what should be an ongoing exchange between practice and science, with each influencing the other in an unending cycle. Indeed, it is important to note that the first step in the cycle, historically, has often been one in which practice influences science. That is, some of the most prominent EBTs are treatments originally developed by clinicians treating referred individuals in practice settings; only later were written protocols developed for these treatments to document the clinical procedures for training purposes and to permit tests of treatment effects by researchers. Moreover, after the initial tests under controlled conditions, more clinical wisdom is likely to be required to adapt treatment protocols for use and testing in new practice contexts, as proposed in a recent "deployment-focused model" of treatment development and testing (Weisz, 2004).

Clinicians continue to develop strategies for helping specific target groups in clinical practice (e.g., child alert programs for sexually abused children) that may well warrant documentation and empirical testing, after which more clinical input will likely be needed to adapt these strategies for various practice settings. In addition to their role in creating and refining specific treatment procedures and protocols, many clinicians have developed skills in engaging and motivating their clients that may well warrant codifying to test their ease in dissemination and impact on client care. Finally, as we have stressed in much of this chapter, clinical practitioners have much to teach researchers about the clients and context of real-world clinical care, about the conditions within which science and practice may collaborate most fruitfully, and about the research questions that matter most to those on the front lines of clinical care. So, for a variety of reasons, the most promising form of science–practice collaboration is bidirectional.

CONCLUSION

Professionals in clinical practice and in clinical research share important goals related to understanding and ameliorating dysfunction and distress. However, the worlds of clinical practice and clinical research differ in regard to short-term objectives, incentive systems, constraints, work pressures, work products, and the nature of daily activity. The shared goals offer broad common ground and a platform for cooperation. The differences between the worlds of practice and research mean that considerable bridging is required to create shared understanding and to build collaborations that meet the needs of both participants.

In this chapter, we have described two efforts to bridge practice and science in the treatment of children, adolescents, and adults. These efforts, involving effectiveness research in outpatient community clinics, conveyed lessons about the engagement of key participants. Clients and families approach practitioners seeking help, not research; they are likely to be engaged in research only to the extent that it emphasizes quality care. Practitioners chose their careers to provide clinical care, not to do studies; their engagement may depend on the extent to which the research emphasizes respect for their skills, provides opportunities for professional growth, and does not add unduly to time and financial pressures. Clinical administrators have important oversight responsibilities; their engagement will likely depend on the extent to which research can fit into ongoing clinic operations, coexist with current contracts and mandates, and avoid adverse financial impact. Research personnel are apt to begin practice–research collaboration focused mainly on scientific integrity of their project; their research goals may depend on their ability to learn from clinical practitioners and administrators, appreciate their perspectives and work requirements, and engage in collaborative planning and problem solving.

Our experience in research–practice collaboration suggests significant challenges for the future. These challenges include reaching out to nonpsychologist practitioners, working toward consensus—across and within professions—regarding ways of identifying best practices, linking evidence-based practice to evidence-based assessment, finding ways to cover the costs associated with changing practice, moving from rote use of EBTs to thoughtful alternation of assessment and intervention refinement throughout episodes of care, building an evidence base on EBTs in relation to usual clinical care, and continually complementing science $\rightarrow$ practice collaboration with practice $\rightarrow$ science collaboration.

Clinical science uninformed by practice may risk sterility—the creation of knowledge that will not survive reality checks or relevance tests in the world of clinical care. Practice uninformed by science may risk uncritical repetition of familiar patterns, some of which could be improved through close scrutiny and empirical testing. Thus, the long-standing insularity of clinical research and clinical practice may pose significant risks to both enterprises, and a closer, ongoing linkage could generate genuine benefits for both. The work we have described in this chapter represents only one approach to bringing practice and science closer together. The array of other methods for meeting this challenge is potentially as rich as the collective wisdom and creativity of the many practitioners and investigators. To the extent that these groups can find bigger and better ways to work together, both research and practice are likely to improve, to the ultimate benefit of those they seek to help.

REFERENCES

Achenbach, T. M., & Rescorla, L. A. (2001). *Manual for the ASEBA School-Age Form & Profiles*. Burlington: University of Vermont Research Center for Children, Youth, and Families.

Addis, M. E. (2002). Methods for disseminating research products and increasing evidence-based practice: Promises, obstacles, and future directions. *Clinical Psychology: Science and Practice, 9,* 381–392.

Addis, M. E., Hatgis, C., Krasnow, A. D., Jacob, K., Bourne, L., & Mansfield, A. (2004). Effectiveness of cognitive–behavioral treatment for panic disorder versus treatment as usual in a managed care setting. *Journal of Consulting and Clinical Psychology, 72,* 625–635.

Addis, M. E., & Krasnow, A. D. (2000). A national survey of practicing psychologists' attitudes toward psychotherapy treatment manuals. *Journal of Consulting and Clinical Psychology, 68,* 331–339.

Addis, M. E., & Waltz, J. (2002). Implicit and untested assumptions about the role of psychotherapy treatment manuals in evidence-based mental health practice. *Clinical Psychology: Science and Practice, 9,* 435–438.

Allness, D. J., & Knoedler, W. H. (2003). *A manual for ACT start-up.* Arlington, VA: National Alliance for the Mentally Ill.

American Psychiatric Association. (1994). *Diagnostic and statistical manual of mental disorders* (4th ed.). Washington, DC: Author.

Borkovec, T. D. (2004). Research in training clinics and practice research networks: A route to the integration of science and practice. *Clinical Psychology: Science and Practice, 11,* 211–215.

Budney, A. J., & Higgins, S. T. (1998). *A community reinforcement plus vouchers approach: Treating cocaine addiction.* Rockville, MD: U.S. Department of Health and Human Services, National Institutes of Health, National Institute on Drug Abuse.

Chamberlain, P. (1998). *Family connections: A treatment foster care model for adolescents with delinquency.* Eugene, OR: Northwest Media.

Chorpita, B., Delaiden, E., & Weisz, J. R. (in press). Modularity in the design and application of therapeutic interventions. *Applied and Preventive Psychology.*

Chorpita, B., Delaiden, E., & Weisz, J. R. (2005). Identifying and selecting the common elements of evidence-based interventions: A distillation and matching model. *Mental Health Services Research, 7,* 5–20.

Connor-Smith, J. K., & Weisz, J. R. (2003). Applying treatment outcome research in clinical practice: Techniques for adapting interventions to the real world. *Child and Adolescent Mental Health, 8,* 3–10.

Craske, M. G., Meadows, E., & Barlow, D. H. (1994). *Therapist's guide for the mastery of your anxiety and panic II & agoraphobia supplement.* Albany, NY: Graywind Publications.

Fensterheim, H., & Raw, S. D. (1996). Psychotherapy research is not psychotherapy practice. *Clinical Psychology: Science and Practice, 3,* 168–171.

Flynn, L. (2005). Family perspectives on evidence-based practices. *Child and Adolescent Psychiatric Clinics of North America, 14,* 217–224.

Garb, H. N. (1998). *Studying the clinician: Judgment research and psychological assessment.* Washington DC: American Psychological Association.

Goisman, R. M., Warshaw, M. G., & Keller, M. B. (1999). Psychosocial treatment prescriptions for generalized anxiety disorder, panic disorder, and social phobia, 1991–1996. *American Journal of Psychiatry, 156,* 1819–1821.

Hatgis, C., Addis, M. E., Krasnow, A. D., Khazan, I. Z., Jacob, K. L., Chiancola, S., et al. (2001). Cross-fertilization versus transmission: Recommendations for developing a bidirectional approach to psychotherapy dissemination research. *Applied and Preventive Psychology, 10,* 37–49.

Hawley, K. M., & Weisz, J. R. (2003). Child, parent, and therapist (dis)agreement on target problems in outpatient therapy: The therapist's dilemma and its implications. *Journal of Consulting and Clinical Psychology, 71,* 62–70.

Henggeler, S. W., Schoenwald, S. K., Borduin, C. M., Rowland, M. D., & Cunningham, P. B. (1998). *Multisystemic treatment of antisocial behavior in children and adolescents.* New York: Guilford Press.

Hoagwood, K. (2005). Family-based services in children's mental health: A research review and synthesis. *Journal of Child Psychology and Psychiatry: Annual Research Review, 46,* 690–713.

Jensen, A. L., & Weisz, J. R. (2002). Assessing match and mismatch between practitioner-generated and standardized interview-generated diagnoses for clinic-referred children and adolescents. *Journal of Consulting and Clinical Psychology, 70,* 158–168.

Kazdin, A. E. (2000). *Psychotherapy for children and adolescents: Directions for research and practice.* Oxford, England: Oxford University Press.

Kazdin, A. E., Bass, D., Ayers, W. A., & Rodgers, A. (1990). Empirical and clinical focus of child and adolescent psychotherapy research. *Journal of Consulting and Clinical Psychology, 58,* 729–740.

Kazdin, A. E., & Weisz, J. W. (1998). Identifying and developing empirically supported child and adolescent treatments. *Journal of Consulting and Clinical Psychology, 66,* 19–36.

Kendall, P. C. (1994). Treating anxiety disorders in children: Results of a randomized clinical trial. *Journal of Consulting and Clinical Psychology, 62,* 100–110.

Lucas, C. P., Xhang, H., Fisher, P., Shaffer, D., Regier, D., Narrow, W., et al. (2001). The DISC Predictive Scales (DPS): Efficiently predicting diagnoses. *Journal of the American Academy of Child and Adolescent Psychiatry, 40,* 443–449.

McLeod, B. M., & Weisz, J. R. (2005). The Therapy Process Observational Coding System Alliance scale: Measure characteristics and prediction of outcome in usual clinical practice. *Journal of Consulting and Clinical Psychology, 73,* 323–333.

Morgenstern, J., Morgan, T. J., McCrady, B. S., Keller, D. S., & Carroll, K. M. (2001). Manual-guided cognitive behavioral therapy training: A promising method for disseminating empirically supported substance abuse treatments to the practice community. *Psychology of Addictive Behaviors, 15,* 83–88.

Mufson, L., Dorta, K. P., Wickramaratue, P., Nomura, Y., Olfson, M., & Weissman, M. M. (2004). A randomized effectiveness trial of interpersonal therapy for depressed adolescents. *Archives of General Psychiatry, 61,* 577–584.

Najavits, L. M., Ghinassi, F., Van Horn, A., Weiss, R. D., Siqueland, L., Frank, A., et al. (2004). Therapist satisfaction with four manual-based treatments on a national multisite trial: An exploratory study. *Psychotherapy: Theory, Research, Practice, Training, 41*, 26–37.

Najavits, L. M., Weiss, R. D., Shaw, S. R., & Dierberger, A. E. (2000). Psychotherapists' view of treatment manuals. *Professional Psychology: Research and Practice, 31*, 404–408.

National Alliance for the Mentally Ill. (2003, Fall). An update on evidence-based practices in children's mental health [Special issue]. *NAMI Beginnings, 3*.

National Association of State Mental Health Program Directors. (2004). *NASMHPD Web site listings.* Retrieved November 9, 2005, from http://www.nasmhpd.org_programs

National Institute of Mental Health. (2001). *Blueprint for change: Research on child and adolescent mental health. Report of the National Advisory Mental Health Council's Workgroup on Child and Adolescent Mental Health Intervention Development and Deployment.* Rockville, MD: U.S. Department of Health and Human Services.

National Mental Health Information Center. (2003). *Key elements of the national statistical picture: Chapter 20. Mental health practitioners and trainees.* Washington, DC: Substance Abuse and Mental Health Services Administration.

Office of the Surgeon General. (1999). *Mental health: A report of the Surgeon General.* Rockville, MD: U.S. Department of Health and Human Services.

President's New Freedom Commission on Mental Health. (2003). *Achieving the promise: Transforming mental health care in America. Final Report.* Rockville, MD: U.S. Department of Health and Human Services.

Sexton, T. L., & Alexander, J. F. (2004). *Functional Family Therapy clinical training manual.* Seattle, WA: FFTLLC.

Shakow, D. (1976). What is clinical psychology? *American Psychologist, 31*, 553–560.

Silverman, W. H. (1996). Cookbooks, manuals, and paint-by-numbers: Psychotherapy in the 90s. *Psychotherapy, 33*, 207–215.

Southam-Gerow, M. A., Weisz, J. R., & Kendall, P. C. (2003). Youth with anxiety disorders in research and service clinics: Examining client differences and similarities. *Journal of Clinical Child and Adolescent Psychology, 32*, 375–385.

Stein, L. I., & Santos, A. B. (1998). *Assertive community treatment of persons with severe mental illness.* New York: Norton.

Stricker, G., & Trierweiler, S. J. (1995). The local clinical scientist: A bridge between science and practice. *American Psychologist, 50*, 995–1002.

Stuart, G. L., Treat, T. A., & Wade, W. A. (2000). Effectiveness of an empirically based treatment for panic disorder delivered in a service clinic setting: 1-year follow-up. *Journal of Consulting and Clinical Psychology, 68*, 506–512.

Tuschen-Caffier, B., Pook, M., & Frank, M. (2001). Evaluation of manual-based cognitive–behavioral therapy for bulimia nervosa in a service setting. *Behaviour Research and Therapy, 39*, 299–308.

U.S. Department of Health and Human Services. (2004a). *National training and technical assistance center for child and adolescent mental health cooperative agreement* (Publication No. SM 04-002). Retrieved March 17, 2004, from http://alt.samhsa.gov/grants/2004/nofa/sm04-002_inf_NTTAC.asp

U.S. Department of Health and Human Services. (2004b, June 7). *State implementation of evidence-based practices II—Bridging science and service* (Publication No. RFA-MH-05-004). Retrieved June 7, 2004, from http://grants1.nih.gov/grants/fuide/rfa-files/RFA-MH-05-004.html

Wade, W. A., Treat, T. A., & Stuart, G. L. (1998). Transporting an empirically supported treatment for panic disorder to a service clinic setting: A benchmarking strategy. *Journal of Consulting and Clinical Psychology, 66,* 231–239.

Wampold, B. E., & Bhati, K. S. (2004). Attending to the omissions: A historical examination of evidence-based practice. *Professional Psychology: Research and Practice, 35,* 563–570.

Weersing, V. R., & Weisz, J. R. (2002). Mechanisms of action in youth psychotherapy. *Journal of Child Psychology and Psychiatry, 43,* 3–29.

Weersing, V. R., Weisz, J. R., & Donenberg, G. R. (2002). Development of the Therapy Procedures Checklist: A therapist-report measure of technique use in child and adolescent treatment. *Journal of Clinical Child and Adolescent Psychology, 31,* 168–180.

Weisz, J. R. (2004). *Psychotherapy for children and adolescents: Evidence-based treatments and case examples.* Cambridge, England: Cambridge University Press.

Weisz, J. R., Doss, A. J., & Hawley, K. M. (2005). Youth psychotherapy outcome research: A review and critique of the evidence base. *Annual Review of Psychology, 56,* 337–363.

Weisz, J. R., Southam-Gerow, M. A., Gordis, E. B., & Connor-Smith, J. (2003). Primary and secondary control enhancement training for youth depression: Applying the deployment-focused model of treatment development and testing. In A. E. Kazdin & J. R. Weisz (Eds.), *Evidence-based psychotherapies for children and adolescents* (pp. 165–183). New York: Guilford Press.

Weisz, J. R., Thurber, C. A., Sweeney, L., Proffitt, V. D., & LeGagnoux, G. L. (1997). Brief treatment of mild to moderate child depression using primary and secondary control enhancement training. *Journal of Consulting and Clinical Psychology, 65,* 703–707.

Westen, D., Novotny, C. M., & Thompson-Brenner, H. (2004). Empirical status of empirically supported psychotherapies: Assumptions, findings, and reporting in controlled clinical trials. *Psychological Bulletin, 130,* 631–663.

Woody, S. R., Weisz, J. R., & McLean, C. (in press). Empirically supported treatments: 10 years later. *The Clinical Psychologist.*

Yeh, M., & Weisz, J. R. (2001). Why are we here at the clinic? Parent–child (dis)agreement on referral problems at treatment entry. *Journal of Consulting and Clinical Psychology, 69,* 1018–1025.

EDITORS' COMMENTS

Part II reported findings on the effectiveness, efficacy, and clinical utility of psychotherapy and raised questions about what is needed next to add to the knowledge relevant to clinical practice, such as enhanced feedback mechanisms for both clinicians and for researchers. Contributors explored the importance of understanding and operationalizing the constructs that inform treatment approaches; discussed alternative research designs to better capture the individual client, the therapist–client dyad, and the psychotherapy process; and reiterated the science imperative to test interventions and measure the results.

Part III presents issues related to training, public policy, and the need for caution when considering different points of view about evidence-based practice (EBP). These discussions encompass large perspectives, including the implications of EBP concepts for graduate education and public policy and the reciprocal impact of education and policy on the mental health professions and quality care. Training integrates the needs of practice as discussed in Part I and the canons of science as described in Part II. Good judgment and methodological realism are core concepts for preparing the next generation of practitioners, as is a sophisticated understanding of the scientific attitudes and clinical skills needed for practice. Expansion of the premises of the EBP movement is explored in relation to public policy, from psychological scientism to psychological pluralism, from a one-way translation of science into practice to a full-circuit path of science to practice and back again, and from assumptions that a straight application of narrowly defined EBP makes good policy to the wider societal considerations beyond effectiveness, such as justice. These recommendations are echoed, at least in part, by some of the contributors in both Parts I and II. Finally, Part III offers a stimulating discussion on the context of practice, the design of research, and the search for panaceas. The differences between practice and science are acknowledged throughout Part III, as are the opportunities for bridging differences in a meaningful way.

III

TRAINING, POLICY, AND CAUTIONS

9

TRAINING THE NEXT GENERATION OF PSYCHOLOGIST CLINICIANS: GOOD JUDGMENT AND METHODOLOGICAL REALISM AT THE INTERFACE BETWEEN SCIENCE AND PRACTICE

STEVEN J. TRIERWEILER

A scientific approach to psychotherapy requires an appreciation of psychological science not only as it is but also as it should be. In a similar way, a scientific approach to psychotherapy requires an appreciation of the various forms of psychotherapy not only as they are but also as they should be. The integration of science and practice is a goal that originally defined the discipline of clinical psychology. This goal cannot be achieved if science is thought to be perfected in ways that are remote from practice, or if practice is thought to be perfected in ways forever outside the grasp of science. Unfortunately, in over 50 years of clinical psychology, the methods of science and practice have been conceptualized to be so far apart that the hoped-for integration has failed to materialize. Instead, there is detrimental infighting about which group, academic scientists or clinicians, has the correct approach to knowledge production in the field. For scientists, the concern is that psychological practice represents as closely as possible the state of scientifically based psychological knowledge and avoids straying too far from that knowledge. For the practitioner, the concern is that scientifically based psychological knowledge become sufficiently linked to everyday reality to significantly influence the clinical situation. Are the methods by which scientific knowledge is validated even applicable to the problems clinicians face? Who gets to decide if so, and how?

Having been involved in the study of scientific psychology and some form of psychological practice for over 30 years, and having observed the political ways of the discipline, I have no illusions that psychology's institutional, economic, and guild rivalries will soon be resolved in favor of science–practice integration. However, because both contemporary psychological science and practice are rooted in strong intellectual traditions that are fundamentally scientific, I believe it is possible to push the underlying methodological ideas of each into new territory until it becomes increasingly strained to see them as separate. Integration is a state of mind linked rigorously to the logical and empirical underpinnings of method for both science and practice. It involves a thorough grasp of how methods identify and yet limit knowledge such that the domain of applicability of any given fact may be narrower and more indirect than it may appear. The integrative state of mind draws attention to the scientific understanding and analysis of psychological phenomena as they exist and unfold in the real world. That world is a complex and ever-changing open system of information within which psychological knowledge, at best, offers up working hypotheses to be tested in specific local circumstances (Cronbach, 1975). To accommodate this complexity, both sides of the integration equation must attend to the empirical realities of the psychological phenomena clinicians confront, be they behaviors, cognitions, emotions, or other human processes not so easily classified. Integration lies in the intellectual process of figuring out how scientific facts and real local situations fit together and, ultimately, in what to do about it that might be helpful to the client.

This chapter contributes to the ongoing discussion of the issues that the integration of science and practice raises for clinical psychology (Chwalisz, 2003; Goodheart, 2004; Henriques & Sternberg, 2004; Lampropoulos & Spengler, 2002; D. R. Peterson, 2004; Stricker, 2003). Focusing on fundamental methodological concerns, I argue that practitioners need to demonstrate good judgment and methodological realism to bridge science into practice settings. The local clinical scientist training model, proposed by Trierweiler and Stricker (1991), describes attitude, critical thinking, and methodological competencies relevant to training in good judgment and methodological realism. This perspective on science–practice integration has larger implications for science and scholarship in psychology.

GOOD CLINICAL SCIENCE EQUALS GOOD CLINICAL JUDGMENT

The successful integration of scientific facts with local situations, in essence, is the exercise of good judgment in clinical inquiry—that is, the ability to elicit information in face-to-face interactions with clients, sift through that information identifying what is important, develop the inquiry so that still more relevant information comes to light, and interpret the information in a cautious, well-grounded, scientifically sound fashion. Good judgment is not an easy thing to teach. It is not simple and operational. It takes knowledge and time. It is the larger interpretive context for good scientific operations. Scientific operations are at their best when good judgment is exercised in selecting and implementing those operations. The goal is nothing less than to recognize the truth of a situation and to intervene in a manner that is consistent with that truth. Good judgment distinguishes what might be true from what cannot be true and then, with appropriate humility, dismantles those might-be truths until they either give way to better ones or hold their ground in the face of the strongest empirical tests.

I would be delighted if good judgment were simply the implementation of precise operations found in a well-designed, comprehensive, and incisive treatment outcomes literature. I would be even more delighted if good judgment were the inevitable consequence of the technical application of theory that is well established in mathematical logic and strong empirical testing, like, for example, using calculus to identify the arched trajectory of a cannonball on its way to the target. It is unfortunate that the science of psychology has not achieved this level of precision, and I believe it is highly inappropriate and misleading to act as if it has. Psychology's science offers clues as to what might be happening in the clinical situation, but they are imprecise clues at best. In contrast to the natural sciences, psychology's methods carry less of the theory–empirical observation linkage workload than does psychologists' own good judgment. Thus, psychologists must find, organize, and interpret empirical information to the extent logic, mathematics, and pre-established methods do not do it for them. As research scientists, psychologists have a sizable interpretive burden to bear; as clinicians, the burden is even greater.

Now I know there is nothing new in saying that psychology is not as highly developed a science as is, say, physics, but the proverbial devil is in the details. Just how developed is psychology? Is there not justification for implementing taxonomies such as the *Diagnostic and Statistical Manual of Mental Disorders* (4th ed., DSM–IV; American Psychiatric Association, 1994) or structured approaches to treatment that can be uniformly applied and evaluated? Should psychologists not stick to practice modalities that have been validated with controlled empirical studies? My answers to such questions are inevitably equivocal: yes and no. Psychology is rather developed as a science, particularly in its experimental design and data analysis capacities. Psychologists know more about genetics, neurochemistry, behavior, cognition, interpersonal interaction, and culture and ethnicity than ever before. Yes, psychologists should use the scientific tools that are available judiciously as aids in achieving desirable outcomes for their clients. But, at the same time, there is no psychological science currently available that assures psychologists that their interpretations of events and intervention responses based on those interpretations will be appropriate for the next case they see.

What about the material in peer-reviewed journals? Unfortunately, using such material is not simple. Even the most reliable and valid empirical findings must be assessed comparatively for their fit and applicability within a local clinical context. The local clinical context is a situation in which immediate recognition of what is going on and judgment about its meaning are required. The implications of empirical findings are no longer abstractions and generalities in such situations. Peer review deals with the scientific integrity and generalizability of empirical findings as reported in the published literature. Peer review does not routinely deal with specific applications of findings. Empirical findings from the literature always must be carefully linked to local realities if they are to be useful to the practitioner.

In addition, peer review always involves interpretation of empirical findings, and there is little other than logic (an aspect of science) and acquiescence to authority (decidedly unscientific, though perhaps pragmatic) to ensure that those interpretations are accurate and the best for the local situation (Trierweiler & Stricker, 1998). Although the psychology literature is rich in peer-reviewed theory and empirical findings, it also is rich in trenchant peer-reviewed critique of the implementation of science in psychology (e.g., Gergen, 1985; Hoshmond & Polkinghorne, 1992; Koch, 1959; Lamiell, 1981; Manicas & Secord, 1983). There are ample reasons to doubt the universality of any given finding and its interpretation in the literature. In addition, psychology does not have a generally agreed on interpretive framework (*paradigm*, in the language of Kuhn, 1970) for establishing intervention responses based on any given finding. No finding and its accompanying interpretation in the journals is enough, on its own merits, to carry fully the interpretive load into the clinical situation. Only skilled scientist–clinicians can bridge the journals and the natural settings of professional practice. This was the spirit of the scientist–practitioner training model and its precursor, the so-called Shakow report (American Psychological Association [APA], 1947), and it remains a reasonable aspirational goal for training to this day (Raimy, 1950; Stricker, 1997; Trierweiler & Stricker, 1998).

PUTTING SCIENCE INTO PRACTICE

One thing science could do is to help clinicians understand better how to observe behavior and self-report in the face-to-face clinical situation. Psychologists have information about nonverbal behavior and know that self-report can be flawed, but there is little direct scientific information that describes how a clinician should go about conducting scientific observation. This deficit in the scientific knowledge base results, in part, from the professional separation of clinicians and academic scientists that has developed in the half-century of the scientist–practitioner model in clinical psychology. However, I believe it also is due to insufficient merging of the methods of the practitioner and the scientist. Put simply, psychology has practice methodologies that deal solely with individuals and scientific methodologies that deal solely with groups of individuals. This problem has barely been recognized in the psychological literature, let alone solved (Lamiell, 1981). Yet I believe that addressing it is essential to the future of the scientific approach to psychotherapy or to any other scheme of intervention, be it psychological or biological, that addresses human behavior and experience.

To address this deficit, psychologists need two things: First, we need a realistic understanding of what aggregated, statistical, so-called nomothetic information gives us and how it might be applied to the specific local clinical situation. Second, psychologists need to begin to develop a methodological understanding of the clinical situation. I believe these goals can best be addressed in the ways scientific methods are taught. We need to be explicit about the logical underpinnings of our research design, measurement, and statistical description and inference methodologies, about what these methodologies do and do not tell us about the empirical world.

Because methods are derived from mathematical conceptions, they inevitably require a level of precise thought if students are to understand them. Over the years I have been unhappy with the tendency in the field to present research methods as taken-for-granted stepping-stones to unquestionable truth; they simply are not. Attempts to make complex material easier to understand for nonmathematically oriented students are fine so long as the presentation is rigorous and appropriately critical. However, students must understand that methods work primarily because they link good theory to trustworthy empirical observation. If research does not provide this link in a way that is interpretable to psychological science, it is not worth the effort, however advanced or fashionable the methods used appear to be at a particular time.

In the case of the typical questionnaire study, the summary statistics and reliability and validity estimates for a set of questions initially are rarely more than descriptions of the aggregate (sample) characteristics of simplified answers to (usually) simple questions. Their scientific value cannot rest solely on logical or statistical criteria. If the questions are good ones, they will have face validity, and the basic summary results will be informative about the world in their own right. The results may or may not describe universal properties of human individual differences in nature, or underlying cognitive structures, or the operation of hidden organizing principles such as stereotypes. There is nothing in even the best of statistical studies to ensure that such interpretations are meaningful. Rather, it is only an accumulation of knowledge that involves additional studies and cultural, historical, and ethical or values considerations that offer such legitimacy (Cronbach, 1975; Cronbach & Meehl, 1955; Messick, 1980).

For example, intelligence tests have shown a moderate ability to predict a certain type of school performance in the aggregate. Of this we can be reasonably assured. Certain other low-level inferences follow from this repeatedly established finding, such as that high performance on such a test usually indicates facility with a certain kind of cognitive problem solving. However, most other inferences from such data—for example, about the universality of IQ, its cultural applicability, its predictive value in the next application, or its ultimate cultural value—are subject to debate, opinion, further empirical inquiry, and often policymaking decisions that are heavily loaded in nonscientific considerations (Cronbach, 1984). Statistical studies cannot on their own merits overcome this need for interpretation. I do not mind that psychologists must make theoretical conjectures and policy decisions are inevitable, but I believe a great disservice has been done in scholarly circles to the hoped-for science–practice linkage by the failure to distinguish empirically rooted information from theoretical conjecture, however difficult such a distinction is to unravel. It is a failure to solve difficult scientific theory and rhetoric problems in the presentation of statistical and clinical case-level findings. Both psychological scientists and clinicians are guilty of this error, and only marked changes in the ways they speak about, teach, and work to fund their science will improve matters. I am not calling for nihilism about the prospects for scientific psychology, but I am saying that there is a layer of reasoned and explicit recognition of the limitations of psychological science that must be at the center of any attempt to link science and practice.

METHODOLOGICAL REALISM

Methodological realism, in this context, refers to the need for explicit recognition, in all discussions of scientific findings and their applicability in professional practice, of the true nature and limits of the empirical evidence being discussed. Scientific-sounding phrases that might mislead others about the certainty of a finding should be avoided. For example, a statement like "We now know that early aggression in boys leads to problems later in life" would be more realistically presented as "Evidence suggests that observations of early aggressive behavior in some boys may be associated with problems later in life." I understand that this can be difficult and even controversial, and I cannot say that I have always successfully heeded this concern in my own writing; everyone wants their constructs to have universality and importance. The problem, however, is that the rhetoric of science, particularly as portrayed to the media and funding agencies, can obscure weakness in the evidence and obfuscate any discussion of how such evidence pertains to a specific clinical situation. This is perhaps less a problem with published studies, which usually discuss the limitations of a project. But it definitely is a problem in discussions based on political and self-interest in the field, where science often is presented as the provenance of only a select few. The problem is no less conspicuous on the clinical side: Exercise of the rhetoric of scientific certainty based on successes with a few clinical cases in a few clinical settings disables dialogue about what precisely was observed and its potential generalizability to other cases and settings. Methodological realism requires that we psychologists modify our rhetoric to be more careful about the empirical elements of our science and clinical practice and more transparent about our beliefs and the limits on certainty of our knowledge and expertise. We are entitled to beliefs and we have the right to assert them convincingly, but we should take responsibility for them rather than implying that scientific methods carry their veracity for us.

Returning to the idea of good judgment and how it can be taught, one important focus for developing clinical science will be the scientific task of linking concepts, which includes unraveling the consequences of published empirical findings, to the local empirical data available to a psychotherapist. Other aspects of a scientific approach, such as explicit treatment planning, implementation, and outcomes evaluation, also are important. However, the basic task of recognizing links between well-selected scientific concepts (hypotheses) and empirical data (observations) within a specific clinical situation has received too little attention in the literature. This task involves a whole complex of evidence-gathering and interpretive skills that are central to the best of science and psychotherapy, that play a role in all aspects of intervention and evaluation, and that address directly the larger concern for bridging academic research and practice in psychology.

In the remainder of this chapter, I outline some of the attitude, knowledge, and judgment skills I believe are needed in training future clinician–scientists. The presentation is based on the local clinical scientist model that George Stricker and I developed as a contextual tool for rigorous training in scientific methods for professionally oriented psychologists (Stricker & Trierweiler, 1995; Trierweiler & Stricker, 1991, 1998). The model is intended to provide an interpretive context for relating the philosophy, logic, and methods of research to the local clinical situation—that is, for teaching the scientific issues surrounding the exercise of good judgment in a specific space and time context.

The basic idea appears to be simple: If science produces veridical knowledge, then that knowledge should inform empirical observation in the practice setting, called the *local clinical situation*. A bit of reflection, however, suggests that this is not a simple idea at all. The problem is not with the overarching strategy; the tasks of bringing science to the local clinical situation have been well described in terms of sequential strategies (Kanfer, 1990; D. R. Peterson, 1991). Roughly, the sequence is to identify the problem, develop an intervention plan, implement the plan, and then assess outcome, revising the plan as needed. This sort of scientific strategy is fine, in principle. The problem lies in implementing the strategy in light of the actual empirical complexity of the clinical situation. In particular, I do not believe that enough attention has been paid to the difficult initial task of identifying the problems for intervention and how they are linked to the empirical realities of clients.

THE LOCAL CLINICAL SCIENTIST TRAINING MODEL

The local clinical scientist training model springs from three premises. First, the model assumes that the integration of science and practice cannot be formulaic. Rather, in a more traditional educational sense, addressing the problem involves attitude and critical thinking skills, as well as systematic methodological knowledge. Second, the model recognizes explicitly that there are differences between the information domain of a science based in statistical methods, even when it is experimental research, and the information domain of clinical science, which is based in direct face-to-face interactions in the clinical situation. These differences are one source of the difficulty in bridging science and practice in psychology. Third, there is a need to expand scholarship to include new methods that address clinical issues in a scientific fashion, make explicit the kinds of details in statistical research that are needed to successfully link a particular statistical finding to the local clinical situation, and expand theory such that the realities of behavior and self-report actually existing in the clinical situation become part of the scientific discourse.

Several background concepts describe the educational and practice elements of the model. First, the local clinical situation is viewed to be an open system; clinicians do not have prior knowledge about what will be presented as they conduct an inquiry in that situation. Also, the boundaries of the system to be interpreted are not always apparent at the outset, and the clinician cannot be sure that all relevant information has been gathered by any given inquiry. This perspective presents a stark contrast to the typical presentation of science as involving the control of variance (Kerlinger, 1986). Local scientists do not control variance, because they are not studying variance in the same way as statistical scientists. Rather, in the traditional sense of scientific fieldwork, local scientists gather and interpret (classify) specific information within a specific space–time context. If successful, such actions would serve to control variance—and reduce error as defined in terms of the structure of the inquiry—across many cases, but that domain of discourse is usually secondary to managing the particulars of the local inquiry. Control resides in the careful and thorough way in which the data are gathered; control is something to be achieved within the clinical situation based on developing adequate knowledge of that situation.

Because the information field a clinician must interpret is an open system, local clinical science is more naturalistic, observational, and descriptive than it is experimental. Psychologists have failed to heed this fundamental distinction between the science of clinicians and that of experiments for too long, although the psychology literature has long pointed to the need to do so (Harré & Secord, 1973; Hoshmond & Polkinghorne, 1992; Shakow, 1976). When they are understood to complement one another, even though they differ in fundamental ways, both forms of scientific inquiry can contribute to the work of both psychological scientists and practitioners (Stricker, 1997). In any case, it is important to recognize that we will not always have systematic data gathering tools, like the questionnaires found in research studies, available to us in the clinical setting. Even when these tools are available, they will be incomplete descriptions of all the relevant facts of the case. Statistical data offer information about an individual's possible relationship to a hypothetical population. Such information must always be carefully integrated with the data of the local clinical situation. To this end, scientific clinicians must work with the observation base actually available in the clinical situation so as to effectively interpret the case, apply relevant scientific concepts, and frame appropriate interventions. The biggest mistake practitioners make is to assume that they already know what is happening after only brief contact with the situation (Elstein, Shulman, & Sprafka, 1978).

There are two basic sources of observations available in the psychotherapeutic situation: (a) the behavior of the client, including actions, nonverbal behavior, vocal tone, and the like, and (b) self-report, including the self-reports of significant others. Usually these observation sources are restricted to relatively brief contacts in an interview setting. Because behavioral observation is limited in such settings, a large portion of the available information will come through self-report. Some of the self-reports will focus on events within the therapeutic setting, but most will refer to events, situations, and experiences outside of the face-to-face contact.

Clinicians do not classify objects that stand still on a laboratory shelf; individuals are in a constant state of flux that clinicians periodically access through observation and verbal report. Thus, during the assessment and throughout an intervention, the self-reports of a client must be conceptualized not as static indicators, but as descriptive references to a continuous stream of behavior and experience that predates any contact with the therapist and that continues during and after such contact. All self-reports reflect ideographically specific meanings within this empirically realistic, though not directly observable, stream. Not only are the individuals themselves changing; as they do so, their reports will change. Even the simplest memory narrative may change in important ways as new insights are brought into the treatment context (Trierweiler & Donovan, 1994). Clinicians must be alert to this fluidity of the information field, particularly in the early stages of an assessment when their knowledge of the client is minimal and they are most prone to use stereotypes or cognitive heuristics to overcome uncertainty by jumping to conclusions that may be incorrect (Turk & Salovey, 1988). Within a given time frame, self-reports can describe only part of the large open information system that may be relevant to the problems the client faces. Psychologists must learn to organize the inquiry and judiciously select information for scientific interpretation. Most important, we must remain constantly alert to the inherent limits on the empirical information that can be accessed within the local clinical situation and the implications of these limits for assessment, intervention, and therapeutic outcomes.

The openness of the information system and the limits on direct empirical observation available to the clinician make it necessary for the clinician to attend to the following four different categories of information to attach a scientific concept accurately to a particular observation.

1. *The available pool of theoretical and scientific concepts:* What concepts does the clinician have available that are relevant to this situation? How probingly well do these concepts describe the empirical data (including the actual self-reports obtained, not necessarily the clinician's interpretations of those reports)? What do the concepts not describe? Are there relevant empirical findings in the scientific literature, which come to the clinician essentially as conceptual hypotheses to be attached to the local situation?

2. *Knowledge of the sociocultural circumstances of the individual:* Because clinicians depend so heavily on language and communication for empirical data, sociocultural circumstances may influence the way the client views the local clinical situation and the ways he or she remembers and describes events. An otherwise open and forthright individual can become silent about a topic if family mores have treated communication about it as a sign of weakness. In a similar way, racial, ethnic, and national identities can affect tacit perspectives on therapy and the healing process that the clinician must understand. For example, when a client from a nondominant ethnicity talks about employment in the United States, it may be necessary to assess how that minority status fits into the client's employment setting, however successful or nonchalant about the topic the individual has appeared in previous interactions.

3. *The available information about the unique life circumstances of the individual:* This idiographic assessment realm potentially includes all knowledge of all previous experience, were such comprehensive data available—which, of course, it is not. One

can only imagine how grounded clinical inquiry would be if a clinician actually had a database of well-described life events and experiences relevant to a clinical problem along with extensive idiographic measurement of relevant scientific constructs (e.g., a complete history of depressive episodes, mild to severe). Not having such an empirical tool, clinicians must approximate it with judicious idiographic inquiry.

4. *Recognition on the part of the clinician of the unique space–time local circumstances that may impact how information is elicited and interpreted:* The space–time local information setting includes all aspects of particular moments in the therapeutic interaction, including the current state of the therapist at the time the information becomes available. In many ways, psychotherapy is a performance art. However well-practiced one is, there are always special conditions existing at unique points in time when the clinical situation can be affected in unexpected or potentially misleading ways. For example, a fatigued therapist may have difficulty listening to a complex story; a therapist who has recently read an article about a theorized cause of depression may tend to look for evidence of that cause at the expense of other possible evidence; something a client says may provoke a thought process in the therapist about his or her own life that needs to be explored; or a national event in the news media may set a context for an unusually probing discussion of an individual's family relationships. A scientific clinician must be ever alert to the ways specific uncontrolled aspects of the clinical situation may affect information gathering and treatment implementation.

Of course, I am aware that what I am describing is a tall order to fill for any therapist, even for one who is highly skilled and experienced. Nonetheless, I think the scientific acuity that the local clinical scientist model describes is achievable with practice and awareness of scientific issues from the earliest stages of training. In the next section I describe some competencies of a local clinical scientist as they pertain to good judgment and methodological realism in psychological practice.

THE ATTITUDE OF A SCIENTIST IN THE CLINICAL SITUATION

Trierweiler and Stricker (1991) described several components of a scientific attitude relevant to a local clinical scientist. In this section I discuss two: (a) openness and (b) a healthy, albeit skeptical, respect for empirical evidence from both the scientific literature and the local clinical situation.

To accommodate the lack of a priori control over the available information field, local clinical science requires an attitude of openness to empirical information in the clinical situation. Openness involves an avoidance of premature conclusions about what is observed in the local clinical situation. Geiger (1941/1992) described the quality of openness associated with the experimental method as follows:

> It stands for provisionalism and tentativeness, the reliance upon working hypotheses rather than upon immutable principles. In this way, science . . . represents an attitude that can function in any area of experience, an attitude of free and effective intelligence. (p. 20; see also Cronbach, 1975, for more information)

Openness is a means to the end of ensuring that empirical information receives at least as much attention in the assessment as does the application of scientifically sound concepts or theories. In turn, theories better linked to empirical data have a better chance of actually informing an intervention in the way that was originally intended. This formulation differs from standard thinking about applying scientific information, which typically involves scientific classification based on limited behavioral samples—usually based on answers to a few simple questions, as is most clearly illustrated in the process of psychiatric diagnosis (Wakefield, 1992). There is nothing wrong with good diagnosis. But diagnosis divorced from careful empirical observation is prone to error, even though it might be gathered reliably. For example, if a patient answers a question in a manner different from the original intent of the question, it does not matter how reliable the answer is, the validity of the empirical observation described by the answer is flawed, as are any conclusions drawn from that answer. This is one problem with the relative lack of attention to validity matters in the *DSM–IV* nomenclature (Follette & Houts, 1996).

Noticing an empirical event is the first step. Many confuse noticing an event with interpreting (in effect, linguistically classifying) a noticed event. By adopting an attitude of openness that is tentative, careful, and slow to draw conclusions about what is happening, clinicians have a chance of avoiding this confusion. For example, during an interview, a man says he has been "angry all the time" and "not getting along" with his wife. An interviewer who pursues a line of questioning based on the assumption that these phrases (which are empirical events) mean that there are arguments going on within the marriage is jumping to an inferential conclusion about the meaning of the statements. A follow-up question such as "Tell me about the arguments with your wife" can throw off the inquiry if "arguments" is not a term that accurately captures the client's meaning. It also creates an undesirable situation in which the client has to be assertive with the therapist to correct the misconception. More careful and tentative openness to the ambiguities associated with self-reports would avoid these pitfalls. Consider how the request

"Tell me about 'not getting along' with your wife" keeps the observation field open to potential empirical surprises. An attitude of practiced openness helps to ensure that observations are classified carefully and repeatedly tested against new observational evidence in the clinical interaction.

Again, this is not to say that good categorization cannot be used when it makes sense, which brings us to the second desirable attitude for the local clinical scientist: respect for the empirical data of the local clinical situation. For example, if one suspects that a new client is depressed, then certainly it makes sense to assess the presence of relevant symptoms. However, if clinicians are to avoid a potentially misleading overdependence on a conception of depression (the representativeness heuristic), then they must also attend carefully to the client's behavior and self-reports so that other potentially important data have the opportunity to present themselves and, possibly, cause the clinician to modify the conceptualization. The scientific clinician must recognize the total complexity of the presentations that clients actually produce. Local empirical data take precedence over clinicians' preferences and predilections. Once local data are well understood, then new possibilities for interpreting that data emerge. Some of these possibilities may involve extrapolations from the results of published empirical studies as pertinent to the situation at hand. For example, an observation that depression and anxiety seem to coexist may lead to inquiry into "fear of being crazy," which has been shown to coincide frequently with the depression–anxiety mix (Taylor, Koch, Woody, & McLean, 1996). Scientific clinicians always treat interpretations of local empirical data as working hypotheses subject to revision as needed based on the emergence of new empirical information.

Respect for empirical data extends also to scientific studies. Well-constructed data always must be given appropriate attention, however indirectly they seem to address the problems at hand. For example, scientific clinicians must heed evidence that memory is fallible, but in a way appropriate to the exigencies of the clinical situation. Examining with the client the material details of events, as directly perceived within the client's real life circumstances as they are recollected, can clarify the limits on certainty surrounding specific memory narratives and deepen the therapist's grasp of the client's experience (Trierweiler & Donovan, 1994). Research suggests the possibility for fallibility in the details of memory; therefore, the clinician must assess the potential for fallibility about important memories. At the same time, the research in no way suggests that all details of memory are flawed, and it has not yet clarified precisely the conditions under which flawed memories should be of concern in clinical applications. Therefore, the clinician must invoke such research findings and the working hypotheses they present carefully in each new clinical situation.

I can further illustrate the problem of generalization from research findings with an example from a research article. Hammen and Brennan (2001) posited that depressed children whose mothers also were depressed would present different sorts of interpersonal problems than depressed children who did not have depressed mothers. In one finding, such children showed a difference of two points on a scale measuring perceived ability to make close friends. What does this mean for the psychotherapist working with a depressed individual? Certainly, it suggests that if the individual has a depressed mother, there may be some issue with comfort with friendships. How can this be assessed? And what might the implication be? Often it is suggested that clinicians should merely follow what the peer-reviewed literature suggests. However, close inspection shows that it is not all that clear exactly what the literature is saying. If the depressed client whose mother was depressed does not report problems with friends, should the clinician accept the negative indication, in effect running against the gist of the scientific finding? Might the client not be telling the full story? But how is the clinician to read the scientific finding? The standard deviations on the variable suggest that the average effect size falls within 1 standard deviation for either group. What does a two-point difference in average mean? What self-reports characterize the differences?

The clinician cannot know based on the report exactly what numerical values were reported for either group mean. They might be able to find out by reviewing the relevant literature more broadly, but there is no assurance even then. They know only that one group was more elevated in the positive direction than the other. Now, this is only one of a large number of findings in the study. It is an excellent study by any standards. The imprecision of the effects is discussed, and the study is well deserving of publication and the careful attention of clinicians. However, the level of detail that would be required to answer a psychotherapist's question about even one finding is not available. Nor is there a simple rule the therapist can follow to achieve such an answer. The same situation applies to studies demonstrating the effectiveness of interventions. This is a fundamental problem for clinicians in realistically interpreting published statistical findings.

CRITICAL THINKING

An open attitude is the beginning and surrounding context for careful inquiry. Critical thinking is the tool for verifying observations and testing working hypotheses about what might be going on for the client. The goal of critical thinking is no less than the revelation of the truth of the situation. I am well aware that the idea that a scientist can achieve the truth of a situation has been severely questioned in the past few decades of psychological science (Gergen, 1985; Manicas & Secord, 1983). However, the broader philosophical problems with knowing what is true should not be confused with the aspiration to achieve good enough truth in a specific clinical situation, particularly for interventions that depend on adequate knowledge of the empirical facts of the communications, lives, behavior, and experiences of clients. The goal of critical thinking is the tenacious pursuit of local truth. Even if that pursuit falls short of the ideal, clinicians can strive to develop an empirically grounded and communicable understanding of the local clinical situation that will inform their interventions.

Critical thinking in local clinical science is different from that needed for general science as currently practiced in psychology insofar as most of the primary tools used to legitimate scientific data in published scientific reports— aggregation, randomization, replication, and consensual interpretation—are unavailable in the local clinical situation. In their place, clinicians substitute skills in uncovering relevant information (as in effective interviewing), careful selection of evidence for interpretation, concepts relevant to interpreting the information (as in clinical theories and interpretation of research studies pertaining to a case), and the ability to tie all the various pieces together logically. There may be some consensus establishing operations involved, as in supervision when both clinician and supervisor come to share a view of the clinical situation, but no claims are made to the universality of such perspectives. As with any science, tacit acceptance of the veridicality of a favored perspective needs to be understood and controlled.

In this context, critical thinking involves managing carefully the various alternative possibilities available to the clinician as the inquiry unfolds. Skills in face-to-face interviewing and rapport building are critical to maximizing the information available about events extending outside the time frame of the treatment or about situations that are deeply subjective and difficult for a client to discuss. Knowledge of relevant questions and of effective ways of presenting such questions can be useful (e.g., assessing depression or discrimination in the workplace). The clinician selects reports and behaviors that are crucial to understanding the case for further inquiry and interpretation. He or she then generates working hypotheses and links these to the available empirical evidence, and the whole complex of information is tied together in a tentative case conceptualization. Each of these broad steps requires the ability to recognize and make choices; critical thinking involves uncovering empirically the crucial elements of the case and distinguishing those elements from information that may be less crucial (Trierweiler & Stricker, 1998).

Consider a male client who describes a problematic inability to stick with close relationships. Initially, the problem may seem to reside in common gender-based issues, such as an alleged inability of many men to make relationship commitments. Depression and personality issues also may be pertinent. During discussion of the relationship and various related matters, the client may reveal that a recent partner made him aware of his deficit. Further inquiry may reveal that, in fact, the description of his problem was, indeed, rooted in "feedback" from his partner about his "inability" and that this deficit was not something he had considered before these discussions.

This small self-report "fact," revealed amid many more extensive and complex descriptions of the relationship problems, may be the key to an incisive discussion of how the client came to accept this characterization of his behavior and how his compliance relates to his feelings about the relationship and the actions of his partner. Such revelations can greatly enhance the clinician's understanding of the total picture, particularly if they involve feelings that the client was unable to discuss with his partner or that he has never spoken about before. For example, additional inquiry into the alleged relational deficit may suggest that other clinical observations indicating depressed affect, interpersonal avoidance, and outbursts of anger within his relationship can be understood in light of past experiences that have led the client to fear that he will have no enduring, close relationship in his lifetime. This fear, in turn, may feed a tacit interpersonal strategy to correct the situation silently by tolerating any shortcomings he sees in his partner so as to not "push her away," which he does dutifully until the partner asks him to accept aspects of their relationship that he is unable to accept.

In my experience, simple explanations for problematic clinical behaviors (e.g., the client needs skills training) often are shallow and misleading until such hidden complexities are understood; unfortunately, such understanding rarely comes easily because of the difficulties inherent in translating that complexity into descriptive narratives that a clinician can grasp (Bruner, 1986; Polkinghorne, 1988; Trierweiler & Donovan, 1994). On the positive side, once such complexities are understood, the intervention (e.g., addressing self-esteem and communication skills) can proceed smoothly because it is well grounded in the client's experience. The point is that a local clinical scientist takes nothing for granted, and being unable to inquire immediately into every passing detail, he or she flags situations in which understanding is incomplete so that the relevant communications can be examined in the future. In this way, a conceptual portrait of the client's behavioral and subjective reality can emerge that can be linked to more general characterizations of psychopathology, maladaptive behavior, or the complexities of interpersonal relationships.

METHODOLOGICAL COMPETENCE

The development of sound scientific methodologies stands out as one of the great accomplishments of psychology's scholarly and scientific traditions. Scientific methods offer models for critical thinking and problem solving. They were designed to link empirical observations with meaningful theory and to rule out plausible rival interpretations not germane to the scientific problem at hand (Cook & Campbell, 1979). I believe that local application questions raised by a few methodological concepts are central to the ways scientific methods and the scientific attitude should be conveyed to psychologists in training. Many more suggestions along these lines are available in Trierweiler and Stricker (1998).

For this discussion it is useful to view the problem for the clinician attempting to use scientific findings as twofold, involving (a) a top-down problem of determining how to make individual inferences from statistical studies and (b) a bottom-up problem of empirically identifying characteristics of a client and determining how to interpret those characteristics in light of the population or populations the client may be from. Neither of these goals can be easily achieved. In the section that follows, I look at the top-down problem first, on the basis of an analysis of how statistical methods and aggregated empirical findings relate to an individual circumstance. Then I illustrate the bottom-up problem using applied logic as a method for critical thought and analysis in the clinical situation.

Some Methodological Realities:
The Case of Sampling and Randomization

Statistical techniques were developed to make inferences about hypothetical populations based on samples from those populations. The key issue in sampling is the achievement of representativeness of the underlying population. If samples are large enough and representativeness has been achieved, then the numerically descriptive characteristics of samples (e.g., means and variances) will closely correspond to those of the population, thus lending empirical support to inferences about those populations. Sampling and randomization are central methodological concepts in statistical research; what issues do they present for analysis of a specific clinical situation?

If, as is typical, one believes that a given individual is well represented by the research sample finding, what does this mean? At best, it indicates that the individual is like the sample mean (average). In a normal distribution, depending on the size of the group residing at or very near the mean (the modal frequency), this can be a great many individuals or relatively few. One might consider anyone with scores between 1 standard deviation below the mean and 1 standard deviation above the mean to be "like" the mean. This covers about 68% of the cases or, by inference, 68% of the population. Sixty-eight percent is a sizable number of individuals in the distribution, so the chances of being right in this conjecture will be high across many decisions. If the client comes from the remaining 32% of the sample (or the population), however, this assumption of similarity to the mean would be wrong. But let us make the assumption anyway.

If the mean reflects a numerical score on a 10-point scale with each item contributing one point to the score, then we would know that our client probably scores somewhere in the middle depending on where the distribution of scores is located on the 10-point scale (e.g., a distribution with a mean at 7 would necessarily be different qualitatively in terms of characteristics of self-report than one with a mean of 4—with the importance of the difference depending on the self-reports assessed). Unfortunately, researchers rarely characterize the mean, which is the anchor for theorizing about the meaning of scores on an instrument. Occasionally they provide characterizations of extreme scores of various kinds when tests are widely researched and designed for clinical decision making, as in high scale scores on the Minnesota Multiphasic Personality Inventory (Graham, 1993). Usually, however, qualitative characterization of the mean and even high or low scores is left to the reader of a research article. If one assumes that a relationship between the scale and some other instrument, say, a correlation, is applicable, then one is assuming that another average is descriptive of the individual, namely the average cross product of the deviation scores. The average cross product of the deviation scores determines the magnitude of the correlation coefficient between the distributions of scores on the two instruments. What expectations for relatedness between two properties measured on the scores on the two instruments can be expected when the correlation is, say, .65 (high for the psychology field)? Again, it typically is up to the reader to construct such qualitative characterizations of quantitative values. Interpreting a correlation at the individual level is complicated in any case (see Trierweiler & Stricker, 1998).

Speaking of the reader, I am undoubtedly losing some readers of this chapter in this discussion of inferences about statistical averages and individual cases. This illustrates the problem: Discussions such as this one and all their attendant complexities are too rare in the psychology field. Somehow, the field has assumed that everyone knows how to translate statistics into meaningful conjectures about individuals and, more specifically, that they know what the mean (average) of a given characteristic is like (i.e., the mean is equated with a tacit understanding of normal or typical; Wakefield, 1992). Psychology researchers wonder that professionals and scientists do not think like statisticians in everyday judgments, and yet they do not consider the possibility that no one has ever experienced the actual range and typicality of most human descriptive dimensions adequately to develop an accurate intuitive sense of the average. In fact, people's understanding of aggregate concepts is likely to be seriously restricted to the range of people and events they have experienced in their own lives, with education perhaps serving to expand that range somewhat. If so, then it is possible that no two people have the same conception of the average, so that the hypothetical anchor for judgments is essentially a moving target across judges. This is a very real problem for a statistical science: A true empirical average exists, in principle, in a population, whether one measures it or not. In a similar way, that true average can be correctly described, in principle, whether one knows the correct interpretation or not. To be sure, clinicians would benefit from scientific assistance in this area. I am purposely not providing qualitative examples to make the point that the problems being discussed are inherent in the methods psychologists use, regardless of empirical substance. The problem with substantive characterizations is that clinicians are led to believe that they understand phenomena based on their experience and whatever theoretical definitions they choose to adhere to, rather than because they have a precise grasp of the operationalizations involved in the research. Until psychologists are trained to examine carefully this problematic interface between the aggregate and the individual, psychological science and practice will necessarily be less precise and thoughtful than it needs to be.

Each time clinicians attempt to use research results, and each time they assign a category to an individual (discussed in the next section), they must assess carefully the fit between the sample characteristics of the study and the population from which the individual might be drawn. What population is a clinician sampling? How homogeneous or uniform on relevant dimensions are members of that population (Kiesler, 1966)? How close to the samples described in empirical studies is a particular member of the sample associated with a particular clinical setting? If there are obvious differences between the local sample and a relevant empirical study (e.g., if the study involves college students and the local sample involves a subgroup of patients within a clinical setting), how are the differences to be resolved? These questions cannot easily be answered. The population sampled in the caseload of particular individual clinician may not be like that of any existing research study. Substantive differences between local samples and study samples, however, may not matter all that much. The problem is, one cannot know if differences matter or not.

What about randomization? Randomization is a tool for ensuring that a sample has a high probability of representing the population from which it was selected. It is not a guarantee of such representation, but rather a device for making departures from representativeness unlikely. Randomization cannot ensure that a broadly representative study sample adequately represents the characteristics of any particular case within it. Minority populations, for example, may not be well represented in otherwise representative samples not designed specifically with their demographic characteristics in mind (Jackson et al., 2004). For the local clinical scientist, this means that the best of representative samples randomly selected from relevant populations may not produce results that translate easily and directly into the characteristics of any particular individual; in effect, descriptions of populations, however good they are, do not necessarily describe individuals (Lamiell, 1981).

What am I doing here? I am looking at the details of sampling as a research concept and asking a question about how a particular individual case might fit with the common descriptions of findings from aggregated sample information. Other research and applied statistical concepts such as variance, covariance, standard error, and so on can similarly be analyzed. What, for example, is the implication of an assessment that is at the high end of an individual's personal standard error on, say, depression (i.e., the variability of that individual's scores around his or her true score over many comparable testings)? Assuming that all the assumptions of test theory apply, one implication is that the next assessment will have a high probability of showing improvement due to regression to the true score that is based entirely on errors of measurement rather than on changes in the true score. True improvement would be conceptualized as a change in the true score on depression for the individual.

Observations, Interpretations, and Logic

Now I turn to the bottom-up question that the clinician must address: Given an interpretation (categorization) of an observation made in the clinical setting, what populations are relevant to the observation? This question is the converse of trying to relate an aggregate finding to an individual case; that is, any categorization of an object or event implies a grouping (population) of similarly categorized entities. Observations feed into categorical interpretations that, in turn, feed into constructs that may have been formally measured in scientific research studies.

Because communication in the local clinical situation inevitably involves the use of language, it inevitably involves the use of categories. Cognitive science has provided a basic generic understanding of how categories organize themselves in language. This science has described how people use heuristics to make decisions under conditions of uncertainty, which usually involves a lack of information. The problem is that too little is known about how people use categories in their day-to-day lives, particularly as categories pertain to the conditions of mental health stress and coping that arise in communications during psychotherapy.

It is easy for categorization to take place automatically on the basis of seemingly direct observations. Thus, it is important that clinicians recognize categorical thinking in both themselves and the self-reports of clients, assess the empirical support for the categorization, and use the tools of logic to ensure that these categorical inferences are not undermining accurate understanding. For example, in hospital settings, a patient's story about a life event may appear odd and implausible and, therefore, delusional. That is, a seemingly empirical-level categorical interpretation (oddness and implausibility) of an empirical event (the story as stated by the patient) becomes the "evidence" for the assignment of a symptom that then feeds into a diagnosis. As I noted in a previous section, it is important for clinicians to recognize this categorical inference and not confuse it with raw empirical observation.

Many of the problems clinicians observe in clinical situations can be thought of in categorical terms that are often in defiance of logical sensibility. For example, in logic an assertion cannot be both true and false at the same time. This claim seems trivial, particularly for categories that describe the physical world. It may not be so trivial, however, for descriptions of persons and events. For example, one may hear an individual describe herself as smart but later complain of how stupid she was in a particular social situation. If in an interview the clinician acknowledges the simple contradiction existing in her story, new information can emerge about how the client understands the categories *smart* and *stupid* as they pertain to her life experience and behavior. Her smartness, for example, may be confined only to inanimate objects or abstract ideas, but this faculty may seem to be completely disabled in the context of a social situation. By inquiring into the contradiction in the story, the clinician may discover that the client is unable to use her cognitive abilities to understand social situations because of prior assumptions about being unattractive, clumsy, and not fitting in. As the clinician extends the inquiry further, the client may find that, indeed, on reflection she is able to use her cognitive abilities quite well to interpret the past in more accurate and less contradictory ways, ways that do not always support the notion of her unattractiveness contributing to an undesirable outcome. This is an example of cognitive reframing carefully grounded in the details of experience (Safran & Segal, 1990; Trierweiler & Donovan, 1994).

As another example from applied logic, the simple idea that any assertion can be negated is valuable. Reflection on the negation of a categorization offers a possible tool for identifying overly rigid and universalistic thought in a presentation that might otherwise be taken for granted. For example, if a client presented his father as inept and bumbling, and this bumbling nature is perceived to have had an impact on the life of the client, it is important for the therapist not only to accept the characterization but also to work to understand it better. Examination of the negation of the category may reveal pockets of strength in a relationship that otherwise seems destined to failure. Thus, discovery that the bumbling father is a skilled musician, on exploring ways he is not bumbling, may suggest avenues for discussing more promising aspects of the relationship.

Many other tools from both traditional and nontraditional research methods are described in Trierweiler and Stricker (1998). Realistic methodological training addressing the strengths, weaknesses, and range of applicability of all methodologies available to psychological science is the conceptual foundation for the integration of science and practice envisioned for psychology.

SOME BROADER IMPLICATIONS OF METHODOLOGICAL REALISM

If one takes methodological realism seriously, direct attention to the interface between statistical science and the individual case has broader implications for science and the nature of scholarship in psychology. I close the chapter with brief discussions of a few of these implications (see also Trierweiler & Stricker, 1998).

Because research studies cannot typically address the characteristics of the individual case—and despite the fact that many studies can characterize populations quite well—no single research study or body of case material supports strong conclusions about how psychotherapy should be conducted. I am not arguing against strongly held opinions or recommendations, but I am arguing against all suggestion that certainty has been achieved, when it has not. Generalizability of research findings, even from randomized designs, always must be evaluated carefully in terms of the empirical characteristics of the local clinical situation—that is, the four settings of information previously discussed. In part, such assessment will involve the problem of generalizing an aggregated research finding to a specific case. Treatment studies, for example, that offer thorough qualitative descriptions of cases obtaining positive, neutral, and negative scores on measured outcomes will facilitate this endeavor. The problems associated with generalizing from the aggregate to the individual and the inevitable caution that is needed due to the imprecision of statistical findings need to be part of all discussions of the nature of evidence in the psychology field. In turn, it must be recognized that local evidence may be as important or more important than any given recommendation from a scientific study. The lack of attention to these matters is most troublesome in situations in which there is strong motivation to overgeneralize preliminary results from studies that support one's political or self-interest perspective (Antonuccio, Danton, & McClanahan, 2003). Of course, confidence in the generalizability of a finding is facilitated by multiple samples performing similarly across several studies or effects that can be readily observed at the level of the individual case.

Statistical Results Always Require Local Translation

Psychologist scientists and practitioners must recognize that most scientific questions related to observations of individual behavior cannot be completely answered by statistical findings. This is the problem of never being able to achieve point predictions in "soft science" that Meehl (1978) pointed out many years ago. Statistical findings are inevitably imprecise. However, by focusing on smaller and smaller subpopulations, the range of contexts for interpreting findings can be narrowed. In this sense, advancement as a statistical science should not be considered simply in terms of direct relationships between variables, which often are presented as if causal determinism has been established, when it has not (e.g., irrational thought tends to cause depression), but rather in terms of the description in greater and greater detail of the subcontexts that modify the empirical manifestations of those relationships (e.g., subgroups created by the intersection of values on variables, such as social class plus intellectual ability plus personality, will narrow the context for interpreting why an individual is not doing well in school better than does just an intelligence score).

Of course, as a correlational relationship approaches 1.0, this need to seek out and manage the subcontexts created by mediator and moderator variables is lessened. Departures from 1.0, particularly with correlationally small relationships (.20 to .40), would require relatively more such research to be useful to clinicians. Once described, these subcontexts provide the clinician with richer, more probing working hypotheses about what might be true in the local clinical situation. It is appropriate to use subcontext-related hypotheses accordingly. Even large bodies of statistical research, however, do not necessarily support strong assertions about what is true (e.g., persons with depressed mothers will have interpersonal problems, memory blocks indicate prior abuse) without careful and extensive assessment of case specifics.

Values on Variables Are Working Hypotheses

When deterministic relationships have not been established, values on variables need to be understood as identifying potential contexts for behavior rather than determinants of behavior. By explicitly framing values on variables as context identifiers (as opposed to tacit construct quantity indicators), one is allowing for the reality of statistical imprecision, a reality not always apparent when quantification is invoked as a justification for confidence in an assertion. In this way, for example, one would understand that a score residing at the 75th percentile on a measure of conscientiousness does not necessarily imply behaviors normative at that level, nor that the individual necessarily exhibits 75% of the possible quantity of the construct available in the population. The score is a context for identifying normatively what is possible, not for certainty.

To support the notion that values on variables are probabilistic contexts for behavior, psychologists need a body of scientific work that generates qualitative descriptions of the kinds of situations clinicians observe for various values on measurements on research scales in the psychology field. For example, if one has measured a personality characteristic such as conscientiousness, what types of observations, qualitatively speaking, might be observed at the 50th percentile or at the 75th percentile? The best descriptions would include both those fitting well with the ostensive quantitative description—that is, showing a moderate or high level of conscientiousness—and those not fitting the quantitative descriptions so well—for example, scoring high but not necessarily manifesting the characteristic in an obvious way. Consider that in the physical realm, where quantity characterizes physical phenomena quite effectively and can be referenced to a palpable physical standard (in a bureau of weights and measurements), if one knows that an object weighs 100 pounds, one also knows something about the effort needed to carry the object. What does one need to know about the 75th percentile of conscientiousness relative to a local clinical goal—such as the achievement of an accurate self-report—where the quantitative characterization is more indirect and bound to a sample and an implied population that cannot be observed directly? A body of scholarship that combines quantification with qualitative description would facilitate psychologists' grasp of how information about particular measurements might inform potential observation of the individual case.

Client Self-Report Is Central to Scientific Clinical Inquiry

Research is needed that explores how various phenomena may manifest themselves in clients' self-reports. The client's own understanding of his or her life is an important standard, in addition to typical reliability and validity considerations, against which reports need to be evaluated as they feed into clinical inferences about a case. For example, if a client's report of depression is based on an understanding of the concept of depression that he or she has obtained from a television commercial for a psychotropic medication, the clinician, having identified this situation, will quickly understand that the client's preliminary description may be incomplete and that more information is needed before the diagnosis can be rendered. Simple answers to simple questions about a symptom, like depressed mood, may offer incomplete understanding of the true nature of the report unless the clinician expands the inquiry. At the same time, however, clinicians must understand that if they do not ask certain questions, it is possible that important material will not be assessed in the interactions with clients.

The Scientific Attitude Must Be Taught to All Students of Psychology

There is a need to expand the body of scientific methods taught to students, the theory of how methods contribute to an understanding of the nature of local evidence, and the discussion of the requirement that ideas from research and clinical theories must be tested against behavior and self-report information available in the local clinical situation (Trierweiler & Stricker, 1998). If young psychologists are to pursue their own interests, they must understand that there is a requirement that those interests be coordinated with empirical data that are actually available in a clinical situation. For science, this means that there is no magic in statistical studies that would justify broad generalizations from limited samples or from indirectly representative populations (e.g., college students to clinical cases). Meaningful generalization is possible, but it must be done tentatively until local data become available to justify top-down inference. Similarly, clinicians need to understand that their most solid observations in the clinical situation may not generalize to the next case or to any other case. Ideas developed in the clinical situation need to be tested broadly before they are presented as the truth of the matter.

CONCLUSION

Ultimately, the future of psychological training depends on the development of theory and rhetoric consistent with the methods available, both for scientific research and for scientific clinical inquiry. Effective substantive description of the ways statistical findings offer useful working hypotheses for local examination should be at the center of this endeavor. Indeed, I believe that an entire body of literature could be developed devoted to elaborating the bridges between statistical findings and clinical theory and inquiry. This literature—perhaps including an Internet-accessible database of consensually interpreted findings—could extend beyond just outcome studies to contain substantive material from other areas of psychological science, such as cognitive studies, that clinicians could elaborate in ways directly pertinent to the tasks and decisions that they confront. Of course, this would require considerable development and improvement of the scientific literature, beyond the common reports of one-shot findings and into the actual intricacies that exist in using statistical technologies to answer substantive psychological questions that have implications for the assessment of individuals (R. L. Peterson & Trierweiler, 1999). I am not critical of psychology's scientific methods, but I am critical of the rhetoric that pushes scientific products beyond their reasonable range of applicability and that inhibits serious examination of the complexities psychologists face in extending their science beyond research article production. In like fashion, clinical theories need to be properly framed as hypotheses in need of explicit connection to the raw material of the practice setting, namely, the behavior and self-reports about experience that clients actually present to clinicians. Such linkages are needed to establish the empirical integrity of scientific practice and, in so doing, will demonstrate how the larger project of psychological science can inform practice.

The local clinical science model is not sanction for the status quo; it highlights the need for renewed open dialogue and significant change in the ways the science–practice interface is discussed. Good judgment and methodological realism are at the core of this vision. It is ironic that they were arguably at the core of the vision for training described in the Shakow Report (APA, 1947) report as well. I believe it is time to move this vision forward and properly locate psychology at the center of mental health science and practice.

REFERENCES

American Psychiatric Association. (1994). *Diagnostic and statistical manual of mental disorders* (4th ed.). Washington, DC: Author.

American Psychological Association, Committee on Training in Clinical Psychology. (1947). Recommended graduate training program in clinical psychology. *American Psychologist, 2,* 539–558.

Antonuccio, D. O., Danton, W. G., & McClanahan, T. M. (2003). Psychology in the prescription era: Building a firewall between marketing and science. *American Psychologist, 58,* 1028–1043.

Bruner, J. (1986). *Actual minds, possible worlds.* Cambridge, MA: Harvard University Press.

Chwalisz, K. (2003). Evidence-based practice: A framework for twenty-first-century scientist–practitioner training. *The Counseling Psychologist, 31,* 497–528.

Cook, T. D., & Campbell, D. T. (1979). *Quasi-experimentation: Design and analysis issues for field settings.* Boston: Houghton Mifflin.

Cronbach, L. J. (1975). Beyond the two disciplines of scientific psychology. *American Psychologist, 30,* 116–127.

Cronbach, L. J. (1984). *Essentials of psychological testing* (4th ed.). New York: HarperCollins.

Cronbach, L. J., & Meehl, P. E. (1955). Construct validity in psychological tests. *Psychological Bulletin, 52,* 281–302.

Elstein, A. S., Shulman, L. S., & Sprafka, S. A. (1978). *Medical problem solving: An analysis of clinical reasoning.* Cambridge, MA: Harvard University Press.

Follette, W. C., & Houts, A. C. (1996). Models of scientific progress and the role of theory in taxonomy development: A case study of the *DSM. Journal of Consulting and Clinical Psychology, 64,* 1120–1132.

Geiger, G. (1992). Philosophy and social change. *Antioch Review, 50,* 15–27. (Original work published 1941)

Gergen, K. J. (1985). The social constructionist movement in modern psychology. *American Psychologist, 40,* 266–275.

Goodheart, C. (2004). Evidence-based practice and the endeavor of psychotherapy. *The Independent Practitioner, 24.* Retrieved November 8, 2005, from http://www.division42.org/MembersArea/IPfiles/IPWtr_04/prof_practice/goodheart.php

Graham, J. R. (1993). MMPI–2: Assessing personality and psychopathology (2nd ed.). London: Oxford University Press.

Hammen, C., & Brennan, P. A. (2001). Depressed adolescents of depressed and nondepressed mothers: Tests of an interpersonal impairment hypothesis. *Journal of Consulting and Clinical Psychology, 69,* 284–294.

Harré, R., & Secord, P. F. (1973). *The explanation of social behavior.* Totowa, NJ: Littlefield, Adams.

Henriques, G. R., & Sternberg, R. J. (2004). Unified professional psychology: Implications for the combined-integrated model of doctoral training. *Journal of Clinical Psychology, 60,* 1051–1063.

Hoshmond, L. T., & Polkinghorne, D. E. (1992). Redefining the science–practice relationship and professional training. *American Psychologist, 47,* 55–66.

Jackson, J. S., Torres, M., Caldwell, C. H., Neighbors, H. W., Nesse, R. M., Taylor, R. J., et al. (2004). The National Survey of American Life: A study of racial, ethnic, and cultural influences on mental disorders and mental health. *International Journal of Methods in Psychiatric Research, 13,* 196–207.

Kanfer, F. H. (1990). The scientist–practitioner connection: A bridge in need of constant attention. *Professional Psychology: Research and Practice, 21,* 264–270.

Kerlinger, F. N. (1986). *Foundations of behavioral research* (3rd ed.). New York: Holt, Rinehart & Winston.

Kiesler, D. J. (1966). Some myths of psychotherapy research and the search for a paradigm. *Psychological Bulletin, 65,* 110–136.

Koch, S. (1959). *Psychology: A study of a science* (Vol. 3). New York: McGraw-Hill.

Kuhn, T. S. (1970). *The structure of scientific revolutions* (2nd ed.). Chicago: University of Chicago Press.

Lamiell, J. T. (1981). Toward an idiothetic psychology of personality. *American Psychologist, 36,* 276–289.

Lampropoulos, G. K., & Spengler, P. M. (2002). Introduction: Reprioritizing the role of science in a realistic version of the scientist–practitioner model. *Journal of Clinical Psychology, 58,* 1195–1197.

Manicas, P. T., & Secord, P. F. (1983). Implications for psychology of the new philosophy of science. *American Psychologist, 38,* 399–413.

Meehl, P. E. (1978). Theoretical risks and tabular asterisks: Sir Karl, Sir Ronald, and the slow progress of soft psychology. *Journal of Consulting and Clinical Psychology, 46,* 806–834.

Messick, S. (1980). Test validity and the ethics of assessment. *American Psychologist, 35,* 1012–1027.

Peterson, D. R. (1991). Connection and disconnection of research and practice in the education of professional psychologists. *American Psychologist, 46,* 422–429.

Peterson, D. R. (2004). Science, scientism, and professional responsibility. *Clinical Psychology: Science and Practice, 11,* 196–210.

Peterson, R. L., & Trierweiler, S. J. (1999). Scholarship in psychology: The advantages of an expanded vision. *American Psychologist, 54,* 350–355.

Polkinghorne, D. E. (1988). *Narrative knowing and the human sciences.* Albany: State University of New York Press.

Raimy, V. C. (Ed.). (1950). *Training in clinical psychology.* New York: Prentice Hall.

Safran, J. D., & Segal, Z. V. (1990). *Interpersonal process in cognitive therapy.* New York: Basic Books.

Shakow, D. (1976). What is clinical psychology? *American Psychologist, 31,* 553–560.

Stricker, G. (1997). Are science and practice commensurable? *American Psychologist, 52,* 442–448.

Stricker, G. (2003). Evidence-based practice: The wave of the past. *The Counseling Psychologist, 31,* 546–554.

Stricker, G., & Trierweiler, S. J. (1995). The local clinical scientist: A bridge between science and practice. *American Psychologist, 50,* 995–1002.

Taylor, S., Koch, W. J., Woody, S., & McLean, P. (1996). Anxiety sensitivity and depression: How are they related? *Journal of Abnormal Psychology, 105,* 474–479.

Trierweiler, S. J., & Donovan, C. M. (1994). Exploring the ecological foundations of memory in psychotherapy: Interpersonal affordance, perception, and recollection in real time. *Clinical Psychology Review, 14,* 301–326.

Trierweiler, S. J., & Stricker, G. (1991). The research and evaluation competency area: Training the local clinical scientist. In R. L. Peterson, J. McHolland, R. J. Bent, E. Davis-Russell, G. E. Edwall, E. Magidson, et al. (Eds.), *The core curriculum in professional psychology* (pp. 103–113). Washington, DC: American Psychological Association and National Council of Schools of Professional Psychology.

Trierweiler, S. J., & Stricker, G. (1998). *The scientific practice of professional psychology.* New York: Plenum Press.

Turk, D. C., & Salovey, P. (Eds.). (1988). *Reasoning, inference, and judgment in clinical psychology.* New York: Free Press.

Wakefield, J. C. (1992). The concept of mental disorder: On the boundary between biological facts and social values. *American Psychologist, 47,* 373–388.

10

EXPANDING THE TERMS OF THE DEBATE: EVIDENCE-BASED PRACTICE AND PUBLIC POLICY

SANDRA J. TANENBAUM

Evidence-based practice (EBP), although defined differently by different parties, usually means that clinical practice is answerable to experimental studies, traditionally the findings of randomized controlled trials (RCTs). EBP adheres to an applied science model wherein what are deemed the most scientific research methodologies are used to determine what does and does not "work" in the treatment of individual patients. Practitioners are urged, trained, and sometimes coerced to change their practices accordingly. The EBP movement, furthermore, not only promotes the funding and dissemination of experimental studies but also seeks to supplant the current clinical knowledge regime with its own; thus, the movement equates "evidence" in general with experimental studies in particular and posits a psychological practice reliant on evidence-based manuals and guidelines. From this perspective, the best practice is the most faithful to research (Drake et al., 2001), and practitioners who diverge from the evidence are willfully ineffective and therefore morally culpable (Meehl, 1997).

This stark view of the EBP movement is not meant to paint the many thoughtful proponents of EBP with an unfairly broad brush. It is not to ignore, for example, ongoing efforts within the movement to refine the match of kinds of research evidence to kinds of practice questions (e.g., Beutler & Castonguay, 2005). It does, however, recognize that despite differences in views among its supporters, this influential movement strives to make experimental studies authoritative in psychological practice and mental health policy. Although EBP is sometimes portrayed as an integration of external evidence and individual expertise (e.g., Institute of Medicine, 2001), the knowledge hierarchies that accompany these portrayals consistently put clinical trials at the top (Chambless & Ollendick, 2001; Sackett, Rosenberg, Muir-Gray, Haynes, & Richardson, 1996; University of Oxford, 1998). Moreover, these hierarchies have been implemented to distinguish—for the profession and the polity—unapproved treatments from approved ones (Chambless et al., 1998), that is, treatments that can be counted on to "work." Although psychologists do the important work of disputing what science is good enough for good practice, EBP's continuing emphasis on RCTs and pursuit of specific treatments for specific diagnoses from the *Diagnostic and Statistical Manual of Mental Disorders* (4th ed., *DSM–IV*; American Psychiatric Association, 1994) is creating a gold standard (Timmermans & Berg, 2003) to which patients, practitioners, and policymakers are being held.

As a knowledge regime in psychology, EBP is of academic and professional significance. It also reaches beyond the American Psychological Association (APA) into the American polity because in important ways, professions are creations of the state. Psychologists qua professionals are sheltered, by licensure, from the full force of economic competition; permitted to credential and regulate their peers and training institutions; and paid, by public entities, for services psychologists deem necessary and safe. The EBP movement has the potential to redefine psychological professionalism. If practitioners were once thought to bring erudition and discretion to their work, EBP's applied science model minimizes the distance between research data on the one hand and psychological intervention on the other. The practitioner thereby requires less training and exercises less judgment. The role of practice knowledge is diminished. Psychologists may find that given current pressures for reform of the health care system, the public policies that affect them—licensure and other forms of professional self-regulation, economic viability through market shelter, malpractice litigation, public reimbursement, and the regulation of managed care—respond not only to the power of their guild but to the public understanding of what professionals know (Tanenbaum, 1993).

It is the purpose of this chapter to view EBP with an eye toward public policy. First, it puts the rise of EBP in mental health in the context of developments in the U.S. health care system generally. Second, it describes what seem to be the movement's three working hypotheses for effecting positive change in mental health care and suggests that both the EBP debate and its policy consequences would benefit from a more expansive version of the terms of this debate. Finally, it locates EBP in a number of specific policies and thus demonstrates the ramifications of the current terms of the EBP debate.

THE RISE OF EVIDENCE-BASED PRACTICE

Since the early 1970s, U.S. health policy has been about cost. The United States spent 15.3% of its gross domestic product (GDP) on health care in 2003, and that portion is expected to reach 18.7% by 2014 (Heffler et al., 2005). This figure compares with the current health care spending rate of approximately 8% of GDP in the non-U.S. countries of the Organisation for Economic Co-Operation and Development (Reinhardt, Hussey, & Anderson, 2004). Per capita health care costs increased almost continuously between 1966 and 2000, and health care spending is now growing faster than it was in the late 1980s and early 1990s (Altman, Tompkins, Eilat, & Glavin, 2003). Total expenditures for health care were $1.7 trillion in 2003 (Centers for Medicare and Medicaid Services, 2005).

The cost of mental health care is no exception to the trend. In fact, between 1987 and 2000, only heart disease accounted for a greater percentage of the increase in total health care spending than mental illness (Thorpe, Florence, & Joski, 2004). At the beginning of that period, exemption from the Medicare prospective payment system (which used diagnosis-related groups) encouraged growth in the number of psychiatric hospital bed days (Cummings, 2000), and over time, the treated prevalence rate for mental illness almost doubled, to 8,575 per 100,000, accounting for 59% of the cost increase. Still, 21% of the rise in mental health care spending resulted from cost per treated case (Thorpe et al., 2004), and given the size of the overall increase, mental health remains a target for health care cost cutters. Policymakers will likely round up the usual suspects—technological advance, demographic change, competition (too little or too much), regulation (too little or too much), and, especially in the case of mental health, unlimited demand, unlimited supply, and practice variation among health care providers.

In the early 1980s, Dartmouth physician–researcher John Wennberg conducted a series of what he called "small-area variation" studies. He found large, "unexplained" variation in the rates of common medical procedures among localities in a relatively small geographic area. Wennberg and others concluded that this variability in practitioner behavior resulted from uncertainty about the value of alternative interventions and from clinically superfluous factors such as convenience or tradition (Wennberg, 1984). Presumably, physicians could be made more certain and less distractible through the findings of rigorous research on treatment outcomes. Once there were clear associations between what a clinician did and how the patient fared, the clinician would certainly do what worked. If several interventions proved equally successful, practitioners could be directed to choose the least costly one.

The small-area variation studies were well received. They lent credence to the popular "waste theory" (Mehlman, 1986), which held that uninformed physicians were squandering health care dollars on unnecessary diagnostic tests and ineffective patient care. Wennberg's (1984) call for more research was compatible with the longstanding U.S. policy that funds health care research instead of health care coverage (Rothman, 1997). As a reform agenda, it partook of the American propensity for social problem solving by technical means (Morone, 1994). The "outcomes movement" (Epstein, 1990) promised to contain cost and improve quality in a single blow—and this without resorting to politics or ideology.

Yet the Wennberg (1984) studies and their aftermath were political. Medical outcomes research empowered researchers—specifically those with statistical expertise—relative to practitioners (Armstrong, 1977). Wennberg urged academic medicine to increase its support for disciplines such as clinical epidemiology, biostatistics, and clinical decision making, and the federal Agency for Health Care Policy and Research (now the Agency for Health Care Research and Quality, or AHRQ) was charged with funding extramural outcomes research in the tens of millions of dollars (e.g., the Schizophrenia Patient Outcomes Research Team; Lehman & Steinwachs, 1998). Given the rising cost of health care, effectiveness studies became cost-effectiveness studies. Economists and clinicians who could think like economists received the federal government's "legislative and fiscal blessing on these hitherto arcane callings" (Brown, 1991, p. 12), and outcomes researchers, operating within the "economizing model," "outlived, outtheorized, and outmaneuvered" colleagues who framed health care questions differently (Fox, 1990, p. 496). What health services researchers knew acquired new authority relative to what physicians, and even basic scientists, knew. Statistical knowledge, moreover, could be rendered as practice guidelines. The outcomes movement provided a scientific rationale for the "behavioral regulation" (Brown, 1992, p. 17) of physicians by health insurers, managed care organizations, and government (Tanenbaum, 1994).

By the early 1990s, the outcomes movement had evolved into evidence-based medicine and, by extension, EBP. Adherents aspired to nothing less than a "new paradigm" of clinical practice in which "examination of evidence from clinical research" replaces "intuition, unsystematic clinical experience, and physiologic rationale" (Evidence-Based Medicine Working Group, 1992, p. 2420). The Society for Clinical Psychology (Division 12 of the APA) created a Task Force on the Promotion and Dissemination of Psychological Procedures in 1993. The chair of the initial Task Force located her work squarely in the tradition of evidence-based medicine (Chambless & Ollendick, 2001).

THREE WORKING HYPOTHESES OF THE EVIDENCE-BASED PRACTICE MOVEMENT

EBP is ubiquitous in psychology. It accounts for published volumes like this one (as well as, e.g., Beutler & Castonguay, 2005; Nathan & Gorman, 2002; Wampold, 2001), hundreds of articles in journals such as *Clinical Psychology: Science and Practice* and *Psychotherapy Research,* and at least one profile in *The New York Times* (Carey, 2004). EBP is also controversial (Elliott, 1998) and the cause for "psychological warfare between therapists and scientists" (Tavris, 2003, p. B7). Evidence seems to be at the heart of the controversy, but this is as much rhetorical as real. Both camps practice empiricism—that is, both proponents and opponents of EBP are guided by experience as well as theory—and evidence is the distillation of experience. The dispute, then, is about how to value, study, and use experience in psychological practice. EBP proponents insist that only specified statistical methods can turn experience into evidence. Opponents maintain that evidence can issue from other social scientific methodologies and from the "reflective practitioner" (Schon, 1983) himself or herself. This is a disagreement about *kinds* of evidence and about what is knowable, with what certainty, and at what remove from the patient.

The EBP movement is not monolithic. Proponents of EBP disagree about evidence, practice, and policy. Although Division 12 abides by an RCT-dominated evidence hierarchy (Chambless et al., 1998), there have been more recent efforts to broaden the definition of science for practice (Nathan & Gorman, 2002; Norcross, 2002). Other divisions of the APA have themselves called the Division 12 hierarchy into question. Still, the EBP movement holds three working hypotheses about effecting positive change in mental health care. The first is that whatever the difficulties, it is possible to have good science. The second is that good science, well managed, leads to good practice. The third is that good practice writ large defines good policy. These hypotheses set the terms of the EBP debate and shape the policies that issue from it.

Whatever the Difficulties, It Is Possible to Have Good Science

The EBP debate focuses primarily on what qualifies as evidence. The movement chose brilliantly to name as "evidence" only (more or less restrictive) experimental studies, thereby putting other ways of knowing, say qualitative or personal, on the defensive. One can hardly argue with evidence. EBP's working hypothesis, however, is more than that only science counts as evidence; it is that there is (or will be reasonably soon) enough good science to serve as the bedrock of an effective practice. Proponents of EBP decry the paucity of high-quality research (for a compelling example from EBM, see

Tunis, Stryer, & Clancy, 2003), but they do not consider that scientific knowledge, however well gathered, may not suffice for clinical practice. This possibility, however, should penetrate the EBP debate, because under the EBP model, insufficient science creates a vacuum of authority. Perhaps clinical science as currently conceived can inform clinical practice in a rigorous, timely, and comprehensive way. There are, however, serious obstacles to this end, and what happens to EBP when science defaults? How, then, do practitioners do what is right?

The work of Division 12 epitomizes EBP on this point. The division's Task Force on the Promotion and Dissemination of Psychological Procedures compiled a list of empirically validated (more recently termed *empirically supported* and then *evidence-based*) treatments for which there exists sufficiently rigorous evidence of efficacy—at least two RCTs or 10 single-case experimental studies—with patients fitting specific *DSM–IV* diagnostic categories. A precondition for sufficient rigor was that treatments were administered according to treatment manuals. Division 12 issued its first list of EBTs in 1996; the latest update was published in 1998 (Chambless et al., 1998). On its current Web site, the Division admits that some "beneficial psychotherapies" may not yet have been studied; still, the group advises potential patients to undergo the treatments on the list because these have met "basic scientific standards for effectiveness" (Society for Clinical Psychology, 2000). Division 12 does not have all the science, but it glosses the difference between untested and ineffective treatments.

The Division 12 list reaped both praise and blame. It was widely influential (as discussed later in this chapter), but it also raised serious questions about the science of EBP: whether rigorous science is necessarily the right science; whether research questions that yield rigorous answers are necessarily the right questions; and whether, given the myriad practical limitations on research, rigorous science is as possible—that is, as timely and affordable—as it needs to be. There is little disagreement, for example, that RCTs inform clinicians about efficacy but not effectiveness—that RCTs achieve internal but not external validity (e.g., Garfield, 1966). Like the proponents of "practical clinical trials" in evidence-based medicine (Tunis et al., 2003), some psychological scientists are trying to solve this problem, for example, by designing "hybrid" studies to measure both efficacy and effectiveness (Carroll & Rounsaville, 2003). Because many mental health interventions, as "socially complex services," necessarily violate the assumptions of RCT methodology—precise protocols, equivalent trial conditions, and so forth—they arguably require at least an extensively modified approach to measuring efficacy (Wolff, 2000). Furthermore, psychological investigators do not agree whether the performance of specific treatments for specific diagnoses is even the most valid measure of psychotherapeutic efficacy (Nathan & Gorman, 2002). Some argue that so-called common factors, such as therapeutic alliance, are more determinative of patient benefit and should be the focus of evidence gathering in mental health (e.g., Messer & Wampold, 2002).

Then, there are serious practical issues that cut across research questions and study types. For example, top officials at the Centers for Medicare and Medicaid Services and AHRQ recently acknowledged that to conduct the necessary practical clinical trials, they must secure substantial funding, especially for large sample sizes and long-term follow-up. Given the cost, they report, investigators may resort to "large simple trials," in which data are collected only on the smallest number of elements (Tunis et al., 2003), not enough, perhaps to capture the complexities of mental illnesses. Another strategy for achieving large-scale results is through the meta-analysis, or statistical manipulation, of smaller study findings. Meta-analysis is common in EBP research but has been roundly criticized methodologically (Miettinen, 1998) and for the "authoritative aura" it undeservedly assumes (Feinstein & Horwitz, 1997). Ethical limitations also impinge on study design: Does the trial achieve true therapeutic equipoise? When, and for how long?

In the pursuit of rigor, Division 12 and EBP generally have drawn a putatively bright line between scientific and unscientific knowledge. In EBP, science is privileged as evidence because it is objective rather than subjective, but social studies of science find a "tacit dimension" to scientific knowledge (Polanyi, 1967). The design even of RCTs calls for a series of decisions made by investigators relying on their judgment (Gonzales, Ringeissen, & Chambers, 2002), and the implementation of RCT-based protocols requires clinicians' interpretations of what they read and of their immediate circumstances (Berg, 1997). Assuming that EBP involves choices among research questions to ask and research methods to use, on what grounds are these choices made? There is no purely scientific answer to the question of which science is best. Rather, it would seem, the research enterprise rides on the judgment, as well as the science, of the scientist.

Perhaps most urgently for psychological practice, the EBP movement locates whole schools of psychotherapy on the other side of this not-so-bright line. Because they cannot demonstrate experimentally that they are efficacious vis-à-vis other therapies (or placebo), these treatments do not generally appear on lists such as Division 12's and are thereby delegitimized as psychological practice (Bohart, O'Hara, & Leitner, 1998). Psychodynamic and humanistic psychotherapies have been found effective in nonexperimental research (e.g., Seligman, 1996) but are fundamentally unsuited to the methodology of RCTs and similar studies: They do not focus on a disorder to be alleviated (but rather on a relationship with an individual patient), they do not enlist a predetermined treatment (but rather principles of therapeutic process), and they do not seek uniformity among therapists (but rather each therapist's adherence to a theoretical orientation and set of techniques that are compatible with his or her "interpersonal presence" and the needs of the patient). Psychologists disagree about how experimental is experimental enough, but some therapies invite study by the human sciences rather than the natural sciences, and the human sciences do not count as evidentiary under EBP. Furthermore, the insistence on RCTs has disadvantaged many kinds of psychiatric patients. Those who have significant comorbidities, fall into small or nonobvious subgroups, or suffer from complex disorders such as personality disorders are harder to accommodate in studies of aggregate efficacy. One meta-analysis of high-quality mental health RCTs found that two thirds of the patients who presented for treatment were excluded and that the trials with the most stringent exclusion criteria testified to the greatest efficacy (Westen & Morrison, 2001). It is not surprising that EBP favors cognitive and behavioral psychotherapies (Chambless et al., 1998) whose epistemological foundations—assumptions about what is knowable and how— are the same as the science that studies them.

The EBP movement circumscribes psychological knowledge for practice. An evidence hierarchy based on RCTs may be exclusionary in the extreme, but even at its most liberal, the EBP movement rejects systematic but nonexperimental knowledge in the form of knowledge gathered by practitioners qua practitioners. The relationship of psychological knowledge to psychotherapeutic practice is explored later in this chapter, but it should be noted in this discussion that EBP does not accept as evidentiary, for example, disciplined inquiry by the clinician (Peterson, 1991) nor analysis of large databases of intensive and systematic case studies (Messer, 2004). Psychology, however, seems to know more than EBP imagines. The terms of the debate, then, might expand to consider how good the science is when so much happens outside of its methodological boundaries. As targeted inquiry, science necessarily provides information of some kinds but not others; even high-quality studies are always incomplete. A rigorous but inclusive psychological pluralism, then, might serve the profession better than psychological scientism, which holds that science is authoritative regardless of the objects and objectives of research (Peterson, 2004). Can good science marry other high-quality research to create a more thorough knowledge base for practitioners? Will this render the profession more faithfully in the policymaker's mind's eye?

Good Science, Well Managed, Leads to Good Practice

Applying science to practice is the raison d'être of the EBP movement. Its goal is to improve practice by delivering science to the consulting room. Generally speaking, EBP adopts an applied science or diffusion of technology approach to building its bridge from science to practice. Experimental studies produce evidence that is communicated to or, if necessary, imposed on practitioners. Some attention is paid to the role of clinical judgment and patient values (e.g., Institute of Medicine, 2001) and to practitioner-driven research (Borkovec, Echemendia, Ragusea, & Ruiz, 2001), but proceeding from the complaint that practitioners do not use available evidence of what works (Hayes, 1996), the EBP movement focuses primarily on changing practice with efficacy or effectiveness study results.

The dissemination of research findings to practitioners has not, for the most part, brought practice into line with research (U.S. Department of Health and Human Services, 2000). There is, therefore, a substantial body of work devoted to the bridge from science to practice—to increased practitioner uptake of scientific results. Decision-making tools include manuals, algorithms, protocols, and guidelines; these specify practice behavior with greater or lesser authority. The Cochrane Collaboration, the premier organization for EBM, builds its bridge electronically with an accessible database of RCTs, meta-analyses, and systematic reviews (Haynes & Haines, 1998), including the electronic journal *Evidence-Based Mental Health*. The National Institute of Mental Health sponsors the design of "implementation toolkits" containing information and training resources for distribution to clinicians who do not yet practice EBP (Torrey et al., 2001). Building the bridge from research to practice is portrayed as the management of technological innovation (e.g., Gotham, 2004).

Applied science and diffusion of technology models assume that because practice is primarily technique, clinical science (i.e., the study of aggregates) is immediately useful. Mental health practitioners, however, may view what they do as primarily relational. Therefore, knowledge for their version of practice is necessarily of the patient and then of the population. Attempts to diffuse technical innovation have elicited resistance from practitioners. They resent the implication that the best ideas originate in the "lab" (Southam-Gerow, 2004). The most effective psychotherapists have been shown to depart from treatment manuals (Strupp & Anderson, 1997). At least in the case of medical practitioners, clinicians resist purportedly value-free guidelines whose values remain unexplicated or incompatible with their own or their patients' (Berg, ter Muelen, & van den Burg, 2001).

Because EBP means to change practitioner behavior, its assumptions about clinical decision making are central to its success. According to the applied science model, the practitioner infers from probabilistic data what he or she ought to do in a particular case. This inferential leap is unproblematic for EBP: The deductive reasoning may require some "clinical expertise" but is best done with the greatest possible fidelity to the research. There are, however, other models of science and practice. One combines the Boulder model with the idiographic study of the individual patient and innovation and creativity in the consulting room (Davison, 1998). A more fundamental critique is that "science and practice are not the same, and no monistic ideology can make them the same" (Peterson, 2004, p. 207). Rather, the "reflective practitioner" decides not by deduction from study findings alone but by induction from all of what he or she knows and experiences, including published studies (including but not limited to "evidence"); disciplined consideration of past clinical experience, the clinician's own and others'; and in-depth familiarity with the individual patient and immediate circumstances. There are numerous studies of expert decision making that challenge the deductive model of EBP (e.g., Klein, 1999; Tanenbaum, 1993).

EBP's proposed bridge from science to practice would affect not only practice behavior but also the professional status of practitioners themselves. According to one well-developed scenario (Hayes, Barlow, & Nelson-Gray, 1999), if practice adheres to research-based manuals and guidelines, most psychological treatment can be performed by clinicians with modest training—master's level or less—and not scientist–practitioners. Doctoral-level scientist–practitioners will design systems, conduct research, and manage quality assurance programs and triage networks and, when necessary, take over the care of patients whose treatment was unsuccessful at the guideline level. Even then, however, the scientist–practitioner will concern himself or herself with more than one patient's care; he or she will analyze why the guideline failed to work in a given case and how he or she can feed the successful treatment of the patient back into the system.

This scenario renegotiates psychological professionalism in the polity. Even under proposals to curb professional power (and these have risen to the level of "the third revolution" in health care; Relman, 1988), members of the professions are assumed to use erudition *and* discretion to do their work, where uncertainty and complexity necessarily inhere. The architecture of EBP's bridge from science to practice, however, imagines that research results, well managed, will largely resolve uncertainty and complexity in psychological practice, thereby diminishing the role of discretion. For EBP, as for Wennberg (1984), practitioner discretion is the source of unjustifiable variation; it is the problem rather than the solution. Thus, the EBP movement undertakes an unlikely program: to build a bridge from well-situated research professionals to practitioners whose own professionalism is thereby circumscribed. Proponents of EBP are well equipped with findings of poor practice that flies in the face of good science (e.g., Lehman & Steinwachs, 1998), not to mention the classic studies of (correctable) bias in expert decision making (Kahneman, 2003). Still, applied science is not practice, at the very least because practice requires the "reparticularization" (Cassell, 1991) of scientific knowledge to individual patients. Practice is an act of interpretation—of clinical reasoning answerable to standards of coherence and verisimilitude. It is of course fallible (Gorovitz & MacIntyre, 1976), but "evidence" provides only limited certainty of what is probable (Tanenbaum, 1993). Given the urgent complexity of practice beyond science, EBP risks public policy making for practitioners who do not exist. Applied science can easily devolve to rule reading. Assuming that practice is more, the EBP debate should reconvene, not on the narrow bridge from science to practice but on a well-traveled pathway from science through expertise to practice and back again.

Good Practice Writ Large Is Good Policy

As the science of "what works," EBP bears a moral imperative. It holds that evidence, through practice, achieves therapeutic efficacy and thereby better mental health, which, like physical health, is an uncontested moral good (Gupta, 2003). In other words, EBP occupies the high moral ground because it succeeds in the psychological treatment of afflicted persons. The effort to compile and disseminate evidence for practitioners and policymakers follows from this. The working hypothesis that EBP is good policy is problematic, however, in several regards.

First, there simply is not yet much evidence that EBP works beyond study conditions—neither as practice nor as policy. Second, for the movement and many sympathetic policymakers, effectiveness is a clear and laudatory policy goal: Policy should shape practice behavior to deliver effective treatment for mental illness. Effectiveness, however, is not self-evident. Although the terms of the EBP debate assume a common endpoint called "working," they much less frequently expand to consider what it means for psychological treatment to work. The lessening of behavioral symptoms is a commonly accepted treatment goal, but it may not signal effectiveness for treatment of an underlying psychological condition. In fact, every experimental study defines effectiveness for itself, and the evidence it yields is that that particular end was reached by a particular means.

Designing scientific studies entails the judgment of investigators, who define effectiveness for a given study. Something as simple as choosing the study's endpoint (6 weeks, 6 months, or 6 years) can determine whether a treatment will emerge as effective or ineffective. Investigators may be influenced by funding opportunities; by the availability and affordability of data; and, as evidence is formulated into guidelines, by the missions and dynamics of the sponsoring organizations or firms (Gupta, 2003). Before treatments can be assessed for effectiveness, they must be "assembled" and chosen from among others (Giacomini, 1999). From which assembly will alternative treatments be chosen, and on the basis of what criteria? Division 12 assembled treatments based on existing treatment manuals; this limiting criterion determined the scope of their review. Investigators must also decide which treatment outcomes are worth measuring and how much of a desired outcome is enough to deem the treatment effective. One review of physiotherapy trials found that 31 trials used 12 different outcome measures; only two were common and therefore suitable for meta-analysis (Rogers, 2002). Were these the most significant to patients, the easiest to measure, or the most pertinent to policy?

When public policy takes up treatment effectiveness, it is likely to do so by means of an implicit or explicit decision rule known as *maximizing expected utility* (MEU). This rule holds that the best policy creates the greatest good (sometimes for a given dollar amount), and because effectiveness is a clear societal good, public policy should act in support of effective treatment. MEU, however, is normatively complex because it does not consider utility to whom. In other words, what is the implicit distribution of costs and benefits of a policy that may maximize utility overall—who are the losers, and how badly do they lose? Assuming, for example, that even effective treatment is not effective in every case, what is the cost of enforced treatment protocols to patients who need something else? Further, there may be ethical limits to the utilitarian aspirations of researchers and policymakers. What is impermissible, even for the sake of effectiveness? MEU may not be the appropriate decision rule, but what is (Deber & Goel, 1990)? These questions go to the heart of mental health policy. At least for the EBP movement, the option of local decision making by practitioners and their peers is not an option.

What works, even if achievable, is not the only goal of personal and population health care. Patients forego what works to avoid inhumane side effects or to preserve the personal meanings they give to health and illness. In mental health, especially, efficacy raises the specter of coercion (Faulkner & Thomas, 2002). Even the psychiatric recovery movement parts ways with EBP. Although recovering mental patients are glad for evidence, at least some see the effectiveness criterion as a possible infringement on their freedom (Frese, Stanley, Kress, & Vogel-Scibilia, 2001). To the extent that EBP serves societal ends, furthermore, effectiveness is only one moral imperative. Justice goals may direct health care resources not to their most effective use (especially as defined by researchers and payers) but to one with distributional implications. Good policy is more complicated than good practice writ large. The EBP debate should fully consider that treatment effectiveness is only one among many moving targets; institutionalizing it at the policy level may create moral confusion and patient hardship.

The EBP movement compares effectiveness with ineffectiveness and identifies the former as its moral compass. Until the EBP debate expands, however, to include the issues raised in this chapter, it creates a moral vacuum to be filled by the most powerful parties in the health care system. To be sure, some proponents of EBP consider its amenability to market and political forces a strength (Hayes et al., 1999), but in the absence of debate about effectiveness goals, the means and ends of research and treatment remain vulnerable to pharmaceutical companies (Gupta, 2003), managed care organizations (Bologna, Barlow, Hollon, Mitchell, & Huppert, 1998), and public agencies (Carpinello, Rosenberg, Stone, Schwager, & Felton, 2002), all with their own definitions of what works. These agendas are not transparent; do not invite outside criticism; and cannot significantly further practitioner, patient, or citizen participation in the framing of effectiveness research and effective treatment (Giacomini, Cook, Streiner, & Anand, 2000). Psychology has already permitted a severe evidence hierarchy, and the fruits of early labors have become authoritative in the clinic and the polity.

PUBLIC POLICY AND EVIDENCE-BASED PRACTICE

The EBP movement offers a tonic for the cost crisis in mental health care. EBP is not necessarily less costly than treatment based on custom rather than evidence; it may in fact be more costly. Greater access to EBP will indubitably increase costs, at least in the short run. EBP, however, has both rhetorical and practical strengths in the policy arena. First, by claiming to know "what works" for specific disorders—and by opposing the putatively fuzzy-headed and irresponsible guild—EBP stares down charges that psychological treatment is not scientific—not as scientific as medicine, that is—and that it promises everything to everyone with a problem in living. Whatever is spent, EBP promises, it will be spent wisely. Second, because efficacy research is framed by the investigator, proponents of EBP have been able to focus it on short-term, manualized interventions. These treatments can be implemented by less highly trained mental health workers in private or public managed care environments (Hayes et al., 1999), in which EBP can control costs without appearing to compromise the quality of care.

The core of a profession's identity, however, is control over the content of its work. In the United States, professions such as psychology license and regulate their own members and credential their educational institutions. Licensed professionals, in turn, are sheltered from unfettered economic competition; they compete (more and more) among themselves, but not with unlicensed providers within their scope of practice. At the level of the profession, EBP is a double-edged sword. To the extent that it establishes an expanding scientific base for psychological treatment, EBP confers greater legitimacy on the field and builds its case for self-governance. If practice is something more than science, however, the EBP model constricts psychological professionalism by undercutting discretion based on other ways of knowing. EBP's insistence on manualized interventions, for example, locates professional knowledge outside the practitioner and allows mental health workers of lesser training and independent judgment to deliver services. Who controls the content of these psychologists' work? At best, other psychologists—research psychologists forming, as in the case of evidence-based medicine, a "knowledge elite exerting technical and cognitive power" over a "clinically based rank-and-file" (Hafferty & Light, 1995, p. 138). Moreover, just as general practitioners are empowered vis-à-vis specialist physicians by evidence-based medicine (Lipman, 2000), nonpsychologist mental health workers are empowered by EBP.

Along with credentialing and the accompanying market shelter, professional liability is one policy area in which EBP may have an effect. Little is known about the role of EBP in psychological malpractice specifically, but evidence-based medical practice guidelines are beginning to figure in malpractice policy and law. Historically, malpractice has required negligence, which was defined with reference to a community standard. The standard was established through expert testimony, and defendants were expected to conform only to their peers. Now judges are looking beyond custom to guidelines. In 11 states and the District of Columbia, custom has been explicitly rejected in favor of a reasonableness test; another 9 states have endorsed a reasonableness test without reference to custom. In other words, in these jurisdictions, a malpractice defendant is negligent if he or she did not act in a way that was reasonable, no matter what other practitioners in the community would have done. Reasonableness, in turn, is defined for the court by a practice guideline issuing from a well-respected group (Mello, Studdert, & Brennan, 2003). These developments raise critical questions for the EBP debate. Is psychological science authoritative enough for the courtroom? Are plaintiffs' attorneys to be the foot soldiers of EBP?

The EBP movement has also exerted considerable influence over private and public payers for mental health services. In the public sector, a number of state mental health authorities are using EBP to organize their policy agendas and service delivery systems. New York State, for example, has mounted a "campaign to implement EBPs for people with serious mental disorders" (Carpinello et al., 2002, p. 153). In response to a 1999 consent decree, the state of Hawaii established a panel to review the efficacy and effectiveness of treatments for a range of childhood and adolescent mental health conditions. The Empirical Basis to Services (EBS) Task Force searched and evaluated controlled studies in childhood mental health using criteria for *empirically based* much like the criteria used by Division 12. Hawaii attempted to determine effectiveness as well as efficacy, and the EBS Task Force included health administrators and parents of mentally ill children as well as clinicians and academics. Still, RCTs were the gold standard (Chorpita et al., 2002). At present, an EBS committee continues to review the literature and decide on the content of practice guidelines; these are then appended to the requests for proposals issued by the Child and Adolescent Mental Health Division of the Hawaii Department of Health to service providers seeking contracts with the department (E. Daleiden, personal communication, July 12, 2004).

The District of Columbia Department of Mental Health (DMH) has, as of this writing, proposed a policy (No. 311.2) regarding evidence-based psychotherapy in that system. According to the draft policy, all psychotherapy delivered to adult consumers in the District of Columbia's mental health system will conform to a 1 1/2-page list of evidence-based treatments. The list includes 12 disorders and a maximum of four approved therapies for each. Five of the disorders have only one treatment option; for example, only dialectical behavior therapy is approved for borderline personality disorder. Psychodynamic psychotherapy does not appear on the list; eye-movement desensitization and reprocessing therapy does. The DMH Chief Clinical Officer, in consultation with experts, reviews the list annually. Providers may submit requests to expand it, but they must also be credentialed in the specific therapies they undertake. "Psychotherapists that are not credentialed for a particular psychotherapy should not attempt to provide that evidence-based psychotherapy" (District of Columbia DMH, 2004, p. 1). Credentialing requirements are vague, but the policy makes clear that DMH providers will not be paid unless they abide by the psychotherapies list and qualify for the care they provide.

In August 2003, the state of Oregon took a different approach to EBP in mental health when Senate Bill 267 became law. The act requires that for the biennium beginning July 1, 2005, a number of state agencies, including "that part of the Department of Human Services that deals with mental health and addiction issues," will spend 25% of their program budgets on evidence-based programs. The figure rises to 50% in 2007 and 75% in 2009. Agencies that do not meet this requirement will face budget consequences in the following biennium. According to the legislation, an evidence-based program is one that "(a) incorporates significant and relevant practices based on scientifically based research; and (b) is cost effective" (State of Oregon, 2003, Section 3). The Oregon Office of Mental Health and Addiction Services (2004) offered an operational definition of EBP: RCTs are at the top of the evidence hierarchy, and except at the lowest level of acceptable evidence, implementation must be measured by a fidelity tool.

CONCLUSION

This chapter has viewed EBP in psychology through a public policy lens. The polity creates the professions through licensure, malpractice, and reimbursement policies, and in turn psychology, like other professions, strives for societal ends. EBP is a new knowledge regime in psychology, one that seeks to mold practice to the findings of experimental studies. Its ramifications are being felt by practitioners, patients, and policymakers. EBP promises effective psychological services, and this would seem an unassailable ambition. The movement, however, defines effectiveness for itself and proceeds on three working hypotheses: that whatever the difficulties, it is possible to have good science; that good science, well managed, leads to good practice; and that good practice writ large is good policy.

This chapter has suggested that each of EBP's working hypotheses is unnecessarily restrictive. Experimental science is an insufficient knowledge base for psychological practice. At the very least, other forms of high-quality inquiry fill the gaps left by probabilistic studies. Good practice, moreover, is not an applied science. Practitioners must exercise judgment even in the face of scientific research, and public policy regarding the professions counts on that. Finally, EBP is an insufficient basis for good policy, which must consider the issues of what kind of effectiveness, for whom, and in combination with what other societal ends. None of these matters is beyond consideration by the profession; some of them have already been raised by psychologists. The recommendation of this chapter is simply that psychology expand the terms of the EBP debate to include not only multiple ways of knowing for practice but also an appreciation of the "epistemological politics" (Tanenbaum, 1994) of supplanting one knowledge regime with another.

EBP as public policy is relatively new, and it remains to be seen what precisely will follow from its implementation (Tanenbaum, 2005). There is no doubt, however, that EBP is already public policy in nontrivial ways and that "evidence-based" care of real patients by real practitioners proceeds in tandem with psychologists' scrupulous refinement of EBP definitions and hierarchies. The EBP movement's working hypotheses must expand to consider the policy implications of its certitude. If there is a broader knowledge base, a more complex practice, and a more articulated "effectiveness," politics will eventually find them. Patients, practitioners, and citizens will be spared significant missteps if public policy is made to recognize them from the start.

REFERENCES

Altman, S. H., Tompkins, C. P., Eilat, E., & Glavin, M. P. V. (2003). Escalating health care spending: Is it desirable or inevitable? *Health Affairs Web Exclusive.* Retrieved August 23, 2004, from http://content.healthaffairs.org/cgi/content/full/hlthaff.w3.1v1/DC1?maxtoshow=&HITS=

American Psychiatric Association. (1994). *Diagnostic and statistical manual of mental disorders* (4th ed.). Washington, DC: Author.

Armstrong, D. (1977). Clinical sense and clinical science. *Social Science and Medicine, 11,* 599–601.

Berg, M. (1997). *Rationalizing medical work: Decision-support techniques and medical practices.* Cambridge, MA: MIT Press.

Berg, M., ter Muelen, R., & van den Burg, M. (2001). Guidelines for appropriate care: The importance of empirical normative analysis. *Health Care Analysis, 9,* 77–99.

Beutler, L. E., & Castonguay, L. G. (Eds.). (2005). *What works in psychology, and why.* New York: Oxford University Press.

Bohart, A. C., O'Hara, M., & Leitner, L. M. (1998). Empirically violated treatments: Disenfranchisement of humanistic and other psychotherapies. *Psychotherapy Research, 8,* 141–157.

Bologna, N. C., Barlow, D. H., Hollon, S. D., Mitchell, J. E., & Huppert, J. D. (1998). Behavioral health treatment redesign in managed health care settings. *Clinical Psychology: Science and Practice, 5,* 94–114.

Borkovec, T. D., Echemendia, R. J., Ragusea, S. A., & Ruiz, M. (2001). The Pennsylvania practice research network and future possibilities for clinically meaningful and scientifically rigorous psychotherapy effectiveness research. *Clinical Psychology: Science and Practice, 8,* 155–167.

Brown, L. D. (1991). *Competition and the new accountability: From market incentives to medical outcomes.* Unpublished manuscript, Columbia University, School of Public Health, New York.

Brown, L. D. (1992). Political evolution of federal health care regulation. *Health Affairs, 11,* 17–37.

Carey, B. (2004, August 10). For psychotherapy's claims, skeptics demand proof. *The New York Times,* pp. D1, D4.

Carpinello, S. E., Rosenberg, L., Stone, J., Schwager, M., & Felton, C. J. (2002). Best practices: New York State's campaign to implement evidence-based practices for people with serious mental disorders. *Psychiatric Services, 53,* 153–155.

Carroll, K. M., & Rounsaville, B. R. (2003). Bridging the gap: A hybrid model to link efficacy and effectiveness research in substance abuse treatment. *Psychiatric Services, 54,* 333–339.

Cassell, E. J. (1991). *The nature of suffering and the goals of medicine.* New York: Oxford University Press.

Centers for Medicare and Medicaid Services, Office of the Actuary, National Health Statistics Group. (2005). *Health Accounts.* Retrieved March 1, 2005, from http://www.cms.gov/statistics/nhe/default.asp

Chambless, D. L., Baker, M. J., Baucom, D. H., Beutler, L. E., Calhoun, K. S., Crits-Christoph, P., et al. (1998). An update on empirically validated therapies: II. *The Clinical Psychologist, 49,* 5–18.

Chambless, D. L., & Ollendick, T. H. (2001). Empirically supported psychological interventions: Controversies and evidence. *Annual Review of Psychology, 52,* 685–716.

Chorpita, B. F., Yim, L. M., Dankervoet, J. C., Arensdorf, A., Amundsen, M. J., McGee, C., et al. (2002). Toward large-scale implementation of empirically supported treatments for children: A review and observations by the Hawaii Empirical Bases to Services Task Force. *Clinical Psychology: Science and Practice, 9,* 165–190.

Cummings, N. A. (2000). The first decade of managed behavioral health care: What went right and what went wrong. In R. D. Weitz (Ed.), *Psycho-economics: Managed care in mental health in the new millenium* (pp. 19–38). New York: Haworth Press.

Davison, G. C. (1998). Being bolder with the Boulder model: The challenge of education and training in empirically supported treatments. *Journal of Consulting and Clinical Psychology, 66,* 163–167.

Deber, R. B., & Goel, V. (1990). Using explicit decision-rules to manage issues of justice, risk, and ethics in decision analysis: When is it not rational to maximize expected utility? *Medical Decision Making, 10,* 181–194.

District of Columbia, Department of Mental Health. (2004). *Policy No. 311.2: Evidence-Based Psychotherapy.* Washington, DC: Author.

Drake, R. E., Goldman, H. H., Leff, H. S., Lehman, A. F., Dixon, L., Mueser, K. T., & Torrey, W. C. (2001). Implementing evidence-based practices in routine mental health care settings. *Psychiatric Services, 52,* 179–182.

Elliott, R. (1998). Editor's introduction: A guide to the empirically supported treatments controversy. *Psychotherapy Research, 8,* 115–125.

Epstein, A. M. (1990). The outcomes movement—will it get us where we want to go? *New England Journal of Medicine, 323,* 266–270.

Evidence-Based Medicine Working Group. (1992, November 4). Evidence-based medicine: A new approach to teaching the practice of medicine. *Journal of the American Medical Association, 268,* 2420–2425.

Faulkner, A., & Thomas, P. (2002). User-led research and evidence-based medicine. *British Journal of Psychiatry, 180,* 1–3.

Feinstein, A. R., & Horwitz, R. I. (1997). Problems in the "evidence" of "evidence-based medicine." *American Journal of Medicine, 103,* 529–535.

Fox, D. M. (1990). Health policy and the politics of research in the United States. *Journal of Health Politics, Policy and Law, 15,* 481–499.

Frese, F. J., Stanley, J., Kress, K., & Vogel-Scibilia, S. (2001). Integrating evidence-based practices and the recovery model. *Psychiatric Services, 52,* 1462–1468.

Garfield, S. L. (1996). Some problems associated with "validated" forms of psychotherapy. *Clinical Psychology: Science and Practice, 3,* 218–229.

Giacomini, M. K. (1999). The *which*-hunt: Assembling health technologies for assessment and rationing. *Journal of Health Politics, Policy and Law, 24,* 715–758.

Giacomini, M. K., Cook, D. J., Streiner, D. L., & Anand, S. S. (2000). Using practice guidelines to allocate medical technologies: An ethics framework. *International Journal of Technology Assessment in Health Care, 16,* 987–1002.

Gonzales, J. J., Ringeissen, H. L., & Chambers, D. A. (2002). The tangled and thorny path of science to practice: Tensions in interpreting and applying "evidence." *Clinical Psychology: Science and Practice, 9,* 204–209.

Gorovitz, S., & MacIntyre, A. (1976). Toward a theory of medical fallibility. *Journal of Medical Philosophy, 1,* 51–71.

Gotham, H. J. (2004). Diffusion of mental health and substance abuse treatments: Development, dissemination, and implementation. *Clinical Psychology: Science and Practice, 11,* 160–176.

Gupta, M. (2003). A critical appraisal of evidence-based medicine: Some ethical considerations. *Journal of Evaluation in Clinical Practice, 9,* 111–121.

Hafferty, F. W., & Light, D. W. (1995). Professional dynamics and the changing nature of medical work. *Journal of Health and Social Behavior, 35,* 132–153.

Hayes, S. C. (1996). Creating the empirical clinician. *Clinical Psychology: Science and Practice, 3,* 179–181.

Hayes, S. C., Barlow, D. H., & Nelson-Gray, R. O. (1999). *The scientist–practitioner: Research and accountability in the age of managed care* (2nd ed.). Boston: Allyn & Bacon.

Haynes, B., & Haines, A. (1998). Barriers and bridges to evidence based clinical practice. *British Medical Journal, 317*, 273–276.

Heffler, S., Smith, S., Keehan, S., Borger, C., Clemens, M. K., & Truffer, C. (2005). Trends: U.S. health spending projections for 2004–2014. *Health Affairs Web Exclusives*. Retrieved March 1, 2005, from http://content.healthaffairs.org/cgi/content/full/hlthaff.w5.74/DC1

Institute of Medicine. (2001). *Crossing the quality chasm: A new health system for the 21st century*. Washington, DC: National Academy Press.

Kahneman, D. (2003). A perspective on judgment and choice: Mapping bounded rationality. *American Psychologist, 58*, 697–720.

Klein, G. (1999). *Sources of power: How people make decisions*. Cambridge, MA: MIT Press.

Lehman, A. F., & Steinwachs, D. M. (1998). Translating research into practice: The schizophrenia Patient Outcome Research Team (PORT) treatment recommendations. *Schizophrenia Bulletin, 24*, 1–10.

Lipman, T. (2000). Power and influence in clinical effectiveness and evidence-based medicine. *Family Practice, 17*, 557–563.

Meehl, P. E. (1997). Credentialed persons, credentialed knowledge. *Clinical Psychology: Science and Practice, 4*, 91–98.

Mehlman, M. (1986). Health care cost containment and medical technology: A critique of waste theory. *Case Western Reserve Law Review, 36*, 778–877.

Mello, M. M., Studdert, D. M., & Brennan, T. A. (2003). The leapfrog standards: Ready to jump from marketplace to courtroom? *Health Affairs, 22*, 46–59.

Messer, S. B. (2004). Evidence-based practice: Beyond empirically supported treatments. *Professional Psychology, 35*, 580–588.

Messer, S. B., & Wampold, B. E. (2002). Let's face facts: Common factors are more potent than specific therapy ingredients. *Clinical Psychology: Science and Practice, 9*, 21–25.

Miettinen, O. S. (1998). Evidence in medicine: Invited commentary. *Canadian Medical Association Journal, 158*, 215–221.

Morone, J. A. (1994). The bureaucracy empowered. In J. A. Morone & G. S. Belkin (Eds.), *The politics of health care reform: Lessons from the past, prospects for the future* (pp. 148–164). Durham, NC: Duke University Press.

Nathan, P. E., & Gorman, J. M. (2002). *A guide to treatments that work* (2nd ed.). New York: Oxford University Press.

Norcross, J. C. (Ed.). (2002). *Psychotherapy relationships that work: Therapist contributions and responsiveness to patient needs*. New York: Oxford University Press.

Oregon Office of Mental Health and Addiction Services. (2004). *Proposed operational definition for evidence-based practices*. Retrieved November 10, 2004, from http://www.dhs.state.or.us/mentalhealth/ebp/definition0722.pdf

Peterson, D. R. (1991). Connection and disconnection of research and practice in the education of professional psychologists. *American Psychologist, 46*, 422–429.

Peterson, D. R. (2004). Science, scientism, and professional responsibility. *Clinical Psychology: Science and Practice, 7,* 196–210.

Polanyi, M. (1967). *The tacit dimension.* Garden City, NJ: Doubleday/Anchor Press.

Reinhardt, U. E., Hussey, P. S., & Anderson, G. F. (2004). U.S. health care spending in an international context. *Health Affairs, 23,* 10–25.

Relman, A. S. (1988). Assessment and accountability: The third revolution in medical care. *New England Journal of Medicine, 319,* 1220–1222.

Rogers, W. A. (2002). Evidence-based medicine in practice: Limiting or facilitating patient choice? *Health Expectations, 5,* 95–103.

Rothman, D. J. (1997). *Beginnings count: The technological imperative in U.S. health care.* New York: Oxford University Press.

Sackett, D. L., Rosenberg, W. M. C., Muir-Gray, J. A., Haynes, R. B., & Richardson, W. S. (1996). Evidence-based medicine: What it is and what it isn't. *British Medical Journal, 312,* 71–72.

Schon, D. A. (1983). *The reflective practitioner: Toward a new design for teaching and learning in the professions.* San Francisco: Jossey-Bass.

Seligman, M. E. (1996). The effectiveness of psychotherapy: The *Consumer Reports* study. *American Psychologist, 50,* 965–974.

Society for Clinical Psychology, American Psychological Association. (2000). *A guide to beneficial psychotherapy.* Retrieved April 17, 2003, from http://www.apa.org/divisions/div12/rev_est/index.html

Southam-Gerow, M. A. (2004). Some reasons mental health treatments are not technologies: Toward treatment development and adaptation outside labs. *Clinical Psychology: Science and Practice, 11,* 186–189.

State of Oregon. (2003). *An Act: S.B. 267, Chapter 669 Oregon Laws.* Retrieved July 14, 2004, from http://www.leg.state.or.us/orlaws/sess0600.dir/0669ses.htm

Strupp, H. H., & Anderson, T. (1997). On the limitations of therapy manuals. *Clinical Psychology: Science and Practice, 4,* 76–82.

Tanenbaum, S. J. (1993). What physicians know. *New England Journal of Medicine, 329,* 1268–1271.

Tanenbaum, S. J. (1994). Knowing and acting in medical practice: The epistemological politics of outcomes research. *Journal of Health Politics, Policy and Law, 19,* 27–44.

Tanenbaum, S. J. (2005). Evidence-based practice as mental health policy: Three controversies and a caveat. *Health Affairs, 24,* 163–173.

Tavris, C. (2003). Mind games: Psychological warfare between therapists and scientists. *Chronicle of Higher Education, 49,* B7–B10.

Timmermans, S., & Berg, M. (2003). *The gold standard: The challenge of evidence-based medicine and standardization in health care.* Philadelphia: Temple University Press.

Thorpe, K. E., Florence, C. S., & Joski, P. (2004). Which medical conditions account for the rise in health care spending? *Health Affairs, 23*(Suppl. 2), 437–445.

Torrey, W. C., Drake, R. E., Dixon, L., Burns, B. J., Flynn, L., Rush, A. J., et al. (2001). Implementing evidence-based practices for persons with severe mental illness. *Psychiatric Services, 52*, 45–50.

Tunis, S. R., Stryer, D. B., & Clancy, C. M. (2003, September 24). Practical clinical trials: Increasing the value of clinical research for decision making in clinical and health policy. *Journal of the American Medical Association, 290*, 1624–1632.

University of Oxford, Centre for Evidence-Based Medicine. (1998). *Levels of evidence and grades of recommendations.* Retrieved June 27, 2002, from http://www.jr2.ox.ac.uk/cebm/docs/levels.html

U.S. Department of Health and Human Services, U.S. Public Health Service. (2000). *Mental health: A report of the Surgeon General.* Washington, DC: U.S. Government Printing Office.

Wampold, B. E. (2001). *The great psychotherapy debate: Models, methods, and findings.* Mahwah, NJ: Erlbaum.

Wennberg, J. (1984). Dealing with medical practice variations: A proposal for action. *Health Affairs, 3*, 6–32.

Westen, D., & Morrison, K. (2001). A multi-dimensional meta-analysis of treatments for depression, panic, and generalized anxiety disorder: An empirical examination of the status of empirically supported treatments. *Journal of Consulting and Clinical Psychology, 69*, 875–889.

Wolff, N. (2000). Using randomized controlled trials to evaluate socially complex services: Problems, challenges and recommendations. *Journal of Mental Health Policy and Economics, 3*, 97–109.

11

EVIDENCE-BASED PRACTICE: GOLD STANDARD, GOLD PLATED, OR FOOL'S GOLD?

ROBERT J. STERNBERG

Evidence-based practice has many advantages. How, in principle, could anyone be against practice based on evidence? It is hard to imagine. Yet, this volume suggests cautions in the use of evidence-based practice.

CAUTIONS OF VOLUME AUTHORS REGARDING EMPIRICALLY BASED PRACTICE

What are these cautions? In this section I consider 25 of them, along with the chapters in this volume that cite them. (I do not claim either that the list is complete or that I have necessarily indicated every chapter that made every point!)

1. There is a need to take into account the context of practice (see chaps. 1, 2, and 9, this volume).

This context may be different from that of scientific research and thus lead practitioners in a different direction than that of scientific research.

The context of practice is one of providing service for a fee under conditions that are very far away from a laboratory setting. The psychotherapist is ethically bound to provide the test treatment possible—there is no control group getting a placebo. So the therapist must respond in a way that is appropriate to his or her context, not the scientific and especially laboratory one.

2. There are differences in the way evidence is defined (see chaps. 2, 7, and 9, this volume).

Practicing psychologists may feel that they are using evidence. This evidence may not meet the standards of scientists, but it may meet the standards of the practitioners. Conversely, scientific evidence may not meet the standards of practitioners with regard to practical relevance or completeness of the evidence. For example, case studies may not meet everyone's standards for an evidentiary base, but they may be quite useful to practitioners. Psychotherapists work in an idiographic context. They need to personalize their therapy to each individual client. Scientists more often work in a nomothetic context. They look for group generalities. As a result, psychotherapists and scientists may be trying to attain different goals.

3. Evidence-based practice may not be practical (see chaps. 2, 3, and 4, this volume).

It is one thing to propose a form of treatment that works in a scientific study; it is another to propose one that works practically in everyday clinical settings. A manualized treatment, for example, may work, on average. But who is average? And how does such a treatment take into account the astounding diversity with which psychotherapists must cope every day?

4. Therapist effects are greater than treatment effects, so the practitioner matters more than the particular methods used (see chaps. 1 and 2, this volume).

Some studies suggest that more attention should be paid to who is doing the therapy and how well the therapist fits the client than to the particular method the therapist tends to prefer. Therapists profiting from experience may be of signal importance in psychotherapeutic outcomes. Some therapists may be especially apt in treating certain kinds of problems, such as depression. Others may be among those rare people who have serious success with patients with character disorders. These differences do not come out in studies that look only at group averages.

5. Evidence-based techniques are sometimes impoverished, or at least not sufficiently complex to take into account the realities of clinical practice (see chaps. 2, 3, 7, and 9, this volume).

Although manualized treatments may be useful in some situations (see chap. 6, this volume), in others they may not provide rich enough information to be therapeutically effective. Moreover, on a given day a client may be more or less receptive to treatment. A skilled therapist will take into account not only the client's generalized problems but also his or her moods and states of mind.

6. *Psychotherapy is an art as well as a science, and scientific evidence does not always take into account the artistic side of psychotherapy (see chap. 2, this volume).*

Scientists sometimes tend to look at therapy in what seems, to therapists, like a cold-blooded way. But even science has many characteristics of art. The best scientists have a certain style—a way of doing things. They can submit articles for blind review, but their reviewers can recognize their style, even when their name is removed from the manuscript. The best therapists are the same. Neither the art of science nor the art of psychotherapy is well understood, but both are important. The best scientists and therapists distinguish themselves as much by their art as by their science.

7. *There are many situations in which there are no techniques from evidence-based studies to apply (see chaps. 2 and 3, this volume).*

Psychotherapists who insist on using empirically based treatments might find many clients whom they are unable to treat because nothing is available. Moreover, comorbidity of symptoms makes it hard to use manualized treatments that apply only to single particular disorders. It is not feasible to think of manualized treatments for all of the possible comorbidities and interactions that can occur in real psychotherapy, as opposed to therapy that is idealized in the minds of people who wish it to be less messy.

8. *Experience often is a better teacher than evidence-based studies (see chap. 2, this volume).*

Evidence-based studies are certainly helpful to psychotherapists in their work. But even scientists, if asked which is of more help to their actual day-to-day research and to the tacit knowledge of doing research—what they learned in classrooms or what they learned from experience—would acknowledge that their experience is especially valuable to them in doing their research. Why would psychotherapists be any different?

9. *Psychotherapy works, so it is not clear how much of a problem there is in the first place (see chaps. 1, 3, and 5, this volume).*

Given the evidence that psychotherapy is, on average, successful, it is not clear how empirically based treatment will improve outcomes. In the long run, there is no question that science improves practice and that practice improves science. But some psychotherapists believe they have winning strategies and are eager to maintain the practices that they believe to work effectively.

10. The scientific literature does not make sufficiently clear whom to apply various techniques to and when to apply them (see chaps. 3 and 9, this volume).

The techniques are often presented in the abstract, so it is not clear how they can be used in the realities of an actual therapeutic situation. The truth is, many scientists have the same problem. They have taken courses in, say, data analysis. But when they analyze an actual set of data, what they learned in a statistics course is the beginning, not the end, of what they do. They need to bootstrap their analytic techniques to fit actual situations. Clinicians do the same.

11. There are realities of practice, such as limitations imposed by managed care, about which evidence-based psychotherapeutic principles are silent (see chaps. 1, 3, and 8, this volume).

Even if therapists wanted to give the very best scientifically based treatment possible, managed care companies will not always allow them to do so.

12. Psychotherapy involves a working alliance between therapist and client that scientific research does not adequately capture (see chap. 3, this volume).

Although the working alliance is not everything (see chap. 6, this volume), it is important to the results and may even be crucial. Scientists have been studying teams, alliances, and dyadic relationships for many years. No reasonable scientist would claim that science has provided a clear and unequivocal understanding of how these relationships work. So science can help improve psychotherapy, but it does not, by any means, provide all the answers relevant to the psychotherapeutic situation.

13. When clinical experience leads in a different direction from scientific research, it makes sense that a therapist would go with his or her experience (see chaps. 3 and 5, this volume).

From one point of view, it would be unprofessional to ignore or actively contravene the lessons of one's professional experience. Scientists react no differently. They may learn certain assumptions, say, of analysis of variance or regression analysis. But they regularly and freely violate these assumptions when their experience tells them that the inferences they draw will nevertheless be reliable and valid.

14. Western psychotherapy and the science investigating it are based primarily on a Western White middle-class notion of what psychotherapy is and should be (see chap. 4, this volume).

The appropriate form of psychotherapy can and should differ from one culture to another. If clients believe in the importance of spirits in their life, for example, therapy would have to take these beliefs into account, regardless of the belief system of the therapist.

15. *There is little or no evidence that implementation of evidence-based practice actually will improve psychotherapeutic outcomes (see chaps. 1 and 8, this volume).*

Indeed, it is often assumed rather than demonstrated that this is the case. Some scientists may believe that the evidence is clear on this matter. But others may not see things the same way.

16. *Scientific research, which may be conducted in a decontextualized way, may not be as sensitive to what works in real therapy as its proponents claim it is (see chaps. 1 and 9, this volume).*

Sometimes psychotherapists may apply what they believe is the result of scientific research. If the result is not what they hoped for, they may be skeptical the next time they have the same opportunity.

17. *The requirement of some managed care companies for practitioners to use evidence-based treatment may merely result in practitioners refusing to accept managed care clients (see chap. 1, this volume).*

Ironically, then, the call for empirically based treatment may boomerang. In the end, psychotherapists, like scientists, want to do the best work they can. Within certain broad ethical bounds, scientists can do things as they wish, so long as they have the resources to do them. More and more, psychotherapists are not being allowed to do what they believe is best for their clients.

18. *Results of scientific studies may be biased by the theoretical preferences of the investigators (see chap. 5, this volume).*

Scientists are often oblivious to how their own preferred paradigms affect their results. In the days of behaviorism, research seemed to support behaviorist principles. In the days of cognitivism, research seemed to support the principles of this paradigm. Individuals outside these paradigms may be more skeptical of the objectivity of the research results than are those working within the paradigms.

19. *Practitioners already do, for the most part, use or seek to use treatments that are based on empirical data, even if it is not always data from random-assignment designs, although they may not always succeed in doing so (see chaps. 6, 7, and 8, this volume).*

From the practitioner standpoint, they often are doing what they are being asked to do but nevertheless are criticized for not doing it.

20. *Sometimes results of studies of empirically based treatments are not reported in a way that practitioners can understand or, at least, make use of (see chaps. 6 and 9, this volume).*

In such cases, the advice the studies contain goes unheeded. Scientists are often oblivious to their use of jargon. The same problem arises in education, where teachers find it hard to put into practice what educational scientists recommend. Authors must take into account not only what they want to say but also the audiences they wish to reach.

21. *Scientists and practitioners have different views of the world, and they do what they believe is best according to their own respective worldviews (see chap. 8, this volume).*

People who have one worldview often try to impose it on others. Countries, including the United States, have been susceptible to doing so. No one, least of all people with doctorates and years of experience, want to have types of practices imposed on them.

22. *It is not always clear exactly what constitutes an empirically based treatment (see chaps. 7, 8, and 10, this volume).*

How much evidence counts so that one can say that a treatment is empirically based? What kinds of evidence? With whom? In what situations? It is not always clear what an empirically based treatment is!

23. *Use of empirically based treatment might increase treatment costs (see chaps. 8 and 10, this volume).*

A psychotherapist who feels he or she must do all that his or her training and clinical experience suggest is necessary is likely to be reluctant to abandon techniques he or she believes are needed just because the scientific literature suggests other things to be done. The scientific techniques may be add-ons, making it hard to find funds from the patient or insurer to implement them.

24. *Research often neglects mechanisms and processes that contribute to treatment effects and that are of great concern to therapists (see chap. 7, this volume).*

As in other fields, what is important to theorists and what is important to practitioners is often not the same. The result may be that therapists feel that the processes they need to understand have not been adequately elucidated by the science of clinical research.

25. *Therapists can introduce ongoing assessment into their practice to improve their work that is practice relevant, because it derives from their own work (see chap. 7, this volume).*

In this way, therapists can become their own formative evaluators, rather than waiting for others to do evaluations for them.

RANDOM-ASSIGNMENT DESIGNS: A GOLD STANDARD?

Some investigators view random-assignment designs as the only designs worthy of consideration. But are they? Vioxx was supposed to cure pain. Fen-phen was supposed to help people lose weight. Rezulin was supposed to help people to treat diabetes. Baycol was supposed help people reduce cholesterol levels. These drugs had three things in common. First, all were approved by the FDA after random-assignment controlled experimental studies revealed them to be safe. Second, they all did what they were supposed to do. Third, all were recalled, by the manufacturers, the FDA, or both, after later clinical experience and research revealed them to be anything but safe.

The testing of drugs has been used by advocates of random-assignment controlled experimental studies as a model for how testing should be done for psychological treatments, as well as for educational programs. The idea is that the people exposed to psychotherapeutic or educational treatments deserve no less than the care that is given to those exposed to medical treatments. Care? Hundreds of millions of dollars of lawsuits have been filed against manufacturers of drugs that have been released on the market and then later recalled. The system designed to protect people has been flawed. Is evidence better than no evidence? Always. Is good evidence better than bad evidence? Always. Is any one kind of evidence a "gold standard"? Never.

In this concluding chapter, I try to make further sense of the debate regarding evidence-based practice. Although my focus is on psychotherapy, I hope my comments are general in their implications, because the issue is currently a hot one in educational as well as in medical circles. And it is the same issue: Is there a gold standard to be found? The answer is no.

THE SEARCH FOR PANACEAS

Science and religion have in common the search for answers. Many scientists discount religion as an invalid way of answering scientific questions, and they do so with good reason. In the same way, science has not been shown to be a valid way for answering religious questions. When religion becomes science, as in the present-day fad of "intelligent design," people must watch out. The disguise is often very thin. But when science becomes religion, the results are no better.

Why do scientists search for the certainties that, in the end, only religious faith can provide to those who have it? They seek panaceas for the same reasons that everyone else does. They probably originally entered the field of science hoping it would give them the unique answers they did not find they could obtain elsewhere. Some of them come to realize that these unique answers were not forthcoming. Others continue to search for the holy grail. And they are disappointed when they do not find it.

Random-assignment controlled experimental studies have seemed to some to be the panacea in the same way that, for others, brain-based studies are the answer. At the time this chapter is being written, the U.S. Department of Education has, in many of its programs, decided to grant priority to random-assignment study (RAS) designs. Why are RAS designs not, in fact, panaceas? Why is it wrong to give preference to one kind of design over any other?

Questions That Do Not Lend Themselves to Random-Assignment Study Designs

For example, I might want to know the extent to which a new very brief battery for measuring depression, which I believe will be useful in therapeutic interventions, does in fact measure depression, at least in the sense that other existing assessments measure depression. This is a perfectly sensible question to ask, because I do not want to introduce the new battery as a measure of depression unless it shows convergent validity with existing batteries. I may also want to show at least discriminant validity with respect to measures of other constructs, such as anxiety. The questions I address as I construct–validate the new measure lend themselves to a multimethod, multitrait correlational design. They do not lend themselves to an RAS design.

In a similar way, if I create a more extensive depression battery and want to understand whether it is unifactorial or rather measures different types of depression, the appropriate design is a factor analytic one, not an RAS one. It would not make sense to adjust the question one asks to suit the design. The design should be chosen to answer the question. If I have a prior theory of this factorial structure, then I should use confirmatory factor analysis. But in no case is an RAS design the appropriate way of answering the questions I wish to ask. Forcing one particular design on all research limits the questions that can be asked or leads to inappropriate methods for answering the questions.

Not all alternative designs are correlational. Suppose I wish to investigate Sylvia Plath and how her depression led to her suicide. I cannot use an RAS design, nor should I. I would need to do a retrospective case study. A great deal can be learned from case studies. But studies of the lives of outstanding people cannot be studied by RAS designs. When choosing methods, a researcher should decide what methods to use not on the basis of an illusory gold standard, but rather on the basis of the kind of question being asked.

Small-Sample Problems

Suppose I wish to know whether children with autism are receiving adequate treatment through a program in my relatively small school district.

An RAS design will not help me, because I do not have enough children with autism in my district to assign randomly to experimental and control or alternative treatment groups. But there are other kinds of study designs, such as a quasi-experimental design, that might help me get at least some sense of whether my program is working. One could argue that RAS designs should be used, but only in larger districts. But there are some problems that are so rare, such as hyperlexia (i.e., highly skilled reading by a subset of children with autism), that I probably will not be able to use an RAS design, no matter how large my sample. We should not be forced to forego research entirely when large enough samples are not available for RAS designs.

Investigator Bias

Despite the use of RAS designs, a number of drugs, most recently Vioxx and not much before that Rezulin and Fen-Phen, were pulled from the market. These facts suggest that RAS designs provide no panacea. The reason is that when designers of studies have a vested interest in the outcome, flaws in study designs and interpretations are likely to favor the outcome they hope for. This self-fulfilling prophecy effect occurs in all kinds of supposed RAS designs, not just those for psychotherapies and drugs. It is human nature to want to read data so as to confirm one's prior expectations. Results from any kind of design can be interpreted well or poorly. The issue is often that how cautiously and objectively data are interpreted proves to be more important than the particular design that was used. Even when review panels are commissioned to evaluate retrospective evidence, they are not immune to bias. A recent government panel that recommended that Bextra, Celebrex, and Vioxx be allowed to continue to be marketed was composed of a number of people with ties to the very companies whose products were being evaluated.

The Gap Between Experiments and Clinical Reality

If every client was a textbook-pure case of a particular syndrome, then it might be possible to comfortably generalize the results of many and even most RAS studies to clinical settings. The chapters in this book make clear that the degree of fidelity is, at best, variable. This is not to say that the studies are poorly designed or ecologically invalid. Rather, ecological validity is a matter of degree, and as the universe of therapy situations to which one wishes to generalize expands, one has to be increasingly cautious in interpreting the results of RAS designs. Will the treatment work in other cultures? Will it work for people with comorbid diagnoses? Will it work for people on particular combinations of drugs? How will it work for people who are highly resistant to psychotherapy? In the end, one must ask just how general the results of any given study or set of studies can be.

In my own work in education, I have found a very substantial divide between the concerns of educators in the trenches and educational researchers working out of laboratories. The U.S. Department of Education has attempted to remedy this problem by mandating, through the No Child Left Behind Act, that school interventions must be based on good science. But many view this bill as promoting ideology as well as science. Science can end up serving ideology as much as ideology can serve science.

It might be easier if one could point a finger and say that this administration is the problem, or that government is the problem, or that politicians just cannot be trusted. But how far will this line of reasoning go? To the present day, there is considerable dispute among practicing psychologists over the relative values of different kinds of therapies. Such disputes extend not only to practitioners, but to scientists as well. For example, is Freud all washed up—someone who was wrong in pretty much everything he believed—or was he on the right track in many ways and then subject to scientists who wanted to discredit his work, regardless of whether they were doing so correctly?

Currently, there is a national debate in the United States over whether psychologists who receive special training to prescribe psychoactive drugs should indeed be permitted to prescribe such drugs. Huge volumes have been written both in favor of and against prescription privileges, much of it by people with scientific training in psychology or in psychiatry and other branches of medicine. What is notable about this debate is how little of it is being argued on scientific grounds. Almost none of it is being argued on the basis of RAS trials comparing outcomes for specially trained psychologists versus psychiatrists. This is scarcely surprising, because individuals could not be randomly assigned to psychologist versus psychiatrist groups! Thus, an RAS design would not work to address the reasonable question of the relative efficacy of each of the two types of practitioners, and the hot debate seems to be grounded not in any kind of science but, once again, in ideology. Predictably, many more psychologists than psychiatrists support prescription privileges for trained psychologists, although there is no unanimity in either camp. When economic and strong professional interests are at stake, science may take a back seat at the table, and RAS trials, no seat at all.

In the end, science is a self-correcting process, and one can hope that the truth will out. But practitioners cannot wait for final answers, and so they must go with what they have. Scientific evidence is clearly helpful, but it is not yet sufficiently precise so as to provide an answer to every question that a psychotherapist might need to ask regarding how to treat a client.

But just as scientists sometimes may have a tendency to believe they have definitive answers when they do not, so can some practitioners have a tendency to throw out the baby with the bathwater. Just because scientific evidence cannot answer all questions does not mean it cannot answer any questions. On the contrary, it can be enormously helpful when used to guide one's practice. At least one psychotherapist I knew (now deceased) used tarot cards in practice. There is no scientific theory behind the use of tarot cards, there is no scientific evidence supporting the use of tarot cards, and the use of such a device defies good sense and logic. Scientific training should teach one, at the very least, to avoid quackery that will not help patients, that may harm the patients, and that potentially throws psychologists as a group into ill repute.

In the end, dialogue of the kind promoted in this book seems to be a good means to achieve a rapprochement between scientific researchers, science–practitioners, and practitioners of good will. My coauthors and I hope that our volume has contributed toward that end. There is no gold standard in scientific research, other than to design studies to answer the questions they are supposed to answer and then to interpret the results in an objective and conscientious manner.

AUTHOR INDEX

Numbers in italics refer to listings in the references.

Hollon, S. D., 22, *32–34*, *129*, 144, *149*, 250, *254*

Horner, A. J., 85, *101*

Horowitz, M. J., 81, *103*

Horvath, A. O., 69, 70, 72, *78*, 141, *149*

Horwitz, R. I., 245, *256*

Hoshmond, L. T., 214, 219, *236*

Houck, P. R., 86, *100*

Houts, A. C., 222, *236*

Howard, G. S., 114, *130*

Howard, K. I., 26, *34*, 85, *101*, 120, 122, *128*, 158, 170, *175*, *176*

Howard, R. C., 140, *149*

Hoyle, R. H., 119, *127*

Hubble, M. A., 66, *78*

Hueston, J. D., 89, *101*

Huppert, J. D., 140–143, 145, *148–150*, 250, *254*

Hussey, P. S., 241, *258*

Imber, S. D., *77*

Information Please Database, *101*

Institute of Medicine, 7, *10*, 39, *59*, 240, 246, *257*

Ja, D. Y., 90, *104*

Jackson, J. S., 229, *237*

Jacob, K. L., *146*, *203*, *204*

Jacobsen, F. M., 83, *101*

Jacobson, N. S., 45, *59*, 116, *128*

Jakob, K. S., 95, *102*

Javier, R., 85, *101*

Jensen, A. L., 198, *204*

Jensen, J. P., 73, *78*

Jensen, P. J., 153, *175*

Jin, R., 21, *33*

Jindal, R. D., 114, 115, *130*

Johnson, B., 15, *33*

Johnson, S. B., *32*, 100, *150*

Jordan, J. R., 26, *33*

Jordan, J. V., 96, *101*

Jorgensen, C. R., 68, *78*

Joski, P., 241, *258*

Jumper-Thurman, P., *105*

Juster, H. R., 138, *150*

Kahneman, D., 248, *257*

Kakar, S., 94, *101*

Kanfer, F. H., 217, *237*

Kaplan, A., 96, *102*

Karlsson, R., 98, *102*

Kawachi, I., 44, *57*

Kazdin, A. E., 137, *150*, 153, 156, 159–161, 163, 166, 168, 172, *175*, *176*, 184, 186, 187, 199, *204*

Keckley, P. H., 15, 16, 19, *33*

Keefe, F. J., 139, 148, *152*

Keehan, S., *257*

Keleher, J., *149*

Keller, D. S., 183, *204*

Keller, M. B., 184, *204*

Kendall, P. C., 116, *128*, 139, *152*, 160, *176*, 188, *204*, *205*

Kendjelic, E. M., 52, *58*

Kerlinger, F. N., 218, *237*

Kernberg, O. F., 143, 145, *148*

Kessler, R. C., 21, *33*, *35*

Khazan, I. Z., *204*

Kiesler, D. J., 229, *237*

Kinzie, J. D., 94, *102*

Kiresuk, T. J., 158, 162, *176*

Kleber, R. J., 98, *102*

Klein, D. N., 141, 143, *146*, *150*, *151*

Klein, G., 248, *257*

Klein, L. C., 60

Kleinman, A., 95–97, 99, *102*

Klerman, G. L., 88, *102*, 164, *176*

Knipscheer, J. W., 98, *102*

Knoedler, W. H., *149*, 185, *203*

Koch, S., 214, *237*

Koch, W. J., 223, *238*

Kopta, S. M., *128*

Kordy, H., 168, *176*

Korman, L. M., 141, *151*

Koss-Chioino, J., 90, 95, *102*

Kozak, M. J., 138, 144, *148*, *149*

Krasnow, A. D., *146*, 182, *203*, *204*

Kraus, D. R., 26, *33*

Krause, M. S., 120, *128*

Kress, K., 250, *256*

Krupnick, J. L., 90, *104*

Kuhn, T. S., 214, *237*

Lam, A. G., 66, *79*

Lambert, M. J., 17, 18, 26, 27, *32*, *33*, 41, 42, *59*, 64, 69, 71, 72, 74, 77, *78*, 112, 113, 116, 118, 121–124, *126*, *127–130*, 140–142, 144, *149*, *150*, 155, 158, 161, 171, *176*

Lamiell, J. T., 214, 215, 229, *237*

Lampropoulos, G. K., 16, *33*, 212, *237*

Lane, M., 21, *35*

Latimer, E., 144, *147*

Lau, A., 82, *104*

Mondin, G. W., 79
Montgomery, L. M., 129
Moody, M., 79, 130
Moras, K., 85, 101, 170, 175
Morgan, T. J., 183, 204
Morgenstern, J., 183, 204
Morone, J. A., 242, 257
Morrell, B., 122, 127
Morrison, K., 246, 259
Morton, J. J., 128
Moskowitz, M., 85, 101
Mueser, K. T., 144, 147, 256
Mufson, L., 186, 204
Muir-Gray, J. A., 240, 258
Munoz, R. F., 85, 103, 115, 129, 149
Muran, J. C., 71, 79
Murdock, T. B., 86, 101
Murtagh, D. R. R., 119, 129

Najavits, L. M., 182, 183, 205
Narrow, W., 204
Nath, S. R., 116, 128
Nathan, P., 144, 149
Nathan, P. E., 16, 34, 137, 151, 243, 244, 257
National Alliance for the Mentally Ill, 185, 205
National Association of State Mental Health Program Directors, 185, 205
National Committee for Quality Assurance, 133, 151
National Institute for Clinical Excellence, 23, 34
National Institute of Mental Health, 185, 205
National Institutes of Health, 19, 34
National Mental Health Information Center, 196, 205
Navarro, A. M., 85, 103, 129, 144, 151
Neighbors, H. W., 237
Neimeyer, R. A., 54, 59, 113, 129
Nelson, C., 101
Nelson, R., 146, 147
Nelson, R. O., 156, 175
Nelson-Gray, R. O., 132, 149, 248, 256
Nemeroff, C. B., 143, 151
Nesse, R. M., 237
Neumann, K. F., 117, 118, 127
New York State Department of Health, 141, 151
Newman, R., 14, 34
Nguyen, A. N., 90, 105

Nich, C., 141, 147
Nicholson, R. A., 119, 129
Nielsen, S. L., 128, 130, 176
Nietzel, M. T., 117, 129, 130
Nikelly, A. G., 94, 103
Nomura, Y., 204
Norcross, J. C., 18, 24, 34, 38, 43, 59, 60, 66, 67, 69, 71, 73, 78, 81, 92, 103, 115, 129, 142, 151, 243, 257
Noser, K., 144, 147
Novotny, C., 17, 35, 53, 60, 64, 79, 143, 152, 153, 177, 182, 206
Nunez, J., 85, 105

O'Brien, M., 73, 78
O'Hara, M., 245, 254
O'Mahoney, M. T., 158, 175
O'Reardon, J. P., 33
Oei, T. P. S., 117, 129
Office of the Surgeon General, 185, 205
Ogles, B. M., 17, 33, 41, 59, 112, 113, 116, 123, 124, 128, 129, 140, 142, 150
Okiishi, J., 18, 33, 176
Okwumabua, T., 129
Olfson, M., 22, 34, 35, 137, 151, 204
Ollendick, T. H., 137, 139, 147, 148, 240, 242, 255
Olson, S. E., 83, 99
Onken, L. S., 148
OPTAIO, 168, 177
Oregon Office of Mental Health and Addiction Services, 19, 20, 34, 253, 257
Organista, K. C., 85, 86, 103
Orlinsky, D. E., 120, 128
Otto, M. W., 119, 124, 127, 129

Paniagua, F., 90, 103
Parloff, M. R., 118, 129
Parsonson, B. S., 160, 177
Patel, V., 95, 102
Patenaude, A. F., 44, 59
Pedro-Caroll, J., 44, 60
Perel, J. M., 86, 100
Persons, J. B., 153, 177
Peterson, D. R., 40, 41, 46, 60, 212, 217, 237, 246, 247, 257, 258
Peterson, R. L., 235, 237
Phillips, G., 144, 151
Pi, E. H., 83, 103
Pincus, H. A., 34, 35, 151
Plato, 135, 151
Poland, R. E., 83, 102

Wiser, S., 52, *61*
Wolff, N., 244, *259*
Woods, S. W., 141, *147, 149–150*
Woody, S., 223, *238*
Woody, S. R., 183, *206*
Worell, J., 87, *105*
World Health Organization, 15, 21, *35*

Xhang, H., *204*

Yap, L., 119, *127*
Yates, B. T., 67, *79*
Yeh, M., 189, *206*

Yeomans, F., 143, *148*
Yi, K., 90, *105*
Yim, L. M., *32, 148, 255*
Yorkston, N. J., 64, *79*
Young, J. L., 20, *35*
Young, K., 85, *105*
Young, P. R., *32*

Zachar, P., 40, *61*
Zane, N., 85, 95, *104, 105*
Zarin, D. A., 20, *35*
Zoellner, L. A., 22, *35*
Zuroff, D. C., 90, *104*

SUBJECT INDEX

incentive systems/constraints/work pressures in, 180–181

research vs., 180–182

views on relation between research and, 182–183

work products/nature of daily life in, 181–182

youth/adult effectiveness research themes, 195

Clinical practice guidelines, 135, 136

Clinical prediction, 53

Clinical state and circumstances, 49, 51

Clinical trials, 144

Clinical utility criteria, 136

Clinician factors, 67

Clinicians. *See also* Practitioners

allegiance to theoretical model by, 72–74

cultural variation in role of, 89–93

CMHTF (Children's Mental Health Task Force), 22

Coaching, 92

Cocaine abuse, 141

Cochrane Collaboration, 247

Cognitive–behavioral therapy (CBT), 45, 85–87, 114, 138, 140, 141, 182–184, 188

Cognitive biases, 53

Cognitive empathy, 97

Collaboration, 138, 139

Collaborative practitioner–researcher networks, 44

Collectivistic societies, 90, 93–94

Committee on Science and Practice (CSP), 183

Common factors, 118

Common factors approach, 68

Communication, cultural variation in, 93–94

Community Reinforcement Approach, 185

Comorbidity, 144

COMPASS Outpatient Treatment Assessment System, 158

Competencies, 48

Complexity, 155

Conceptual scheme, 71–75

allegiance, 72–74

patient expectancy, 72

rituals/procedures/techniques, 74–75

Confirmatory bias, 53

Confucian thought, 90

Consolidated Standards of Reporting Trials (CONSORT) guidelines, 144

CONSORT (Consolidated Standards of Reporting Trials) guidelines, 144

Consultant role, 92

Consumers, 4

Content of knowledge, 51

Context-poor communication, 93

Context-rich communication, 93

Contextual model, 37, 38, 67–71

history of, 67–69

therapeutic relationship in, 69–71

Control groups, 145

Convergence of views, 6–7

Coping Cat program, 188

Costs

of empirically based treatments, 198–199

of health care, 132, 241

of mental health care, 241

Counselor role, 92

Credentialing, 252–253

Credibility, 95, 96

Critical thinking, 224–226

CSP (Committee on Science and Practice), 183

Cultural empathy, 97–98

Culturally sensitive psychotherapy, 85

Cultural resonance, 94

Cultural variation in therapeutic relationship, 81–99

adaptation of psychotherapy to, 82–89

clinician's role, 89–93

empathy, 96–98

individual/collective, 93–94

management, 94–96

sociopolitical context, 89

Culture (term), 82

"Culture war," 4

Cytochrome P450 (CYP) enzyme system, 83

Data evaluation, 160–161

Depression, 22, 85, 86

Depth of knowledge, 51

Diagnostic and Statistical Manual of Mental Disorders (DSM–IV), 198

Direct approach, 92

District of Columbia, 252–253

Divergence of views, 7–8

Division 12, 183, 242–244, 249

Dodo bird conclusion, 68

Dose–response statistic, 120

Drug metabolization, 83

Goal Attainment Scaling, 158, 162
Goals
    of clinical practice/research, 180
    psychotherapy, 70, 71, 156
    research vs. practice, 180
"Gold standard" methodology, 17
Gold standards, 267
"Good practice writ large is good policy" hypothesis, 249–250
Grant funding, 181
The Great Psychotherapy Debate (B. E. Wampold), 67

Hawaii, 252
Healers, 95
Health care
    costs of, 132
    quality of, 133–134
    regulation of, 133
    restricting access to, 20
    spending on, 15
Health Maintenance Organization Act (1973), 14
Health maintenance organizations (HMOs), 14
Health professionals
    competence of, 14
    deprofessionalization of, 18–19
    employment implications for, 28–30
    training of, 15, 16
Heart, expert of the, 91
Heuristic processes, 52–53
Heuristics, 53
Hierarchical relationships, 90
Hindsight, 53
Hispanics, 83
HMOs (health maintenance organizations), 14
Holistic techniques, 86
Hope, 72
Humanistic psychotherapies, 245
Human sciences, 246
Hypotheses of EBP, 243–250
    good practice writ large is good policy, 249–250
    well-managed good science leads to good practice, 246–248
    whatever the difficulties, good science is possible, 243–246

Idiographic processes, 41
Implementation toolkits, 247
Incentive systems, 180–181

Individualist cultures, 93
Institute of Medicine (IOM), 7, 39
Integration
    of science and practice, 212
    of subsystems of personality, 68
    technical, 73–74
Intelligence tests, 216
Internal review board (IRB), 188–189
Interpersonal therapy (IPT), 85, 86, 88
Interview, clinical, 46–47
Intuition, 94
Investigator bias, 269
IOM. *See* Institute of Medicine
IPT. *See* Interpersonal therapy
IRB. *See* Internal review board

Judgment, 52–54, 155, 212–214

King, Rodney, 89
Knowledge base, 155

Language, 94–95
Latinos, 83, 85, 87, 91
Legislation, 29
Levitt, H. M., 54
Liability, professional, 251–252
Life circumstances, 220–221
Literature, 44–45
Local clinical scientist training model, 46, 218–221
    attitude of scientist in, 221–224
    critical thinking in, 224–226
    methodological realism in, 226–231
    scientific-attitude training in, 234–235
    self-reports in, 234
    translation of statistical results in, 232–233
    values on variable in, 233–234
Local clinical situation, 217

Magellan Health Services, 26
Maintenance of treatment gains, 119–123
Malpractice, 251–252
Managed behavioral health care organizations (MBHOs), 25–28
Managed care, 13–21
    changes in health care due to, 132–133
    deprofessionalization of professionals in, 18–19
    EBP as basis for health care services in, 19–21
    and EBP as public idea, 15–16

expansion of, 14
and Massachusetts outcomes, 25–28
as movement, 14
professional flight from, 29–30
and selective use of evidence, 16–18
standardization/regulation of care in, 14–15
viability of, 133
"Managed care–free" practices, 30
Manualized treatments, 18
Manuals, treatment. *See* Treatment manuals
Massachusetts
managed care in, 13
outcomes and managed care in, 25–28
pharmacological bias in, 22–23
reimbursement policies in, 19
Massachusetts Behavioral Health Partnership, 23, 25–28
Massachusetts Mental Health Coalition, 26
Massachusetts Psychological Association, 27–28
Maximizing expected utility (MEU), 249–250
MBHOs. *See* Managed behavioral health care organizations
Means (term), 156, 157
Measures, selecting, 158–159
Medicaid, 25, 28
Medical drug model, 37, 38
Medicare, 241
Mental health care
cost of, 241
delays in, 21
pharmacological bias in, 21–23
Mental health professions, 196, 197
Meta-analyses, 114–115
Methodological realism, 216–218
implications of, 231–235
sampling/randomization cases in, 227–231
MEU. *See* Maximizing expected utility
Misestimation of covariance, 53
Missed empathetic opportunities, 84
Multicultural Guideline 1, 84–85
Multicultural Guideline 4, 88
Multicultural Guideline 5, 85
Multicultural Guidelines, 84–85
Multidimensional Treatment Foster Care, 185
Multisystemic Therapy, 185

National Child Traumatic Stress Network, 138

National Health System (NHS), 133–134
National Institute for Clinical Excellence, 23, 134
National Institute of Drug Abuse, 138
National Institute of Mental Health (NIMH), 19, 43, 143, 247
National Institutes of Health (NIH), 15, 43
National Service Framework, 133
Negation of category, 231
Negative outcomes, 123–125
Neimeyer, R. A., 54
Networks, practice research, 143–144
New York State, 252
NHS. *See* National Health System
NIH. *See* National Institutes of Health
NIMH. *See* National Institute of Mental Health
Nomothetic processes, 41
Nonspecific factors, 117–119
Nonverbal communication, 94
Norcross, J. C., 81

Objective observation, 46
Object relations framework, 85
Observation, clinical, 46–47
and categorization, 230–231
information categories in, 220–221
sources of, 219
Obsessive–compulsive disorder (OCD), 117, 140, 141
OCD. *See* Obsessive–compulsive disorder
Ongoing assessment, 159–160
Openness, 222–223
Oppression, 86
OQ. *See* Outcome Questionnaire
Oregon, 19, 20, 253
Organisation for Economic Co-Operation and Development, 241
Outcome Questionnaire (OQ), 124, 125, 158, 171
Outcome research, psychotherapy, 170–171
Outcomes, psychological model of, 139
Outcomes measurement
costs associated with, 27–28
employment-environment implications of, 28–30
in Massachusetts, 25–28
movement toward, 23–25
tracking effectiveness with, 46
variations in, 25–27
"Outcomes movement," 242

and payers for services, 252–253
and professional liability, 251–252
rise of EBP as, 241–242
working hypotheses of EBP as, 243–249
Puerto Ricans, 87–89

QOLI. *See* Quality of Life Inventory
Qualitative research, 9, 171–172
Quality of health care, 133–134
Quality of Life Inventory (QOLI), 164–167
Questionnaire studies, 215

Racial stress inoculation, 86
Racism, 86
Random-assignment study (RAS) designs
    clinical reality vs., 269–271
    examples of failings of, 267
    and investigator bias, 269
    as panaceas, 267–268
    questions not applicable to, 268
    and small samples, 268–269
Randomization, 229
Randomized controlled trials (RCTs)
    exclusion criteria as failing in, 246
    as gold standard, 17, 18
    of psychotherapy, 170
    in research design, 43
    spending on, 21
RAS designs. *See* Random-assignment study
    designs
Rating scales, 87–88, 158–159
Rational-emotive therapies, 92
RCTs. *See* Randomized controlled trials
Realism, methodological. *See* Methodological realism
Reasonableness test, 252
Referral, importance of, 97
Regulation of health care, 133
Reimbursement policies
    and devaluation of mental health professionals, 18–19
    EBP-based, 28–29
    for outcomes tracking, 46
Research, 8, 9
    challenges to collaboration in practice and, 196–201
    clinical-practice contributions to, 200–201
    effectiveness trials, 185–195
    goals/objectives of, 180
    impact of, on clinical practice, 183–185

incentive systems/constraints/work pressures in, 180–181
    process, 143
    psychotherapy's use of, 43–44
    views on, 182–183
    views on relation between practice and, 182–183
    work products/nature of daily life in, 181–182
    youth/adult effectiveness, 195
Research findings on psychotherapy, 111–126
    clinically meaningful change, 116–117
    comparative outcomes, 113–116
    efficacy, 112
    maintenance, 119–123
    negative outcomes, 123
    reducing negative outcomes, 123–125
    support systems/placebo comparison, 117–119
Respect for empirical data, 223–224
Retrieval of knowledge, 52
Rezulin, 267, 269
Rosenzweig, S., 67–69, 74

SAMHSA. *See* Substance Abuse and Mental Health Services Administration
Schizophrenic patients, 20
Scientific attitude, 234–235
Scientific journals, 21
Scientists
    attitudes of, 221–224
    practitioners vs., 8–10, 40–41
Selfhood, 84
Self observation, 46
Self–other relationship, 93–94
Self-reports, 219–220, 234
September 11, 2001 terrorist attacks, 89
Signal-alarm cases, 124, 155
Simpson, O. J., 89
Single-case experimental designs, 172
Small-area variation studies, 241–242
Small-sample problems, 268–269
Society for Clinical Psychology, 242
Sociocultural circumstances, 220–221
Sociopolitical context, 89
Socrates, 135
Space–time local information, 221
Statistical aggregation, 53
Statistical significance, 160n, 232–233
Stereotyping, generalization vs., 47
Structural aspects of clinical situation, 67

ABOUT THE EDITORS

Carol D. Goodheart, EdD, is a psychologist in independent practice in Princeton, New Jersey, and a contributing faculty member and clinical supervisor for the Graduate School of Applied and Professional Psychology, Rutgers University, New Brunswick, New Jersey. She is a fellow of the American Psychological Association (APA) and a Distinguished Practitioner of the National Academy of Psychology. Currently, she serves as treasurer and member of the Board of Directors of the American Psychological Association. Dr. Goodheart chaired the 2005 APA Presidential Initiative Task Force on Evidence-Based Practice, which developed the policy recommendation on Evidence-Based Practice in Psychology adopted by APA. She is an author and editor of seven books and numerous chapters and articles related to health, women, and the practice of psychology. Dr. Goodheart is a consulting editor of *Professional Psychology: Research and Practice* and a member of the editorial board of *Pragmatic Case Studies in Psychotherapy*. She is a past president of Psychologists in Independent Practice and recipient of Psychologist of the Year Award from both the New Jersey Psychological Association and Psychologists in Independent Practice, the largest division of APA. Visit her Web site at http://www.drcarolgoodheart.com.

Alan E. Kazdin, PhD, is director and chairman of the Child Study Center and John M. Musser Professor of Psychology and Child Psychiatry at Yale University School of Medicine and director of Child Psychiatric Services, Yale-New Haven Hospital, New Haven, Connecticut. He also directs the Yale Parenting Center and Child Conduct Clinic, an outpatient treatment service for children referred for aggressive and antisocial behavior and their families. He received his PhD in clinical psychology from Northwestern University (1970). Prior to coming to Yale, he was on the faculty of Northwestern University, Pennsylvania State University, and the University of

Pittsburgh School of Medicine. He has been a fellow of the Center for Advanced Study in the Behavioral Sciences, president of the Association for Advancement of Behavior Therapy, recipient of awards from the American Psychological Association and the Association for Advancement of Behavior Therapy, and chairman of the Department of Psychology at Yale.

Dr. Kazdin has served as editor of various journals: *Journal of Consulting and Clinical Psychology*, *Psychological Assessment*, *Behavior Therapy*, *Clinical Psychology: Science and Practice*, and *Current Directions in Psychological Science*. He was editor-in-chief of the *Encyclopedia of Psychology*, an 8-volume work published in 2000 under the auspices of the American Psychological Association and Oxford University Press. He has also edited a book series on *Developmental Psychopathology* and on *Current Perspectives in Psychology*. Currently, he is an associate editor of the *Annual Review of Psychology*.

His research focuses primarily on the development, treatment, and clinical course of aggressive and antisocial behavior in children and adolescents; child, parent, family, and contextual influences that contribute to child dysfunction; and critical processes within and outside of treatment that contribute to therapeutic changes in children, parents, and families. He is actively involved in clinical work and clinical research with children and families. He is a diplomate of the American Board of Professional Psychology and fellow of the American Psychological Association. He has published approximately 550 articles and chapters and has authored or edited 40 books on treatment, child and adolescent disorders, and methodology and research design.

Robert J. Sternberg, PhD, is dean of the School of Arts and Sciences at Tufts University, Medford, Massachusetts. Prior to that, he was IBM Professor of Psychology and Education in the Department of Psychology, professor of management in the School of Management, and director of the Center for the Psychology of Abilities, Competencies, and Expertise (PACE) at Yale University. He continues to direct the PACE Center from Tufts. Dr. Sternberg also was the 2003 president of the American Psychological Association. He was on the Board of Directors of the American Psychological Association (2002–2004) and of the Board of Trustees of the APA Insurance Trust (2004). Dr. Sternberg is the author of more than 1,000 journal articles, book chapters, and books and has received over $18 million in government and other grants and contracts for his research. The central focus of his research is on intelligence, creativity, and wisdom, and he also has studied love and close relationships as well as hate. This research has been conducted in five different continents.

Dr. Sternberg is also a fellow of the American Academy of Arts and Sciences and several other societies. He has won many awards from the American Psychological Association, the American Educational Research Association, the American Psychological Society, and other organizations.

Dr. Sternberg has been listed in the APA *Monitor on Psychology* as one of the top 100 psychologists of the 20th century and is listed by the Information Sciences Institute as one of its most highly cited authors (top .5%) in psychology and psychiatry. He also was listed in the *Esquire* "Register of Outstanding Men and Women Under 40" and was listed as one of 100 top young scientists by *Science Digest*. He is currently listed in *Who's Who in America*, *Who's Who in the World*, *Who's Who in the East*, *Who's Who in Medicine and Healthcare*, and *Who's Who in Science and Engineering*.

Dr. Sternberg is best known for his theory of successful intelligence; investment theory of creativity (developed with Todd Lubart); theory of thinking styles as mental self-government; balance theory of wisdom; wisdom, intelligence, and creativity theory of leadership; and for his duplex theories of love and hate.